Martin Gross

The Science and Art of Occlusion and Oral Rehabilitation

Martin Gross

The Science and Art of Occlusion and Oral Rehabilitation

with contributions by

Stefano Gracis
Iñaki Gamborena
Konrad Meyenberg
Arie Shifman
Joseph Nissan

QUINTESSENCE PUBLISHING

London · Berlin · Chicago · Tokyo · Barcelona · Beijing · Istanbul · Milan
Moscow · New Delhi · Paris · Prague · São Paulo · Seoul · Singapore and Warsaw

A CIP record for this book is available from the British Library

ISBN: 978-1-85097-215-0

The cover front page uses four pictures (in a digital photo frame) out of the book by Dr Mauro Fradeani, Esthetic Rehabilitation in Fixed Prosthodontics Volume 1: Esthetic Analysis – A Systematic Approach to Prosthetic Treatment. London: Quintessence, 2004, p 237; with permission by the author.

QUINTESSENCE PUBLISHING

Quintessence Publishing Co, Ltd
Grafton Road, New Malden, Surrey KT3 3AB,
United Kingdom
www.quintpub.co.uk

Printed in Germany

Foreword

George Zarb

Paradigm shifts in any aspect of the health sciences tend to enhance collective clinical objectivity as well as encourage more robust scientific inquiry. Dentistry has had its fair share of such scholarship shifts in the past half century; with osseointegration, adhesive restorative materials and occlusion immediately springing to mind. These three compelling changes have profoundly influenced both dental education and practice and continue to alter many of clinical dentistry's traditional patient management protocols.

It should be readily acknowledged, as this outstanding text so lucidly demonstrates, that occlusion is no longer the empirical and controversial topic it used to be for those of us who undertook specialty training four or five decades ago. As a scholarship focus, occlusion gradually outgrew its anecdotal legacy; and thanks to emerging data and insights into neuroplasticity, led to gradual recognition of its complex biological and behavioural framework. This quickly usurped the specialty driven parochial approach to the topic as it became apparent that the scientific method could also be applied to the study of occlusion – a necessity, given the challenges of practising dentistry in an era of unprecedented development in scientific bio-technological information.

I hasten to add that old approaches were certainly not be denigrated since they enabled clinicians of my vintage to respond to our patients' immediate needs. We did our best in the absence of evidence-based determinants of safe treatment outcomes and an inadequate understanding of the pathogenesis of disease processes, which were sometimes manifest at the all-too-visible and tangible occlusion level. As dentists, we treated what we saw and saw what we treated; and our presumably successful clinical management outcomes only reinforced our preconceived insights and associated hypotheses. However, we did welcome the new information that challenged old perceptions and convinced us that all ideas, irrespective of their lineage, need to be questioned and redefined on an ongoing basis if this important branch of dentistry was to not fall between the cracks of objectively derived and replicable data analysis.

This text takes stock of the exciting continuum of occlusion's development as a best-evidenced based synthesis of what is now scientifically rigorous and clinically circumspect. It emphasizes ever so convincingly, the essential clinical message provided by basic and behavioural scientists about the remarkable accommodation potential of the masticatory system to subtle and gross changes in the occlusal status. It is an authoritative and detailed text, in fact exhaustive in the relevance of its contemporary clinical scope and wisdom. I have little more to add other than to encourage its deserved wide readership to enjoy its common sense and prudence; and to respectfully suggest that the word be spread that this is a book that belongs in practising dentists' libraries and on dental schools' recommended reading lists. And above all to congratulate the author on synthesizing a complex body of information in such a sensible and impressive manner.

George Zarb

Contributors and Acknowledments

Special Thanks and acknowledgement

Prof George Zarb
For his kindness in accepting to write a forward for this text.

Professor Nitzan Bichacho
For encouragement and assistance in the conception and development of this work

Dr Arie Shifman
Clinical and intellectual soul mate in the development of ideas, clinical concepts and critiques over the last 15 years. Architect and partner in the development of clinical concepts in diagnosis and treatment planning presented here.
For contribution to Chapters on TMDs and Treatment planning

Invited International Clinicians
Dr Stefano Gracis Milan Italy
Dr Inaki Gamborena San Sebastian Spain
Dr Konrad Meyenberg Zurich Switzerland

For generous contribution of advanced prosthetic cases combining excellence in concept and execution exhibiting their particular flare in esthetics, presentation and case fabrication.

To Professor Joseph Nissan
For contributions of biomechanical studies in implant biomechanics

To Professor Joel Rak Department: Anatomy and Anthropology
faculty of medicine Tel Aviv University,

To the zoological mammalian museum of Tel Aviv University.

Thanks to Dr Limor Avivi-Arbel for reviewing chapters of Neuromusculature and Orofacial Pain. Thanks to Dr Danielle Layton for reviewing Chapter 1 statistics and scientific method. Sincere thanks and acknowledgement for generous contribution of histological material Professor Normal Mohl, Professor Henry Goldman, Professor Edwin Rozenberg, Professor Avital Koslovsky and co-workers, Professor Carlos Nemkovsky. Thanks for material to Professor Arthur Lewin, Professor Avinoam, Jaffe, Professor Ervin Weiss, Professor Esther Gazit, Dr Vidal Serfaty.

Many thanks and acknowledgments to the former graduate students, surgeons and staff in the Prosthodontics and Periodontics departments of the Tel Aviv University School of Dental Medicine and the Hebrew University Jerusalem School of Dental Medicine. Acknowledgments go too to the Dental technologists involved in presented cases and clinical materials. Surgeons Professorr Zwika Artzi, Professor Avital Koslovsky, Professor Shlomo Kalderon. Prosthodontists Dr Jenny Chernobelsky, Dr Gil Asafrana, Dr Eran Zenziper, Dr Orly Berman, Dr Oded Gelfan, Dr Benny OzAry, Dr Amin Bukhari, Dr Henrietta Sagui, Dr Dimitry Nerobai, Dr Ilan Priel, Dr Danny Gordon, Dr Gal Rozen and Dr Pnina Segal. Dental technologists Mr Baruch Indig, Mr Phillip Segal, Mr Ofer Koenig, Mr Ezra Kendell, Mr Israel Raanan, Mr Dudi Roie, Mr Shlomi Silverstein. Computer assistance Mr Salo Kegan. Thanks and appreciation to Dr Barry Marshak, Dr Milka Chesler and Dr Ofir Resnik for their contributions of time and effort in reviewing the texts and providing valuable feedback. Special thanks and acknowledgements go to the Quintessence editorial team, Vicki Williams,Thomas Pricker, Daniel Hecht.

Chapter 1 Thanks to Dr Daniel Clayton for review and modifications of Chapter 1 on scientific method and statistics.

Chapter 3 Ch 3-4
Thanks and acknowledgements for images of clinical cases to: Professor Shlomo Kalderon, Dr Amin Bukhari, Dr Ilan Priel, Dr Gal Rozen, Dr Yaron Blasbalg, Dr Jenny Chernobelsky, Dr Oded Ghelfan, Dr Henrietta Sagui, Dr Gil Asafrana, Dr Eitan Barnea.

Chapter 4
Thanks and acknowledgements for images of clinical cases to
Dr Jenny Chernobelsky.

Chapter 5
Thanks and acknowledgements for images of clinical cases to Dr Eran Zensiper, Dr Ina Zandel, Dr Oded Ghelfan.

Chapter 7
Thanks and acknowledgement to Professor Avital Koslovsky and coworkers for use of histological sections. Implant Biomechanics contributor Professor Joseph Nissan. Acknowledgements for images of clinical cases: Professor Avital Koslovsky, Professor Joseph Nissan, Professor Gabriel Chaushu, Dr Beny Oz Ari, Mr Samuel Relu, Dr Oded Gelfan, Dr Ilan Priel, Dr Jenny Chernobelsky.

Chapter 9
Contributor Dr Arie Shifman. Acknowledgement of clinical case Dr Eran Zensiper.

Chapter 10
Thanks and acknowledgements for images of clinical cases: Dr Oded Ghelfan, Dr Henrietta Sagui, Dr Gal Rozen.

Chapter 11
Thanks and acknowledgements for images of clinical cases: Dr Oded Ghelfan, Dr Danny Gordon, Dr Gil Asafrana, Dr Ilan Priel, Professor Shlomo Kalderon.

Chapter 12
The State of the Art Esthetic perspectives
International Case Presentations
Contributors Case presentations of invited international clinicians:
Dr Stefano Gracis, DMD, MSD Milan, Italy
Dr Iñaki Gamborena DMD, MSD, FID San Sebastian, Spain
Dr Konrad Meyenberg DMD Zurich Switzerland
Acknowledgement of clinical images Dr Orly Berman.

Chapter 13
Thanks and acknowledgements for images of clinical cases: Dr Oded Ghelfan, Dr Jenny Chernobelsky, Dr Sharon Marku-Cohen, Professor Avinoam Yaffe, Professor Ervin Weiss, Professor Avital Koslovsky, Professor Zvi Arzi, Professor Carlos Nemkovsky.

Chapter 14
Thanks and acknowledgements for clinical images: Dr Oded Ghelfan. Dr Gil Asafrana, Dr Henrietta Sagui, Dr Jenny Chernobelsky. Prof Avital Koslovsky, Professor Zvi Artzi, Mr Baruch Indig, Mr Ofer Kenig.

Chapter 15
Thanks and acknowledgements to: Dr Oded Ghelfan, Dr Jenny Chernobelsky, Dr Eran Zenziper, Dr Ina Zandel, Dr Ron Lev, Professor Zvika Arzi, Professor Avital Koslovsky, Dr Benny Oz Ary, Dr Barry Marshak, Professor Shlomo Kalderon, Mr Baruch Indig, Mr Ofer Koenig, Mr Ronen Krauze, Mr Phillip Segal, Mr Salo Kagan.

Chapter 16
Acknowledgements for clinical images: Dr Rafael Himel.

To Fanny

Contents

2 The Human Masticatory System

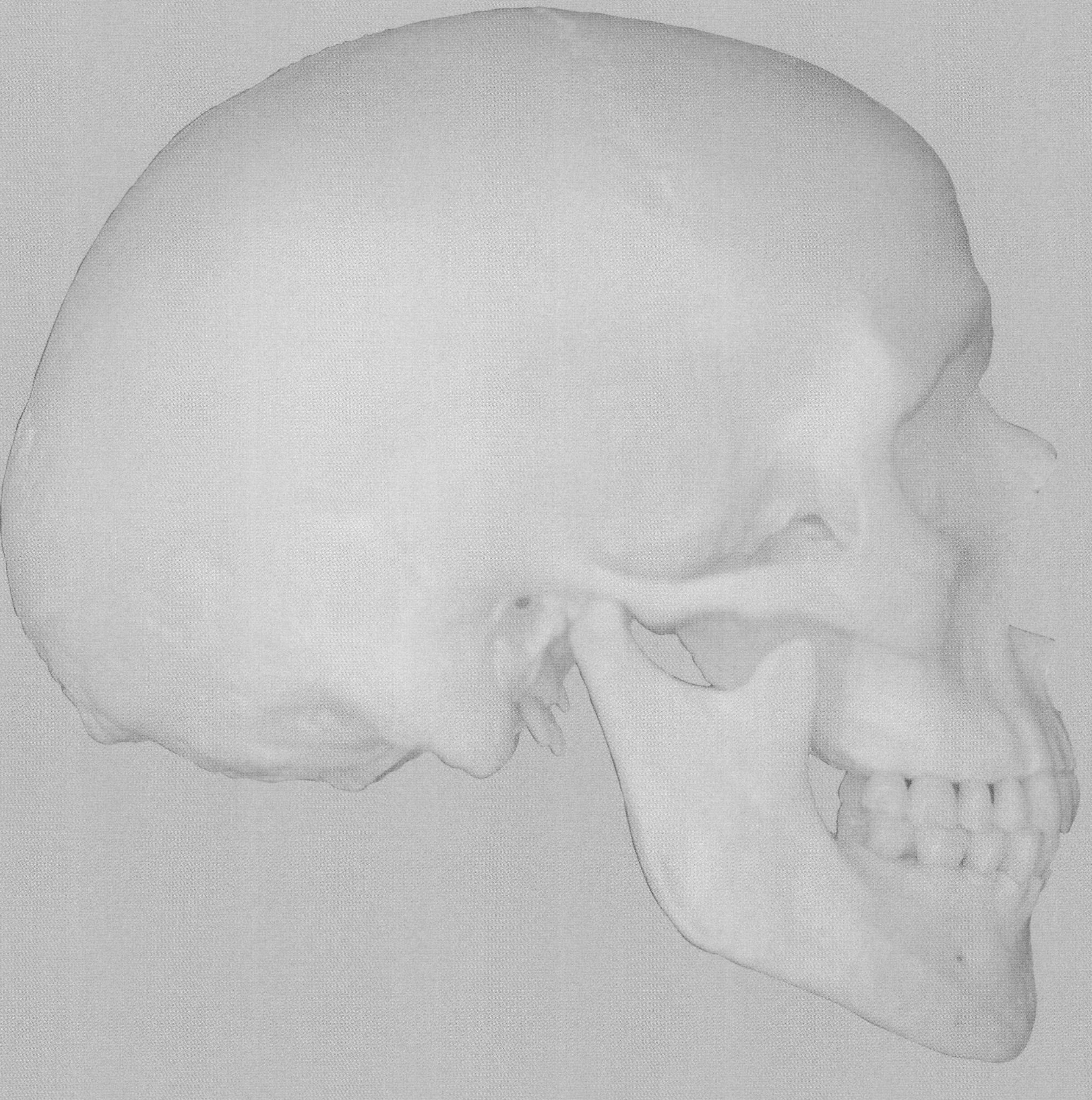

Masticatory system introduction

The following sections presented in Chapter 2 are designed to cover some of the background of knowledge necessary for a fuller appreciation of the subject of occlusion as it relates to clinical dentistry. Evolution and concepts of mammalian evolution through to hominins and modern man provide insight into the nature of the human skull, its functional loading design, and the occlusion of the dentition. This is relevant to clinical concepts of prosthetic loading planning and the concept of mutual protection that implies a specialized role in the mutual relation of the anterior and posterior teeth in the modern human dentition. Growth and development show the deveopmental nature of a normal distribution of skeletal relations and dentitions,which provide a basis for consideration of the normal range and how a clinician should consider deviations from the norm in a restorative perspective. Neuromusculature is covered in some depth to provide the basis for considerations of neuronal transmission, muscle function, dysfunction, and orofacial pain. This provides a better understanding and the ability to evaluate clinical concepts and the many electromyography (EMG) studies quoted in relation to temporomandibular disorders, occlusal parafunction, bruxism, anterior guidance, and vertical dimension of occlusion. Understanding the mechanisms of mastication, deglutition, parafunction, and occlusal traumatism are essential in clinical dentistry for the maintenance and restoration of the dentition. Full knowledge of the complexity and changing concepts of temporomandibular disorders is mandatory together with an understanding of current concepts of orofacial pain and neuronal plasticity. Finally, some considerations on the nature of human skull loading from an evolutionary and current biomechanical perspective is helpful in the understanding and planning of functional and parafunctional occlusal loading of tooth- and implant-supported dental rehabilitations.

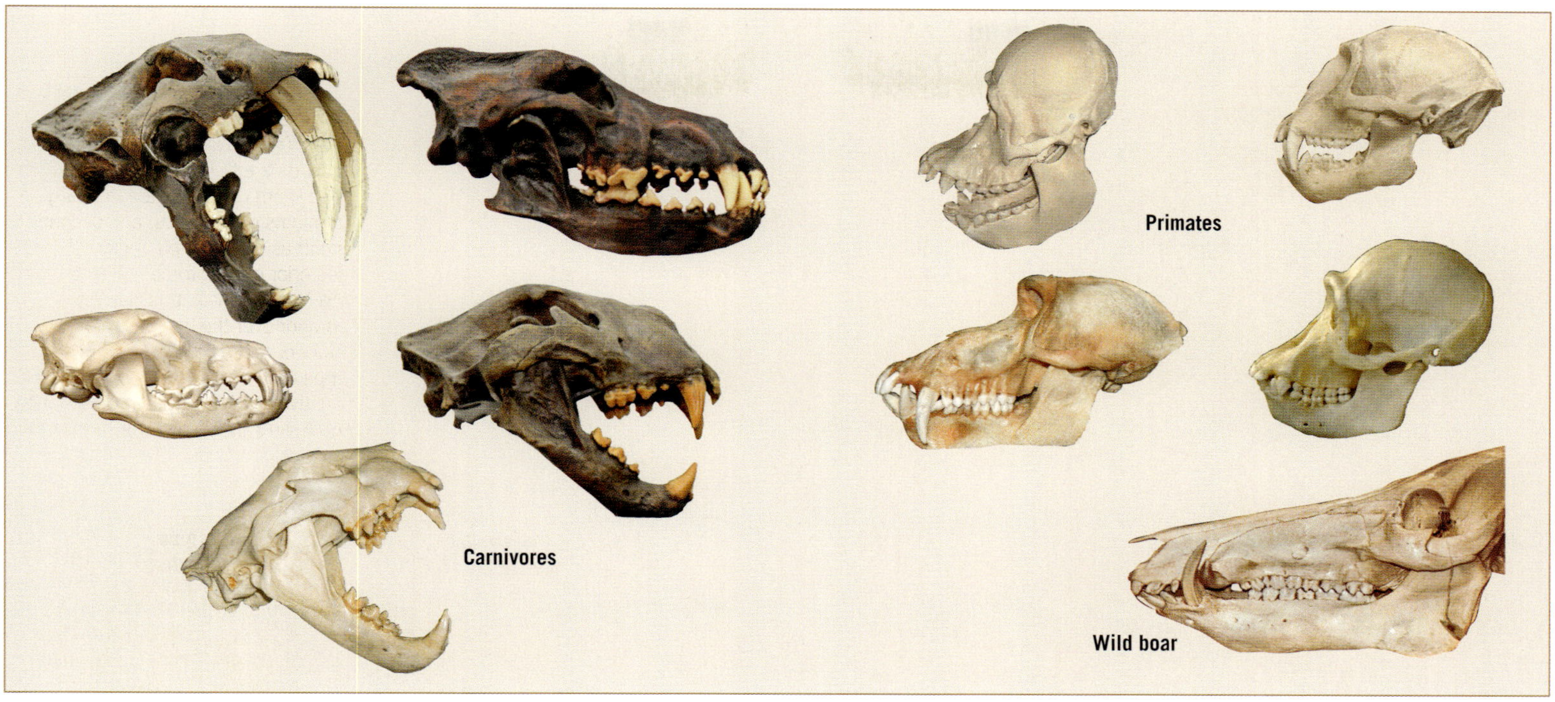

Fig 2-1-21 Canines developed as a distinctive feature of carnivores as tools to catch and debilitate prey (left). They required interlocking mechanisms of the joints which necessitated a large gape with the joints on the same plane as the teeth. Omnivores with large canines (eg, baboons, apes, and pigs) combine the attacking features of the canine for catching prey with an ability to eat foraged trees and grass (right). Canines became smaller with monkeys, apes, and hominins.

transition from hunting and gathering to an agricultural subsistence.[36] Jaw and teeth dimensions in the *Australopithecus afarensis, A. gracile* lineage is more delicate than the robust *Paranthropus robustus* linked to diet and increase in brain size (Figs 2-1-19, 2-1-25, and 2-1-26).

Canine specialization

Mammalian canine specialization is largely seen in terrestrial predatory carnivores. The largest mammalian canines are those of the walrus, which are used in fighting, digging, and locomotion. Some of the most common of the larger land-borne carnivores are dogs, wolves, and bears (*Caniformia);* lions, tigers, leopards, and cougars (*Feliformia*); and hyena and mongoose (*Viverridae*). Sea-borne carnivores include seals, sea lions, walruses, and narwhals.

The walrus forages small marine organisms. Terrestrial predatory carnivores that rely on hunting for food need physical mobility to catch their prey. They require a large gape and use the canines primarily to capture and immobilize their prey until death.

Omnivores with large canines such as baboons apes and pigs combine the attacking features of the canine for catching prey with an ability to eat foraged trees and vegetation (Fig 2-1-21).

Hominin and human canine development

Canines in humans and hominins became progressively smaller than those of the apes. In primates, canines function as both defense weapons and for visual threat. The primates with the largest canines (gorillas and some baboons) both have basically vegetarian diets. They use the canines for defense and as threat devices. Bearing of teeth is in some species seen as a sign of submission and in others as a sign of aggression. Hominin canines are all small and worn equally with the remaining dentition as a result of omnivorous foraging and omnivorous diet (Fig 2-1-24).[37,] Debate over the evolution of primate and hominin canine size has continued over this century. An originally popular concept that the canine in hominids and hominins became reduced (selectively) from a larger size has been questioned. [37] Arguments put forward are that original primate canines were small and remained small in several evolutionary lines. Canines of earlier hominids were smaller than they were in the middle Pleistocene. In contrast to the reductionist theory, the counter hypothesis is presented that "the canine had never been larger than it is in man" and that the retention of a small primitive canine is not necessarily unique to the hominids (Fig 2-1-25). [37]

Incisor specialization

Incisors vary in specialization between orders (Figs 2-1-22 to 2-1-24). Carnivores have small peg-shaped and sometimes serrated incisors used for picking and tearing the flesh of their prey.

Ungulates (hoofed mammals) use the lips, tongue, and incisors for food procurement. They primarily feed on vegetation, with the grazers picking grasses and leaves from ground level (eg, sheep, wildebeest, horses, and rhinoceros). Browsing is the eating of vegetation such as wood twigs and leaves from trees and shrubs. Rodents use the front teeth for gnawing and digging. Many grazers and browsers have missing upper incisors and spatulate proclined lower incisors. They pick the vegetation with lower incisors against upper gum pads. Others such as horses and camels have occluding upper and lower incisors. Few mammals (the aardvark for example) have no incisors at all. The aardvark procures insects with the tongue for consumption (Fig 2-1-22). The elephant (distant relative to the aardvark) has tusks as specialized second upper incisors. A tusk is an extremely long incisor or canine tooth that protrudes when the mouth is closed. Tusk-bearing mammals include elephants, warthogs, walruses, and narwhals.

Primates developed spatulate incisors that are associated with fruit peeling (frugivores) and developed together with color and visual acuity. Frugivorous primates tend to be characterized by relatively small molars with less well-developed features for comminuting leaves, and relatively large incisors that have been linked to incisal preparation of fruits. (Fig 2-1-23)[38-41]

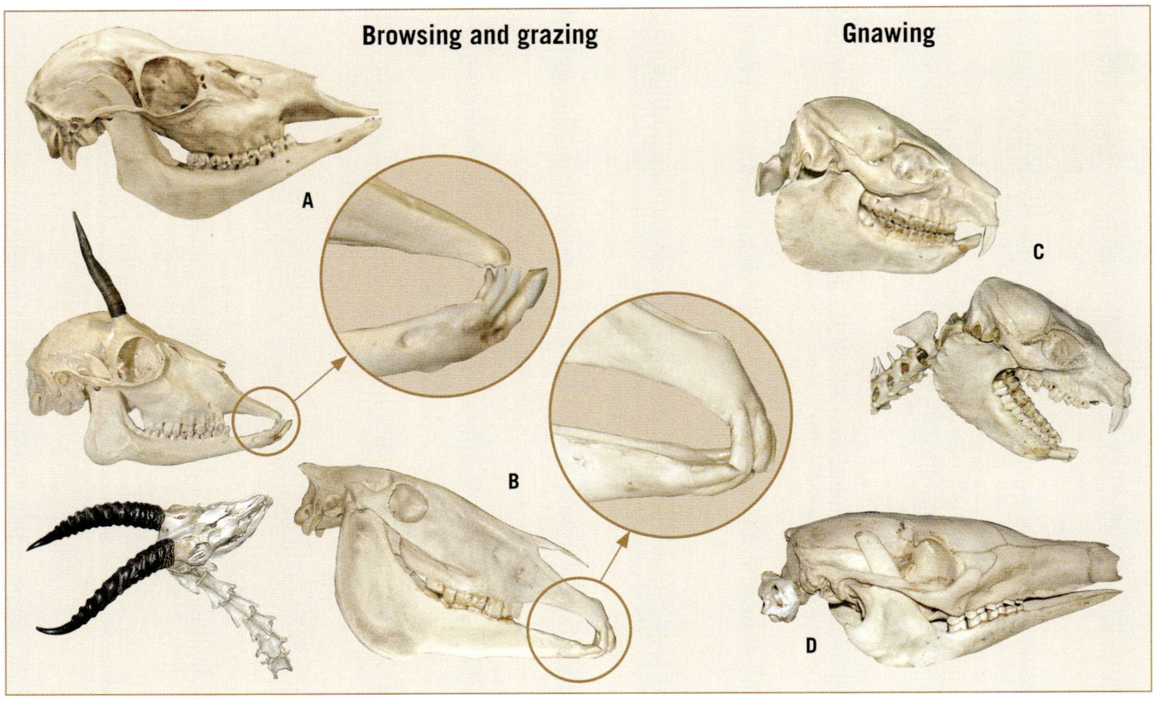

Fig 2-1-22 Incisors in ungulates developed for food procurement. Most ungulates have characteristically long snouts with proclined lower incisors and upper incisors often missing or replaced by gum pads. Grazers use gum pads and lower incisors to pick grass, while browsers use the front teeth to pick twigs and leaves of trees and shrubs for chewing. Rodents have proclined incisors for gnawing. **A**: Gazelle, deer, sheep. **B**: Horse. **C**: Rodent. **D**: Aardvark (anteater with no front teeth at all).

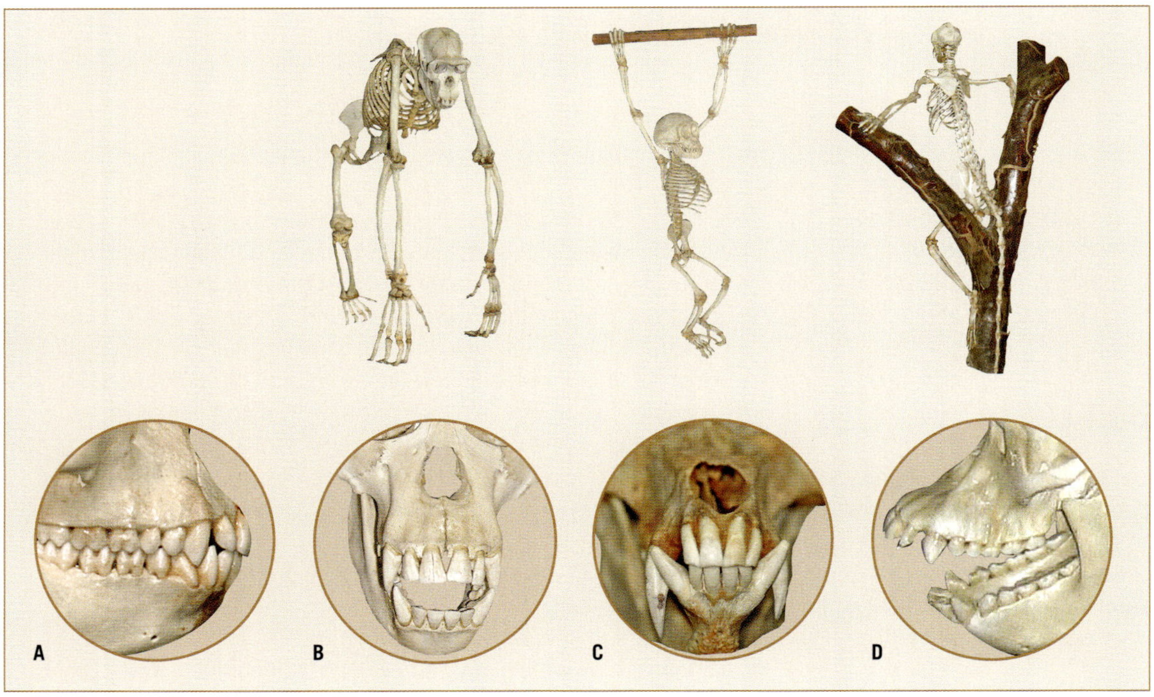

Fig 2-1-23 Incisors developed as primates took to the trees. They developed improved visual acuity, climbing skills, and incisors for the peeling and preparation of fruit. **A**: Macaque. **B**: Chimpanzee. **C**: Baboon. **D**: Orangutan.

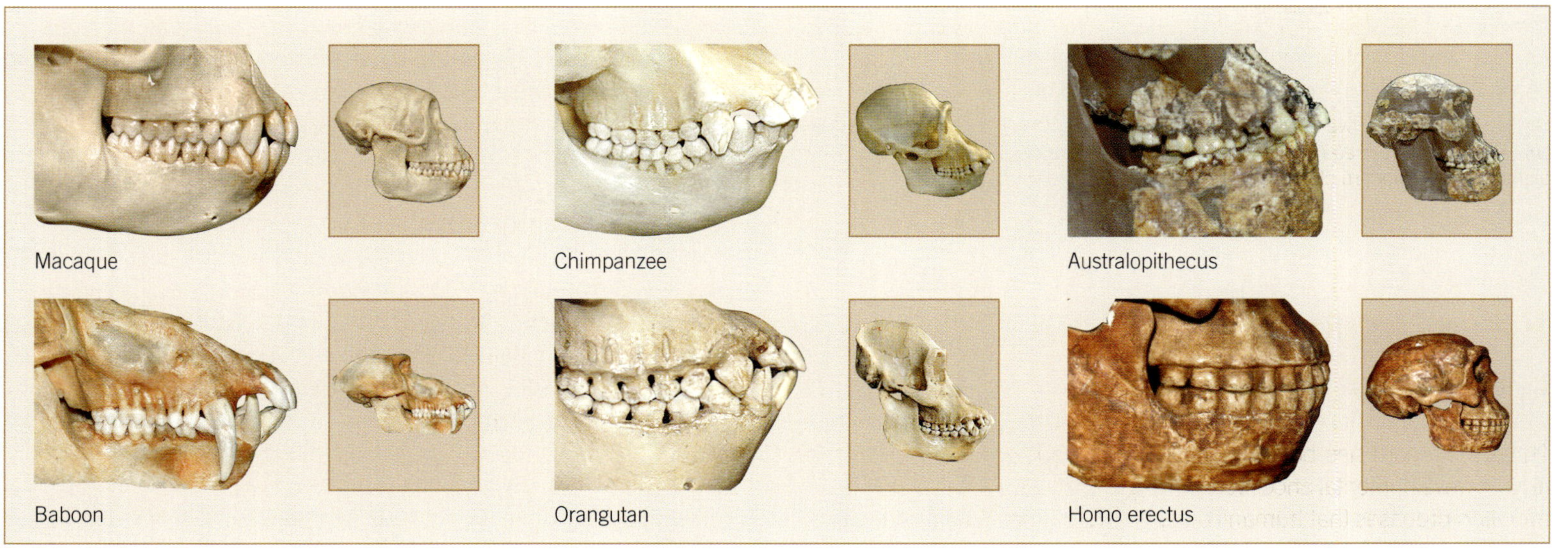

Fig 2-1-24 Monkeys, apes, and hominins. While the premolar and molar anatomy is similar between monkeys, apes, and man, the size of the canine is seen to become progressively smaller. Only the baboon has long recurved canines, while apes have slightly enlarged canines and opposing ape spaces for their interdigitation. Hominins had small canines in proportion with the remaining teeth and exhibited distinctive occlusal wear indicative of a foraging diet.

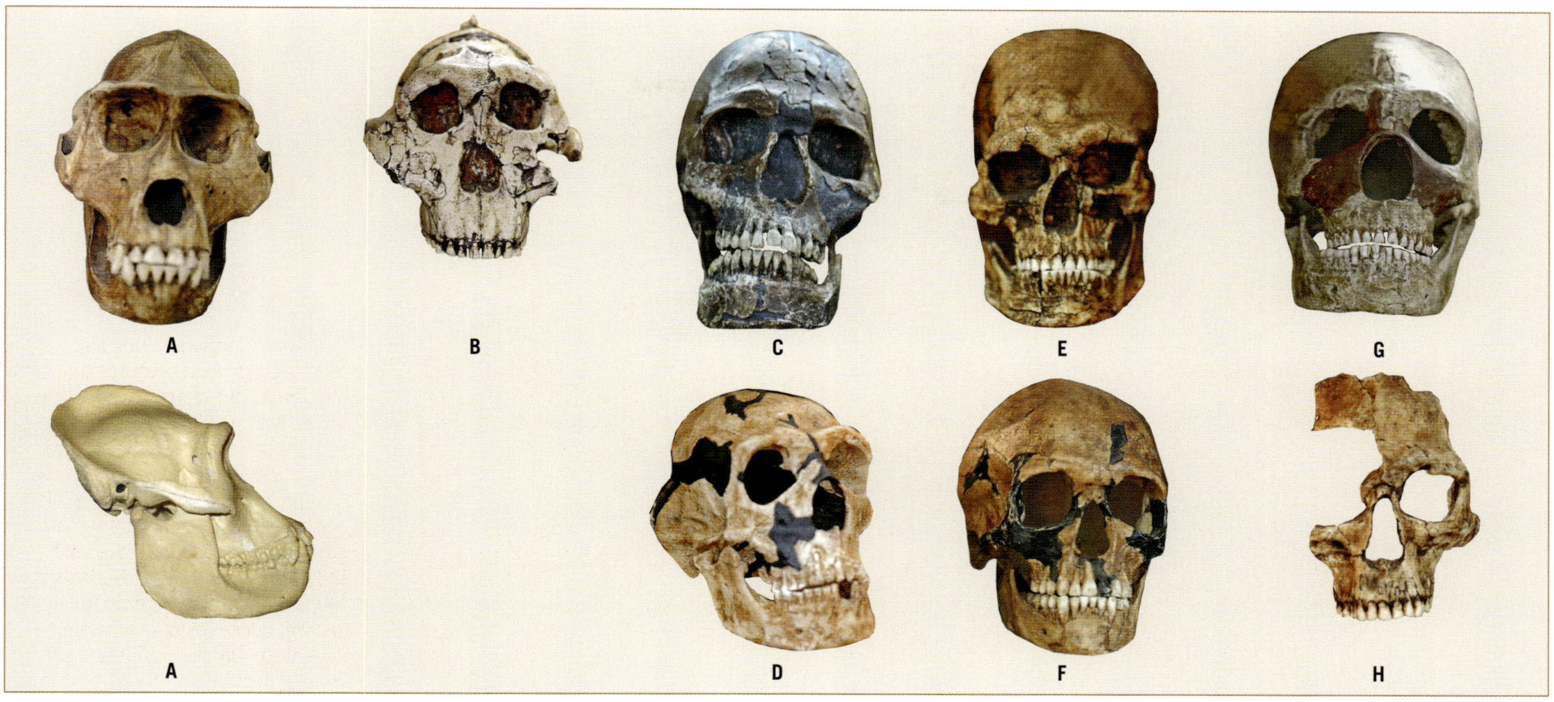

Fig 2-1-25 Hominid and hominin dentitions. As hominins evolved, the canines become smaller. Early Australopithecus had more tooth wear. Homo skulls **C** to **H** show dentitions not dissimilar to the normal range of variation in modern humans. **A**: Ape. **B**: *Australopithecus bosiei* (2 my). **D** and **G**: *Homo neanderthalensis*. **C, E, F**, and **H**: *Homo sapiens* (hominids are all great apes). See Fig 2-1-27 for Hominin classification.

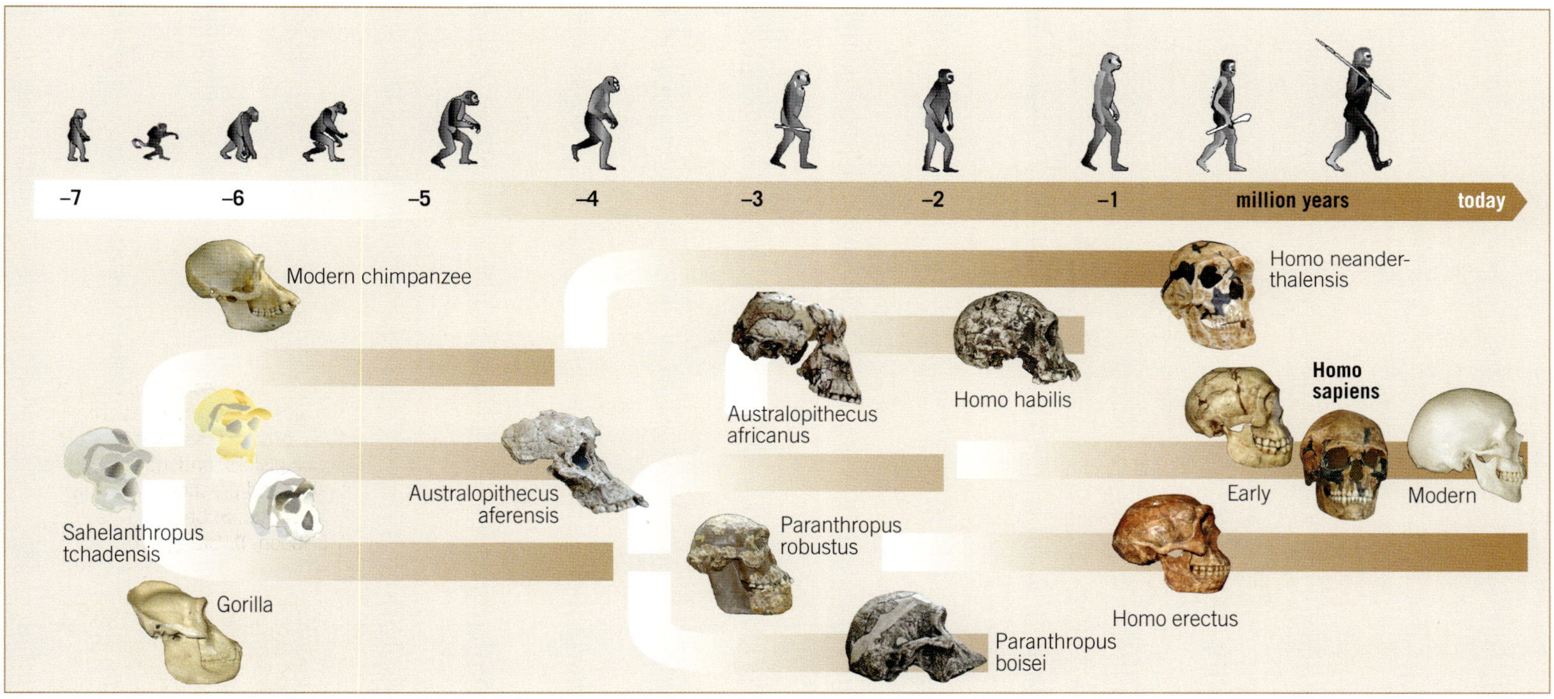

Fig 2-1-26 A speculative family tree of *Homo sapiens*. The oldest fossil finds are from around 7 million years ago. The lineage is traced from apes through chimpanzees and *Australopithecus afarensis* in several branches. The development was a meandering, multifaceted progression rather than a linear progression. Different clades are still being debated. Modern chimpanzee and modern gorilla are shown for comparison (not to scale).

From chimpanzee to *Homo sapiens*

The fossil record has been interpreted into clades or branches of the human developmental ancestral tree (Fig 2-1-26). An account of human evolution proposes that humans arose from a chimpanzee-like ancestor between roughly five million and six million years ago in East Africa and became bipedal on the African savanna.[42,43] Distinguishing hominid characteristics have been defined as bipedalism and canine metamorphism. Since the discovery of Lucy[42] an A. afarensis skeleton dated 3.2 million years old, older hominin fossils have been discovered from Chad, Kenya, and Ethiopia. These have extended the human record back to 7 my.[44]

The fossil record of hominins shows that multiple species existed alongside one another during the later stages of human evolution. Paleoanthropologists are still debating whether this holds true for the first half of our family's existence from 7 to 4.5 my.[43] Some believe that all of the fossils from between 7 and 3 my fit into the same evolutionary lineage. Others view these specimens not only as members of mostly different lineages but also as representatives of an extensive early hominid diversity yet to be discovered.[43]

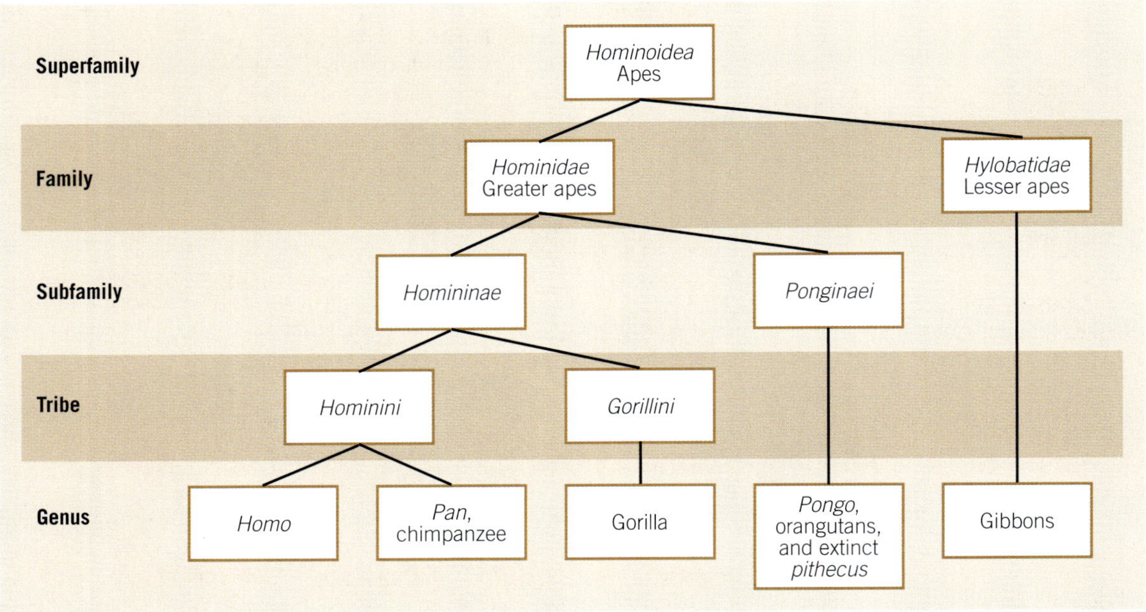

Fig 2-1-27 Taxonomy of hominoids (*Hominoidea*).[45-53]

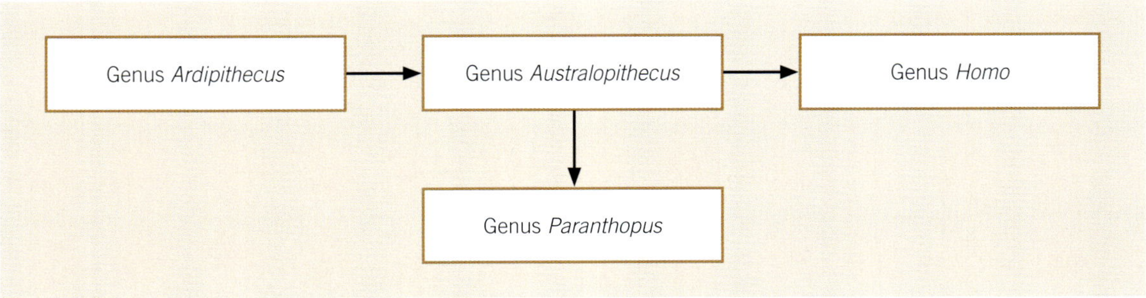

Fig 2-1-28 A current genus grouping. *Australopithecus robustus* became included in a separate genus, *Paranthropus*.

It is now considered that humans developed from apes and specifically from the chimpanzee (*Pan*). Through DNA comparison, it is believed that a Pan/Homo divergence (evolutionary split between chimpanzee and human) occurred between 5.4 to 6.3 my. An initial split was followed by later hybridization called speciation that took 4 million years.[45,46] Speciation is the evolutionary process by which new biological species arise.

Taxonomy changes since the 1980s (*Hominids* to *Hominins*)

Up until the 1980s, paleoanthropologists usually followed the Linnaeus taxonomic system established by the 18th century scientist Carl Linnaeus, in relation to the various species of humans.

The family of *Hominoids* included the subfamily of *Hominids* (humans and their ancestors) and *Anthropoids* (chimps, gorillas, and orangutans). These conventional evolutionary lineages were derived from morphological studies. Molecular DNA studies have led to a revision of the hominoidal taxonomy and is shown in (Fig 2-1-27).[45-53] Molecular studies have shown that humans, chimps, and gorillas are closer to one another than to orangutans and further away from orangutans and gibbons. A subsequent taxonomy was formulated. *Hominoidea* comprises all of the apes including humans (superfamily). These divide into two families, the great apes (*Hominidae*) and the lesser apes (*Hylobatidae*) that contain the gibbons. The hominid (*Hominidae*) family divides into subfamilies of *Homininae* and *Ponginaei*. The *Homininae* divide into tribes of *Hominini* and *Gorillini*. *Hominini* divides to genus *Homo* and genus *Pan* (chimpanzee).[47,48]

A hominin is what was formerly termed a hominid: a creature that paleoanthropologists have agreed is human or a human ancestor. This includes the *Homo/Pan* line and excludes the *Gorilla* line. These include all of the *Homo* species (*Homo erectus, H. ergaster, H. georgicu, H antecessor, H neanderthalensis, H. rudolfensis, H. sapiens,* etc), all of the australopithecines (*Australopithicus africanus, A. boisei,* etc) and other ancient forms like *Paranthropus* and *Ardipithecus* (Fig 2-1-27).[45-53]

Australopithecus robustus and *Australopithecus bosei* have been recently named *Paranthropus robustus* and *Paranthropus bosei*. The genus *Homo* is considered to be derived from the genus *Australopithecus* (Figs 2-1-27 and 2-1-28).[47-51] Orangutans speciated from the ancestors of the other three genera roughly 14 my. The ancestors of the *Hominidae* family had already speciated from those of the *Hylobatidae* family, circa 15 to 20 my.[50,51]

Hominin dentitions

P. robustus (formerly *Australopithecus robustus*) had disproportion between anterior and posterior dentition. Incisors and canines were small while premolars and molars were extremely large.

A. Afarensis showed similar micromorphology in dental wear to extant gorillas and chimpanzees. Less wear was seen in early *Homo.* The *Hominini* showed a reduction of incisors and canines with the appearance of bicuspid premolars. Canines diminished to a spatulate form. Canine spaces disappeared and they developed an even-rounded dental arcade (Figs 2-1-19, 2-1-24, and 2-1-25).

In *Homo habilis,* incisors were more spatulate and molars became smaller. *H. erectus* records exhibit heavy wear patterns, pit scratches, and polished surfaces that indicate an unspecialized omnivorous diet. *H. sapiens* displayed a reduced jaw bone size with dental crowding and reduced size of the third molar.[53-56]

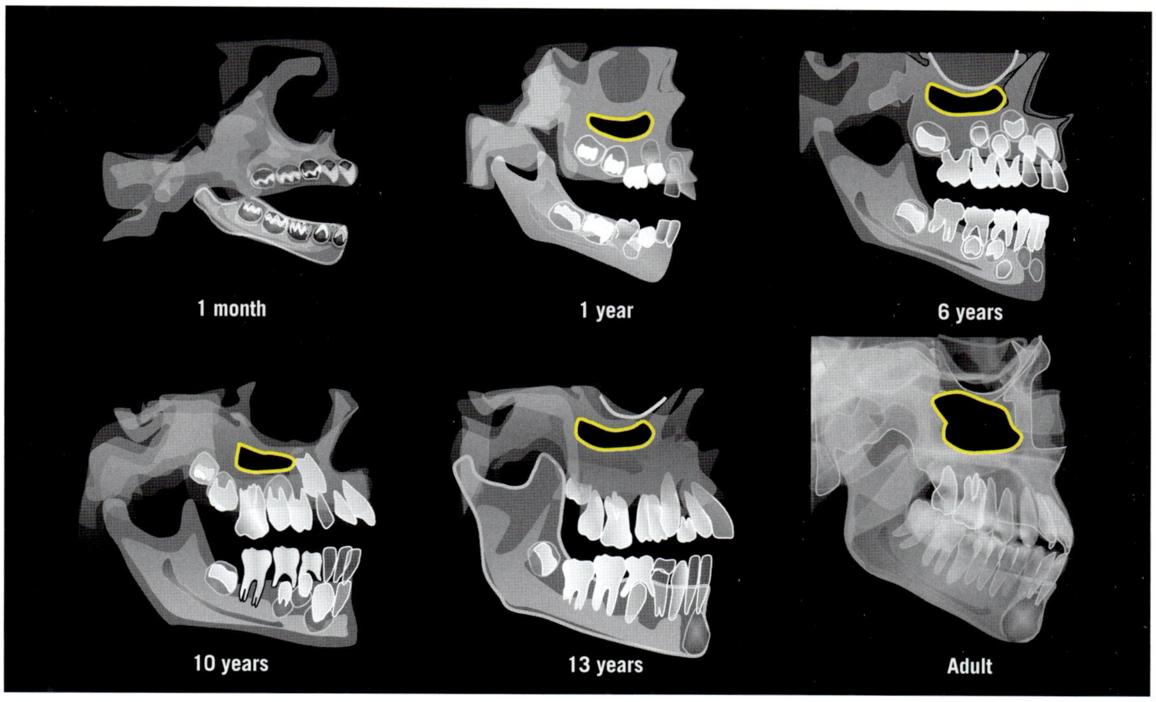

Fig 2-2-15 Development of the maxillary sinus. At birth the sinus is very small (5 × 7 mm). As the alveolus grows inferiorly and the teeth erupt, the sinus grows in anteroposterior vertical and lateral dimensions – at birth: 5 mm high × 7 mm long; at birth: around 5 to 7 mm; at 1 year: 14 mm; at 3 years: around 21 mm; at 7 years: around 28 mm; and in adulthood: around 35 mm.[8,31-35] (Redrawn and adapted from Scott and Symons.[8])

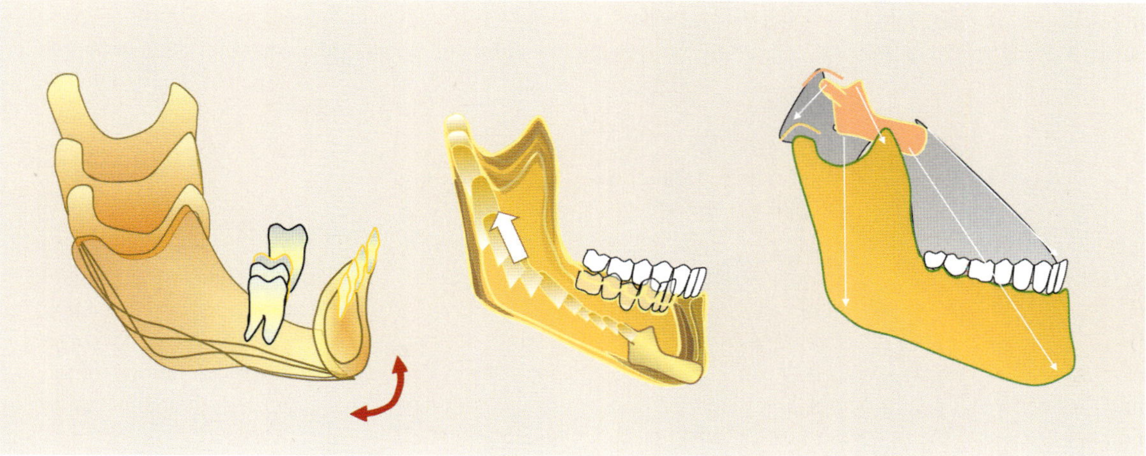

Fig 2-2-16 Growth of the mandible. Downward and forward, and rotation that can be in a forward or backward direction.[42]

some years between tooth descent and the vertical downward growth of the sinus. The periods of most active growth of the sinuses are during the first two years and between 15 and 18 years.[8,32]

The anteroposterior length of the maxillary sinus increases with the forward growth of the maxilla. At birth this is around 7 mm, 14 mm (double) at 1 year, (tripled) 21 mm at 3 years, 28 mm (quadrupled) at 7 years and five times as great in the adult, at 35 mm. The development of the sinus is linked to the development of the surrounding sinus cavities of the middle third of the facial skeleton (Fig 2-2-15) [8,31-35]

Condyle and eminence

The articular eminence grows rapidly to almost half its adult form by the age of 2 years. Bone deposition along the distal incline occurs together with the eruption of the maxillary incisors and first and second molars, increasing in height up to the age of 7 years. Growth has been shown to cease in the mixed dentition and achieve its maximum height by 20 years.[36]

According to skull examinations, children have a shallower slope of the eminence than adults.[37]

As flat condyles become steeper – seen in childhood to adulthood – non-working contact incidence was reported to decrease.[36-41]

Development and postnatal growth of the temporomandibular joints

The growth cartilage of the developed condyle is located at the condylar surface just under the fibrous articular layer. It atrophies in the absence of function but retains its endochondral capacity in response to functional demands. It is active in prenatal mandibular and postnatal craniofacial development, forming the condyles and condylar necks by endochondral bone formation. The rest of the mandible grows by intramembranous growth, stimulated regionally by the muscles. The articular eminence and glenoid fossa also form by intramembranous ossification.

Postnatal growth and development of the craniofacial complex

Mandibular rotational growth path

The mandible grows downwards and forwards by upward growth from the condylar cartilage and peripheral intramembranous modeling from functional muscular forces (Fig 2-2-16). A rotational component is also described based around the pterygomasseteric sling at the angle of the mandible (Fig 2-2-18). The overall form is genetically determined and

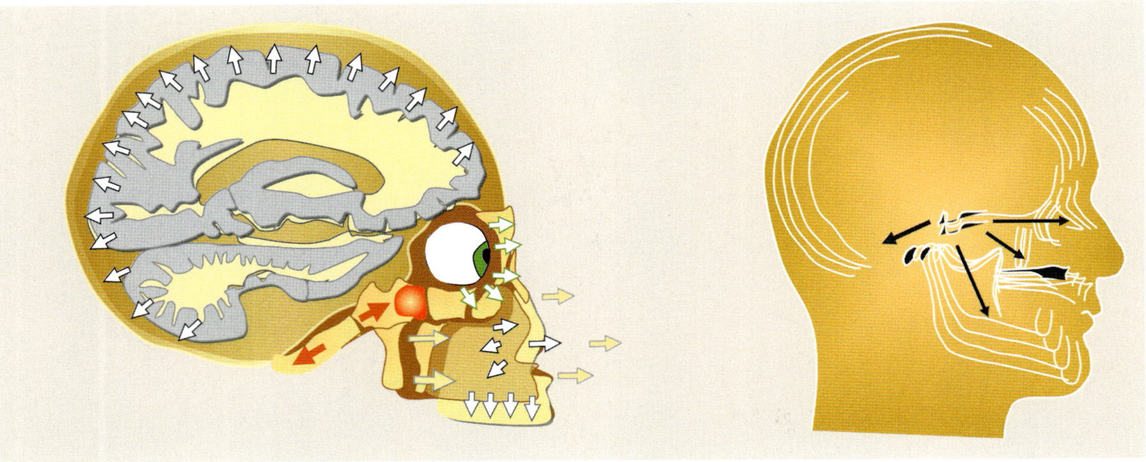

Fig 2-2-17 Growth direction of the craniofacial complex. Various axes of growth have been postulated. One theory purported growth centered in the region around the sella turcica.[42,43,46,47]

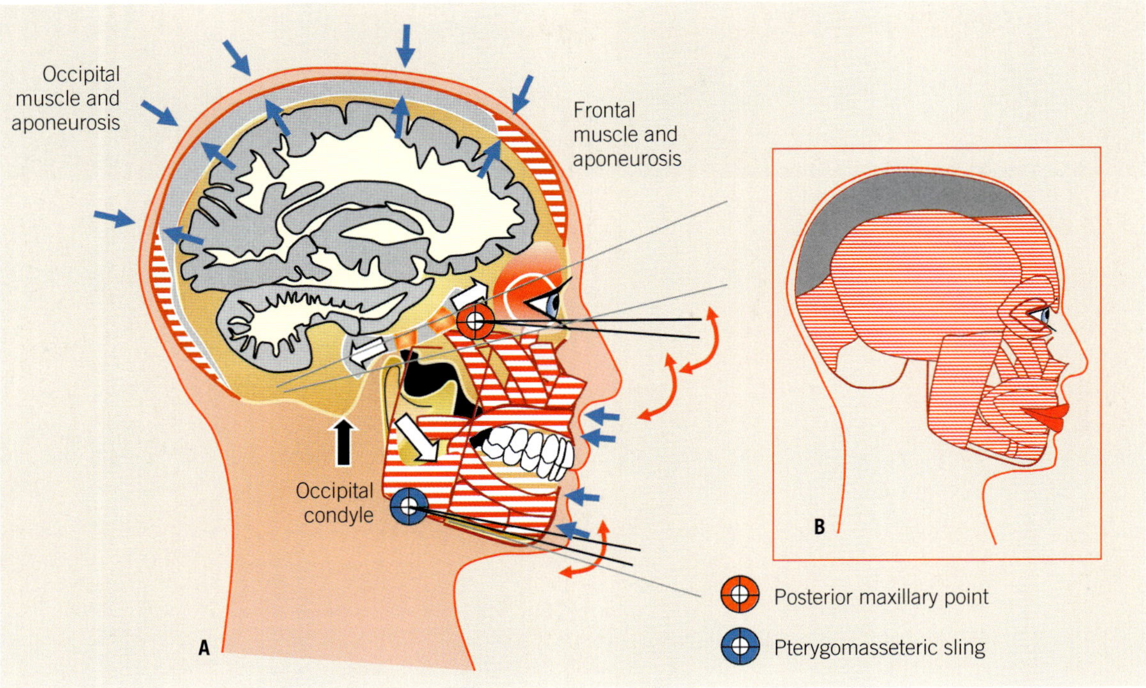

Fig 2-2-18 **A**: The aponeurotic tension model of craniofacial growth: Occipital axis of craniofacial growth. Late brain growth caudally and ventrally together with spheno-occipital growth is resisted and modified by the facial mask of the craniofacial musculoaponeurotic system (CFMAS). Mandibular growth rotation around the pterygomasseteric sling axis (PTM sling). Maxillary growth rotation around posterior maxillary (PM) point. Light gray lines indicate divergence of the facial planes. **B**: The superficial musculoaponeurotic systems (SMAS).[25]

is governed by the individual genetic makeup if uninfluenced by adverse local forces. Disturbed local factors can alter the natural growth potential leading to morphologic variations.[42]

Facial growth patterns and centers

Growth patterns have been postulated in various forms (Figs 2-2-13, 2-2-16, 2-2-17, and 2-2-18).[7,42-48] An axis center or central zone around which growth occurs has been postulated round the sella turcica and region of the spheno-ethmoid growth center.[43,46,47] Theories of growth include the functional matrix theory and the effect of the nasal septum.[45] Separate functional matrices are proposed as developing in response to function, the neurocranial capsular matrix, and the orofacial capsular matrix.[28-30] Growth of the brain and neural structures cause expansion of the neurocranial matrix. Brain growth is the principal force of craniofacial development up to 11 years. Airway enlargement is considered to drive the enlargement of the orofacial matrix. The nasal septum directs prenatal and some postnatal growth to the age of 4 years by when fibrosis of the sutures occurs. Late brain growth has been described with gray matter peak formation for frontal and parietal lobes at 12 years, 16 years for temporal lobes, and around 20 years for the occipital lobe. This growth is considered to occur in an anterior and posterior or caudal and ventral directions.[7,25]

The aponeurotic tension model of craniofacial growth

An additional model for craniofacial growth was proposed, based on continued brain growth resisted by the fronto-occipital musculature and the superficial musculoaponeurotic systems (SMAS).[25] Tension force is transmitted from the frontal and occipital muscles down through the mask of muscles overlying the face, modifying craniofacial rotations of growth direction and adaptation, up to the age of 20. The combined effects of the regional SMAS form a craniofacial musculoaponeurotic system (CFMAS) that is considered to significantly affect maxillary and mandibular development. Variations of CFMAS by strong or weak phenotypes are proposed as being able to vary the maxillomandibular rotational growth pattern between counterclockwise forward rotation and a clockwise posterior rotation.[25]

This theory proposes the occipital condyles as the axis of cranial rotational growth and craniofacial growth due to brain growth, spheno-occipital growth, pneumatization of facial bone, and CMFAS modification. A rotation axis of growth has been proposed for the mandible at the pterygomasseteric sling at the angle of the mandible. A center or axis of rotation of the maxilla is proposed at the convergence of the posterior maxillary (PM) plane and the top of the face, and also at the bottom of the anterior cranial base (Fig 2-2-18).[25] The PM plane demarcates the back of the midface at its junction with the sphenoid, and maintains a 90-degree angle to the neutral horizontal axis of the orbits in primates.[47,48]

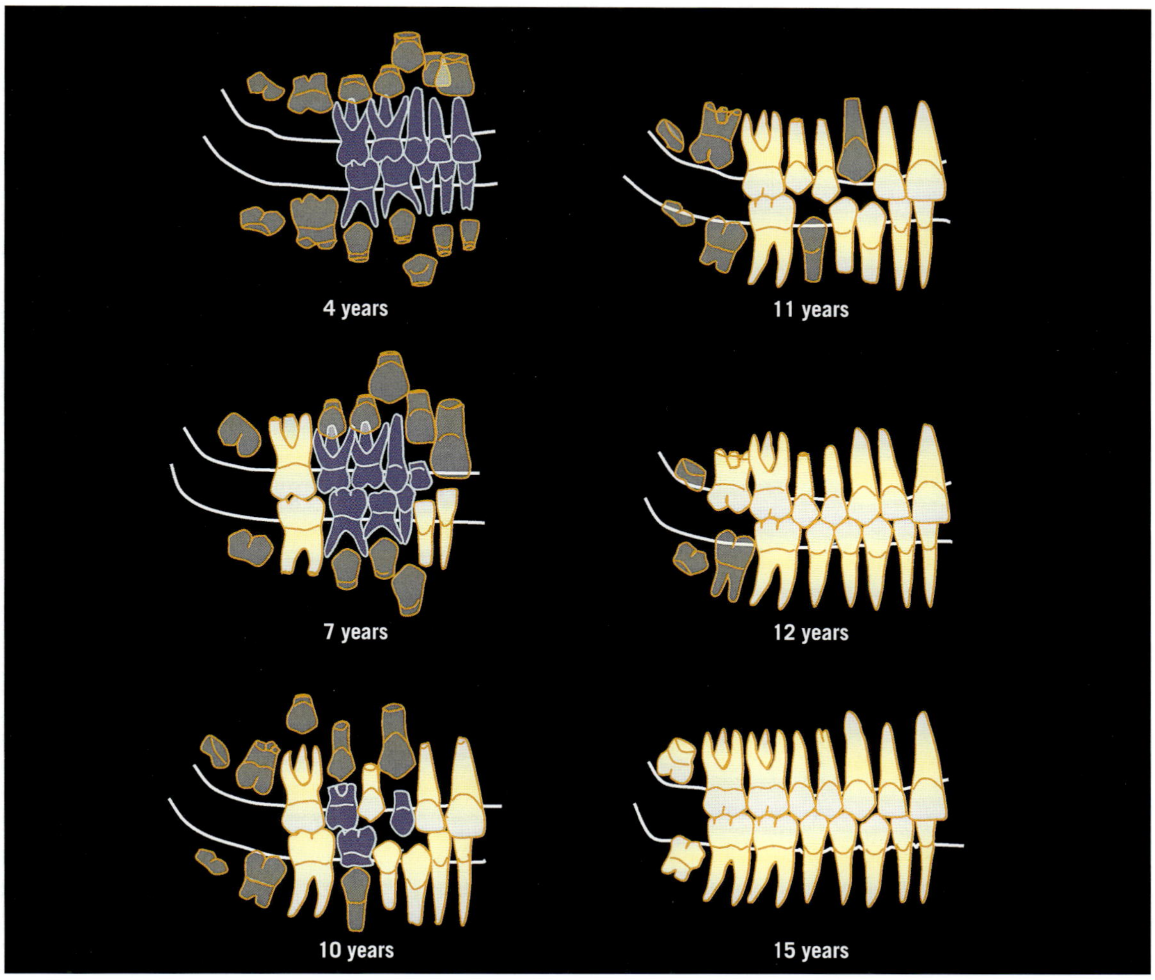

Fig 2-2-19 Normal eruptive sequence from deciduous through mixed to adult dentition.

Normal eruptive process

During the process of facial growth and development, the teeth continue to erupt in a prescribed genetically predetermined sequence, chronologically and directionally. Eruption occurs in six stages:

1. Growth of the tooth follicle.
2. Pre-emergent eruptive spurt.
3. Postemergent eruptive spurt.
4. Juvenile occlusal equilibrium.
5. Circumpubertal occlusal eruptive spurt.
6. Adult occlusal equilibrium (Fig 2-2-19). [49]

The eruptive process

The mechanism of the eruptive process is still not fully understood.[49-55] Initial theories ascribed an effect of the Hertwigs root sheath stimulating the generation of a new tooth substance and resulting in an occlusion direction of the developing tooth bud. [49,50] The dental follicle is necessary for eruption. Bone apposition and resorption ceases on the removal of the follicle. In dog premolars, surgical removal of the follicle from the unerupted tooth prevented the tooth from erupting.[51] Leaving the follicle intact and substituting an inert object for the tooth resulted in the eruption of the inert object.[52] An osteoblast-specific transcription factor, Cbfa1 (Runx2), found in high levels in the dental follicle is considered to play a role in molecular events that regulate tooth eruption.[55]

Requirements for intraosseous tooth eruption are outlined as:

- Intervening bioactive soft tissues, the dental follicle.
- Initiating signals as the developmental program.
- Histological process as bone modeling.
- Oseoclastogenesis CSF-1, VEG, RANK/RANKL/osteoprotegrin.
- Osteogenesis by developmental programming.[50-55]

The continued process of eruption to the prescribed occlusal relation occurs as a combination of eruptive force and soft tissue mediation. The functional matrix influences this prescribed process as the teeth arrive into their prescribed occlusal relationships, and are maintained in a state of equilibrium.

Equilibrium theory

Following eruption, the relations of the teeth are maintained in equilibrium. This is acheived by the interaction of the lips, cheeks, tongue, eruptive process, and dental occlusion. The resting soft tissue plays a significant part in the maintenance of this equilibrium.[50,56-59] The eruptive process also continues to play a role. The eruptive potential remains long after the teeth have reached their initial occlusal level. First molars and incisors must erupt further, after initial occlusal contact to keep pace with vertical jaw growth and the development of the alveolar process. Stretching of oblique periodontal fibers and functional socket deformations have been suggested, but the exact mechanism is still unclear.[50,56-59]

Tongue, lips, and eruptive forces

Equilibrium components include forces of occlusion with very high intensity and very short durations. Lip or tongue pressure in swallowing is of high intensity and short duration. During speech, forces are of low intensity and short duration. Similarly, at rest, forces are of low intensity and long duration. The forces of eruption are very low and of long duration. The primary factors are the resting pressure of the tongue and the lips and eruptive forces. The resting pressure of lips and tongue are more important for vertical positioning of the teeth than pressures during swallowing. This holds true for other spatial relations (Fig 2-2-20).[56,57]

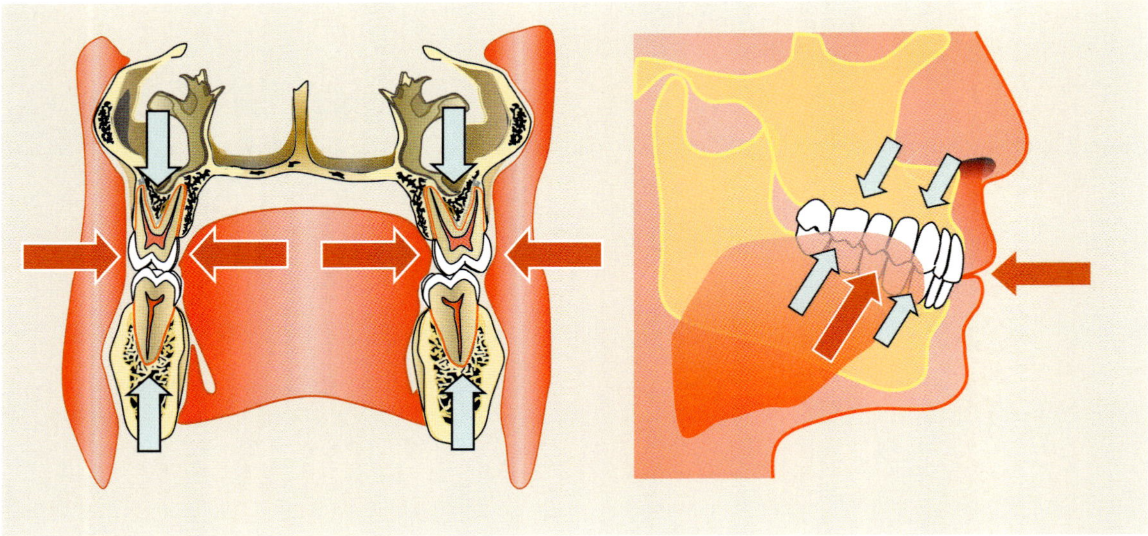

Fig 2-2-20 Forces maintaining tooth equilibrium. Primary equilibrium factors are the cheeks and tongue at rest (red arrows) and the eruptive forces of the teeth (blue arrows).

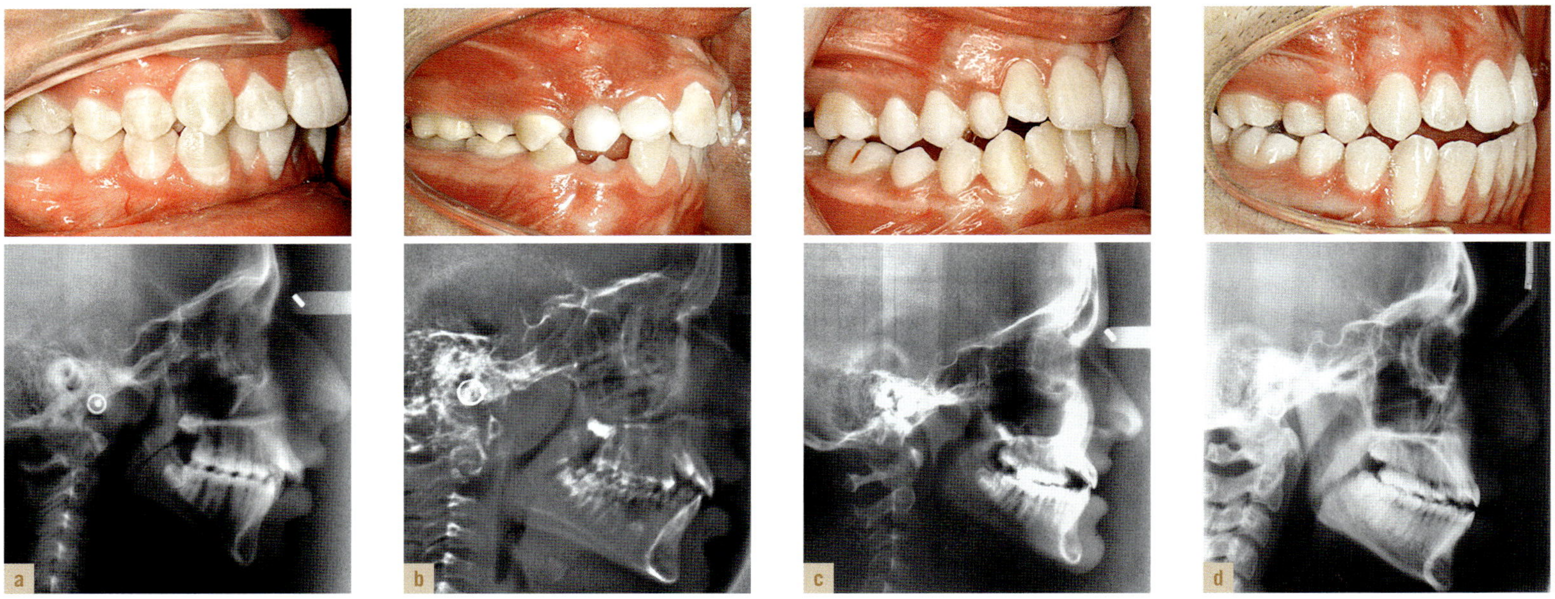

Fig 2-2-21 Varying anteroposterior skeletal relations: (a) retrognathic class II; (b) orthognathic class I; (c) prognathic class III; and (d) anterior open bite with vertical skeletal discrepancy.

Adult growth

Facial growth has been shown to continue during adult life with an increase in all facial dimensions. Vertical changes were seen to occur more than anteroposterior changes, and width changes were less evident. Differences are seen between genders. Adult growth changes were in the magnitude of 1 mm per year. The cumulative effects over decades were large. Rotation of both jaws continued into adult life together with vertical changes and eruption of the teeth. Males showed a net rotation of the jaws forwards, decreasing the mandible plane angle. Females had a tendency to backward rotation, increasing the mandibular plane angle. Occlusal relations were maintained by compensation. Soft tissue changes included an elongation of the nose, flattening of the lips, and an augmentation of the chin.[60]

Adult tooth eruption: compensatory eruption

Adult eruption continues through life. Continued eruption occurs when antagonist contact is lost. Teeth and segments may continue to erupt taking with them the alveolar ridge. Such segmental overeruption can cause significant functional and esthetic difficulties. Why some teeth erupt when unopposed and others do not has not been explained. The role of the tongue in swallowing may play a role. Tooth eruption was reported to compensate for 60% of tooth wear in severe attrition. The supracrestal periodontal fibers play a significant role in the maintenance of tooth position and potential unopposed eruption.[50,61-63]

Normal range of variability

Normal growth and development is reflected in ranges of normal variability, with skeletal relations between class I orthognathic (70%), class II retrognathic (20%), and class III prognathic (10%) (Fig 2-2-21).[2] Ranges are seen within and between ethnic, racial, and international studies.[64-77]

Vertical variations occur with long faces with a high gonial angle or short faces with a flat gonial angle. Extreme vertical transverse and horizontal discrepancies occur in lower percentages and tend to be more aberrant and less common.[66-77]

Anomalies

An anomaly is a marked deviation from normal. Skeletal and dental anomalies in children and adolescents are described from various multiracial, ethnic studies with incidence varying widely from 30 to 93%.[66-77] A classification of anomalies was proposed in categories of:

dentitional anomalies; occlusal anomalies; and space anomalies. Dentitional and occlusal anomalies may be sagittal, vertical, or transversal. Dental anomalies include crowding, spacing, median diastema deviations, and single-tooth anomalies, such as:ectopic eruption; impaction supernumeraries; congenitally missing; inverted; infraocclusion; tipping; tilting; microdontia; and macrodontia.[76] The origin and development of dental and skeletal anomalies may be genetic, developmental or environmental (see Chapter 3.4).[27,77-85]

Crowding

Anomalies are generally either skeletal or dental. Skeletal genetic determinants can result in the dental arches being too small for the size of the teeth, resulting in tooth crowding.

Anterior component of force: interproximal wear

Local factors may also have an effect, including the anterior component of force and interproximal wear. Abrasion of interproxial contacts can reduce arch circumference. Posterior interproximal wear can cause the mesial migration of the posterior teeth, postulated as occurring from the effects of the anterior component of force. The anterior component of force is believed to arise as a result of the mesial axial inclination of the posterior teeth. As a result of teeth inclination and muscle vectors in intercuspation, forces of occlusion are dissipated axially and towards the front of the mouth through the proximal contact points.[86]

References

1. Larsen WJ, Sherman LS, Potter SS, Scott WJ. Human Embryology, ed 3. Edinburgh: Churchill Livingstone, 2001.
2. Mohl N, Zarb G, Carlsson G, Rugh J. A Textbook of Occlusion. Chicago: Quintessence Publishing, 1988.
3. Dechow PC, Carlson DS. Development of mandibular form: phylogeny, ontogeny and function. In: McNeill C (ed). Science and Practice of Occlusion. Chicago: Quintessence Publishing, 1997.
4. Smith SC, Gaveson AC, Hall BK. Evidence for a developmental and evolutionary link between placodal ectoderm and neural crest. J Exp Zool 1995;270:292–301.
5. Gans CM, Northcutt RG. Neural crest and the origin of vertebrates: a new head. Science 1983;220:268–274.
6. Garcia-Fernanez J, Holland PW. Archetypal organization of the amphioxus Hox gene cluster. Nature 1994;370:563–566.
7. Timeline of evolution. Time Tree of Life. Available at: http://www.timetree.org/book.php. Accessed August 2013.
8. Scott JH, Symons NBB. Introduction to Dental Anatomy. London: E & S Livingstone, 1964.
9. Langille RM, Hall BK. Developmental processes, developmental sequences and early vertebrate phylogeny. Biol Rev 1989;64:73–91.
10. Crompton AW, Parker P. Evolution of the mammalian masticatory apparatus. Am Sci 1978;66:192–201.
11. Hall BK. Evolutionary issues in craniofacial biology. Cleft Palate J 1990;27:95–100.
12. Forrey P, Janvier P. Evolution of the early vertebrates: recent discoveries provide clues to the relationships between early vertebrates and their modern relatives. Am Sci 1994;82:554–565.
13. Hall BK. Mandibular morphogenesis and craniofacial malformation. J Caniofac Genet Dev Biol 1982;2:309–322.
14. Frommer J, Margolies MR. Contribution of Meckels cartilage to ossification of the mandible in mice. J Dent Res 1971;50:1260–1267.
15. Durkin JF, Heeley JD, Irving JT. The cartilage of the mandibular condyle. In: Melcher AH, Zarb GA (eds). Temporomandibular Joint: Function and Dysfunction I. Oral Science Reviews Vol 2. Copenhagen: Munksgaard, 1973:29–99.
16. Carstens MH. Development of the facial midline. J Craniofac Surg 2002;13:129–187; discussion 188–190.
17. Jeffery N, Spoor F. Ossification and midline shape changes of the human fetal cranial base. Am J Phys Anthropol 2004;123:78–90.
18. Mohl N. The temporomandibular joint. In: Mohl N, Zarb G, Carlsson G, Rugh J (eds). A Textbook of Occlusion. Chicago: Quintessence Publishing, 1988:81–96.
19. Yuodelis RA. The morphogenesis of the human temporomandibular joint and its associated structures. J Dent Res 1966;45:182–191.
20. Moffett B. The morphogenesis of the temporomandibular joint. Am J Orthod 1966;52:401–415.
21. Thilander B, Carlsson GE, Ingervall B. Postnatal development of the human temporomandibular joint. 1. A histological study. Acta Odontol Scand 1976;34:117–126.
22. Enlow DH, Harris DB. A study of the postnatal growth of the human mandible. Am J Orothod Dentofacial Orthop 1964;50:25–50.
23. Ranly DM. Early orofacial development. J Clin Pediatr Dent 1998;22:267–275.
24. Enlow DH. A comparative study of facial growth in Homo and Maccaca. Am J Phys Anthropol 1966;24:293–308.
25. Standerwick RG, Roberts WE. The aponeurotic tension model of craniofacial growth in man. Open Dent J 2009;3:100–113.
26. Ermolenko AE, Perepada EA. The symmetry of man. Acta Biomed 2007;78(Suppl 1):13–20.
27. Markovic MD. At the crossroads of oral facial genetics. Eur J Orthod 1992;14:469–481.
28. Ingervall B, Thilander B. The human spheno-occipital synchondrosis. I. The time of closure appraised macroscopically. Acta Odontol Scand 1972;30:349–356.
29. Moss ML. The functional matrix hypothesis revisited. 1. The role of mechanotransduction. Am J Orthod Dentofacial Orthop 1997;112:8–11.
30. Moss ML. The functional matrix hypothesis revisited. 2. The role of an osseous connected cellular network. Am J Orthod Dentofacial Orthop 1997;112:221-226.
31. Marquez S. The paranasal sinuses: the last frontier in craniofacial biology. Anat Rec (Hoboken) 2008;261:1350–1361.
32. Shah RK, Dhingra JK, Carter BL, Rebeiz EE. Paranasal sinus development: a radiographic study. Laryngoscope 2003;113: 205–209.
33. Laitman JT, Albertine K. The anatomical record inside the head: A history of reporting findings on the skull, paranasal sinuses, and nose. Anat Rec (Hoboken) 2008;291:1343–1345.
34. House EL, Pansky B, Jacobs MS, Wagner BM. Gross structure of the ear, nasal cavity and paranasal sinuses of the chimpanzee. Anat Rec 1966;155:77–88.
35. Rossie JB. The phylogenetic significance of the anthropoid paranasal sinuses. Anat Rec (Hoboken) 2008;291:1485–1498.
36. Katsavaris EG, Dibbets JM. The growth of articular eminence height during craniofacial growth period. Crainio 2001;19:19:13–20.
37. Katsavrias EG. Changes in articular eminence inclination during the craniofacial growth period. Angle Orthod 2002;72:258–264.
38. Angel JL. Factors in temporomandibular joint form. Am J Anat 1948;83:223–246.
39. Dechow PC, Carlson DS. Occlusal forces and craniofacial biomechanics during growth in rhesus monkeys. Am J Phys Anthropol 1990;83:219–237.
40. Glineburg RW, Laskin DM, Blaustein DI. The effects of immobilization on the primate temporomandibular joint: a histologic and histochemical study. J Oral Maxillofac Surg 1982;40:3–8.
41. Stegenga B, de Bont LGM. TMJ growth, adaptive modeling and remodeling compensatory mechanisms. In: Laskin DM, Greene CD, Hylander WL (eds). TMDs: An Evidence-based Approach to diagnosis and Treatment Planning. Chicago: Quintessence Publishing, 2006:53–67.
42. Bjork A. Variations in the growth pattern of the human mandible: longitudinal radiographic study by the implant method. J Dent Res 1963;42:400–411.
43. Ricketts RM. Planning treatment on the basis of the facial pattern and an estimate of its growth. Angle Orthod 1957;27:14–37.
44. Moss ML, Young RW. A functional approach to craniology. Am J Phys Anthropol 1960;18:281–292.
45. Scott JH. The cartilage of the nasal septum: a contribution to the study of facial growth. Br Dent J 1953;95:37–43.
46. Rickets RM. Divine proportion. In: Goldstein RE (ed). Esthetics in Dentistry, Volume 1, ed 2. Hamilton, Ontario: BC Decker, 1998:187–206.
47. Kosky K. Cranial growth centers: facts or fallacies? Am J Orthod 1968;54:566–583.
48. McCarthy RC, Lieberman DE. Posterior maxillary (PM) plane and anterior cranial architecture in primates. Anat Rec 2001;264:247–260.
49. Proffit WR, Fields HW, Sarver DM. Contemporary Orthdontics. St Louis, MO: Mosby, 2007.
50. Steedle JR, Proffit WR. The pattern and control of eruptive tooth movements. Am J Orthod 1985;87:56–66.
51. Cahill DR, Marks SC Jr. Tooth eruption: evidence for the central role of the dental follicle. J Oral Pathol 1980;9:189–200.
52. Marks SC Jr, Cahill DR. Experimental study in the dog of the non-active role of the tooth in the eruptive process. Arch Oral Biol 1984;29:311–322.
53. Wise GE, King GJ. Mechanisms of tooth eruption and orthodontic tooth movement. J Dent Res 2008;87:414–434.
54. Marks SC Jr. The basic and applied biology of tooth eruption. Connect Tissue Res 1995;32:149–157.
55. Wise GE, Frazier-Bowers S, D'Souza RN. Cellular, molecular, and genetic determinants of tooth eruption. Crit Rev Oral Biol Med 2002;13:323–334.
56. Proffit WR. Equilibrium theory revisited: factors influencing position of the teeth. Angle Orthod 1978;48:175–186.
57. Proffit WR. Equilibrium theory reexamined: To what extent do tongue and lip pressures influence tooth position and thereby the occlusion? In: Perryman JH

(ed). Oral Physiology and Occlusion. An international symposium. New York: Pergamon, 1978:55–77.
58. Gould MS, Picton DC. A study of pressures exerted by the lips and cheeks on the teeth of subjects with angle's class II division 1, class II division 2 and class 3 malocclusions compared with those of subjects with normal occlusions. Arch Oral Biol 1968;13:527–541.
59. Katona TR, Quian H. A mechanism of noncontinuous supraosseous tooth eruption. Am J Orthod Dentofaial Orthop 2001;120:263–271.
60. Behrents RG. A treatise on the continuum of growth in the aging craniofacial skeleton [thesis]. Ann Arbor: University of Michigan Center for Human Growth and Development, 1985.
61. Newman HN. Attrition, eruption and the periodontium. J Dent Res 1999;78:730–734.
62. Milosevic A. Tooth wear and compensatory eruption. Br Dent J 1998;185:209–210.
63. Craddock HL, Youngson CC, Manogue M, Blance A. Occlusal changes following posterior tooth loss in adults. Part I: a study of clinical parameters associated with the extent and type of supraeruption in unopposed posterior teeth. J Prosthodont 2007;16:485–494.
64. Bjork A. Variability and age changes in overjet and overbite. Am J Orthod 1953;39:779–801.
65. Bjork A, Palling M. Adolescent age changes in sagittal jaw relation, alveolar prognathy and incisor inclination. Acta Odontol Scand 1955;12:201–232.
66. Helm S. Malocclusion in Danish children with adolescent dentition: an epidemiological study. Am J Orthod 1968;54:3352–3366.
67. Scaife RR, Holt JE. Natural occurrence of cuspid guidance. J Prosthet Dent 1969;22:225–229.
68. Helm S. Prevalence of malocclusion in relation to development of the dentition. An epidemiological study of Danish schoolchildren. Acta Odontol Scand 1970;28(Suppl 58):1+
69. Ingervall B. Development of the occlusion. In: Mohl ND, Zarb GA , Carlsson G, Rugh JD (eds). A Textbook of Occlusion. Chicago: Quintessence Publishing, 1988:43–56.
70. El-Mangoury NH, Mostafa YA. Epidemiologic panorama of dental occlusion. Angle Orthod 1990;60:207–214.
71. Brunelle JA, Bhat M, Lipton JA. Prevalence and distribution of selected occlusal characteristics in the US population, 1988–1991. J Dent Res 1996;75:706–713.
72. Proffit WR, Fields HW Jr, Moray LJ. Prevalence of malocclusion and orthodontic treatment need in the United States: estimates from NHANES III survey. Int J Adult Orthodon Orthognath Surg 1998;13:97–106.
73. Thilander B, Pena L, Infante C, Parada SS, de Mayorga C. Prevalence of malocclusion and orthodontic treatment need in children and adolescents in Bogotá, Colombia. An epidemiologic study related to different stages of dental development. Eur J Orthod 2001;23:153–167.
74. Onyeaso CO. Prevalence of malocclusion among adolescents in Ibadan, Nigeria. Am J Orthod Dentofacial Orthop 2004;126:604–607.
75. Gelgor IE, Karaman AI, Ercan E. Prevalence of malocclusion among adolescents in central Anatolia. Eur J Dent 2007;1:125–131.
76. Bjork A, Krebs A, Solow B. A method for epidemiological registration of malocclusion. Acta Odontologica Scand 1964;22:27–41.
77. Mossey PA. The heritability of malocclusion: part 2. The influence of genetics in malocclusion. Br J Orothod 1999;26:195–203.
78. Logan WHG, Kronfeld R. Development of the human jaws and surrounding structures from birth to the age of fifteen years. J Am Dent Assoc 1933;20:379–427.
79. Pascoe JJ, Hayward JR, Costich ER. Mandibular prognathism: its etiology and a classification. J Oral Surg Anesth Hosp Dent Serv 1960;18:21–24.
80. van der Linden FP. Genetic and environmental factors in dentofacial morphology. Am J Orthod 1966;52:576–583.
81. Watnick SS. Inheritance of craniofacial morphology. Angle Orthod 1972;42:339–351.
82. Peck S, Peck L, Kataja M. Class II Division 2 malocclusion: a heritable pattern of small teeth in well-developed jaws. Angle Orthod 1988;68:9–17.
83. Turner S, Nattrazz C, Sandy JR. The role of soft tissues in the aetiology of malocclusion. Dent Update 1997;24:209–214.
84. Harpending H, Cochran G. Genetic diversity and genetic burden in humans. Infect Genet Evol 2006;6:154–162.
85. Kraus BS, Wise, WJ, Frie RH. Heredity and the craniofacial complex. Am J Orthod 1959;45:172–217.
86. Southard TE, Behrents RG, Tolley EA. The anterior component of occlusal force. Part 2. Relationship with dental alignment. Am J Orthod Dentofacial Orthop 1990;97:41–44.

2.3 Neuromuscular Physiology

Contents

The neuromuscular system

Understanding of the mechanisms of the neuromusculature has progressed in the past decades.

Neural pathways, neural transmission, and functional associations of the spinal and central neural regions are being discovered with developing technologies, but we are far from fully understanding the intricate workings and mechanisms of this vastly complex system.

Regarding clinical prosthodontics and its related fields of application, a more detailed knowledge of neuromuscular anatomy and physiology is helpful to better evaluate some of the unclear and controversial aspects of clinical science and art. These include an appreciation of the neuromuscular basis of electromyography (EMG) and its application in clinical and research contexts. Fields of direct clinical relevance include EMG of rest position, mandibular posture, neuromuscular implications of anterior guidance, and purported neuromuscular protection of anterior disclusion. The adaptation of masticatory function to occlusal changes, the effects of occlusal parafunction, bruxism, and the interrelations of temporomandibular disorders (TMDs) are all areas of significant diagnostic and therapeutic relevance that can be investigated using EMG. An appreciation of peripheral and central sensitization and modulation is helpful in the understanding of current models of orofacial pain, myofascial pain, and biopsychosocial models.[1,2]

Muscles, psyche, function, parafunction

The functional interactions of the neuromusculature, dentition, temporomandibular joints (TMJs), and the psyche are pertinent to clinical perspectives of restoring lost dental form and function and understanding TMDs. The brain coordinates and controls function through sensory motor systems, some of which are identified by their afferent, efferent, and central neural pathways.[1-3] Proprioceptive, tactile, and nociceptive receptors relay sensory information via primary afferents through spinal and trigeminal neural pathways to the spine, midbrain, thalamus, and cortex via intermediate neurons. Efferent motor pathways from the central nervous system (CNS) to the muscles via motor centers and motor pattern generators are identified and jaw function described in terms of voluntary, reflex, and cyclic neuromuscular systems.

The influence of the psyche in the form of stress, emotion, and mood on function, adaptation, and orofacial pain has become better appreciated. This is seen as having significant clinical relevance in relation to occlusal parafunction, bruxism, occlusal trauma, restorative longevity, and TMDs (Fig 2-3-1).[3-6]

Sensory receptors

Receptors are found in the periodontal ligament (PDL), gingivae, periosteum, oral soft tissues, muscles, tendons, and joint tissues. These provide feedback information that facilitates all aspects of oral function for breathing, drinking, eating, swallowing, and speech. Receptors include taste buds, hot/cold receptors, and position-related (proprioceptive) receptors in the periodontal ligaments, muscle ligaments, and muscles. Golgi tendon organs, Ruffini corpuscles, and stretch reflex receptors pass proprioceptive positional information to spinal reflexes peripherally and for central processing in the cerebellum and higher centers. Current concepts of orofacial pain mechanisms now emphasize the interaction of peripheral and central sensitization, modulation, and the interrelation of the perceptual and emotional response to nociceptive afferent information (Fig 2-3-2).[1-11]

Structure of the central nervous system

The human brain contains around 100 billion neurons and 100 trillion synaptic connections. Gross anatomical structures, neural pathways, and areas of interaction and function have been identified, with the major anatomical components consisting of the spinal cord and the brain.

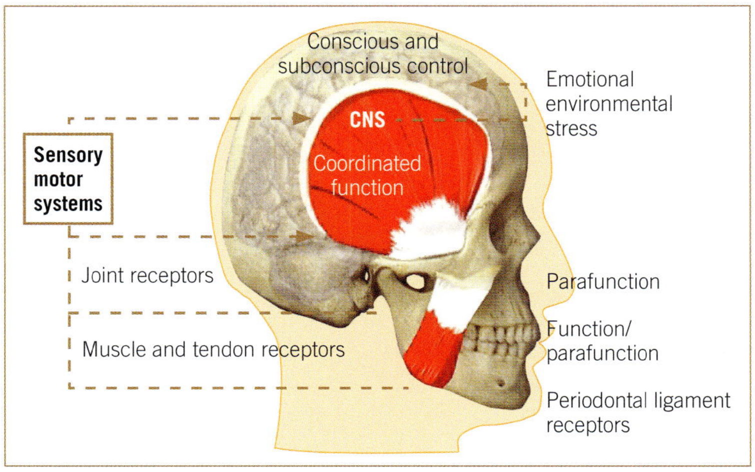

Fig 2-3-1 Jaw function and parafunction are carried out and controlled through the complex interaction of conscious and subconscious control. This is influenced by emotions and environmental stress through sensory motor systems. Function is described as voluntary, reflex, and rhythmic.

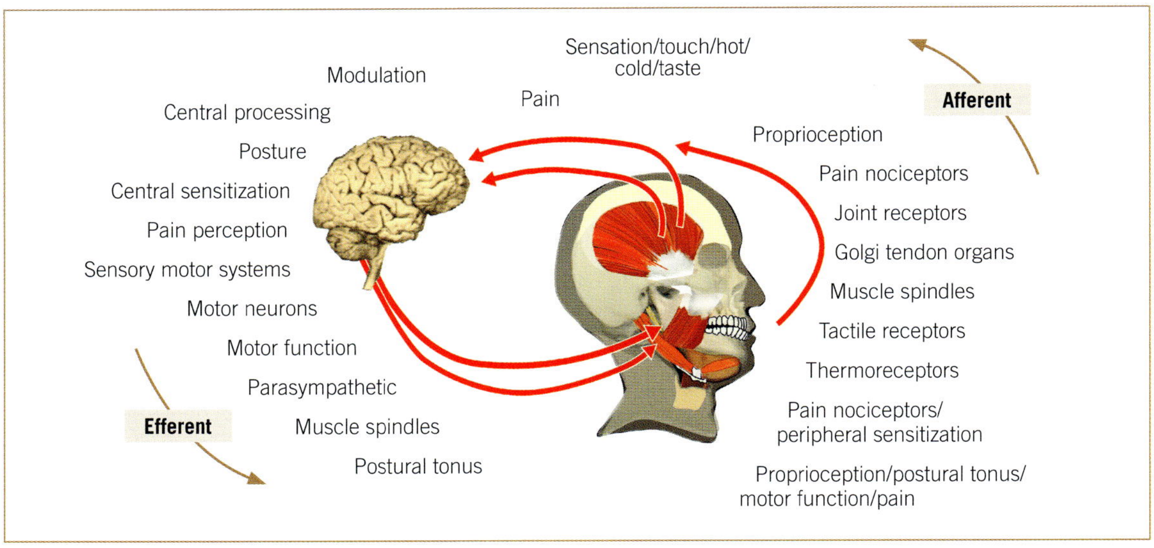

Fig 2-3-2 Afferent sensory neurons pass sensory tactile, proprioceptive (positional), and nociceptive (pain producing) stimuli to the central nervous system. Following central processing, motor efferents pass stimuli to the muscles.

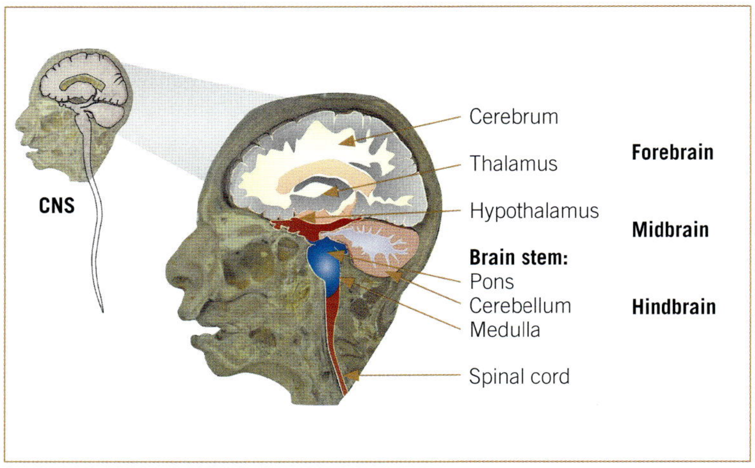

Fig 2-3-3 The central nervous system (CNS) comprises the brain and the spinal column. The brain is composed of the hindbrain, midbrain, and forebrain. The hindbrain contains the medulla, pons, and cerebellum. The midbrain contains the hypothalamus, pituitary, and amygdala, while the forebrain contains the cerebrum with basal ganglia, thalamus, and other structures. The midbrain and the hindbrain constiture the brain stem.

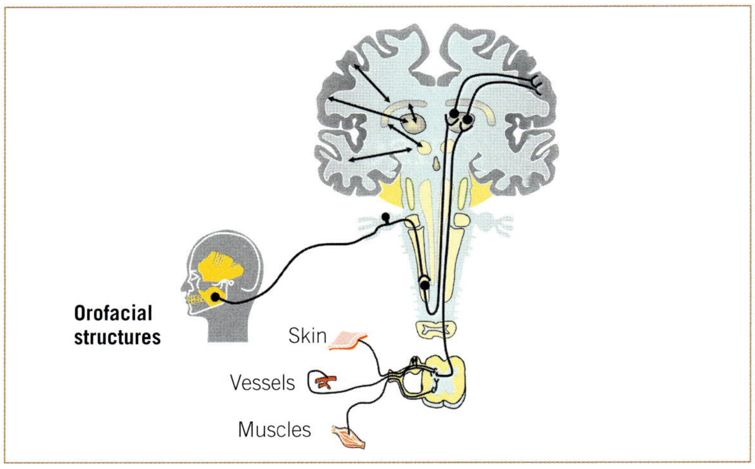

Fig 2-3-4 Sensory information from the teeth, joints, and masticatory muscles passes via primary sensory afferents into the sensory roots of the trigeminal nerve (V) into the main sensory nucleus, spinal tract nucleus of V, and up through ascending sensory pathway to the thalamus and cerebral cortex. Separate ophthalmic, maxillary, and mandibular branches of the trigeminal nerve pass into the three sensory roots of V with their cell bodies in the gasserian ganglion to connect via synapses with second-order neurons at region-specific levels in the spinal tract nucleus. (Redrawn from Okeson.[1])

Structure of the brain

The brain is divided into the forebrain, midbrain, and hindbrain. The midbrain and hindbrain constitute the brain stem and are a continuation of the spinal cord as it connects to the medulla (also called medulla oblongata) (Fig 2-3-3).

Medulla

The medulla contains ascending and descending tracts that communicate between the spinal cord and various parts of the brain. It contains centers regulating heart rate, respiration, and blood vessel diameter and is the origin of cranial nerves XII, XI, X, IX, and VIII.

Pons

The pons contains origins of the trigeminal nerve (V), abducens (VI), facial (VII), and vestibulocochlear (VIII) nerves and houses the respiratory center.

The midbrain houses visual and auditory reflex centers and the origins of the oculomotor (III) and trochlear (IV) nerves.

Spinal cord

The spinal cord extends from the hindbrain down to the lumbar vertebrae. The brain and the spinal cord consist of gray matter and white matter. The gray matter of the spinal cord contains cell bodies and synapses with anterior and posterior horns surrounded by the white matter with myelinated ascending and descending tracts. The ascending tracts contain sensory afferent neurons transmitting sensory impulses from receptors in the skin, skeletal muscles, tendons, joints, and viscera. The descending tracts transmit efferent motor information to

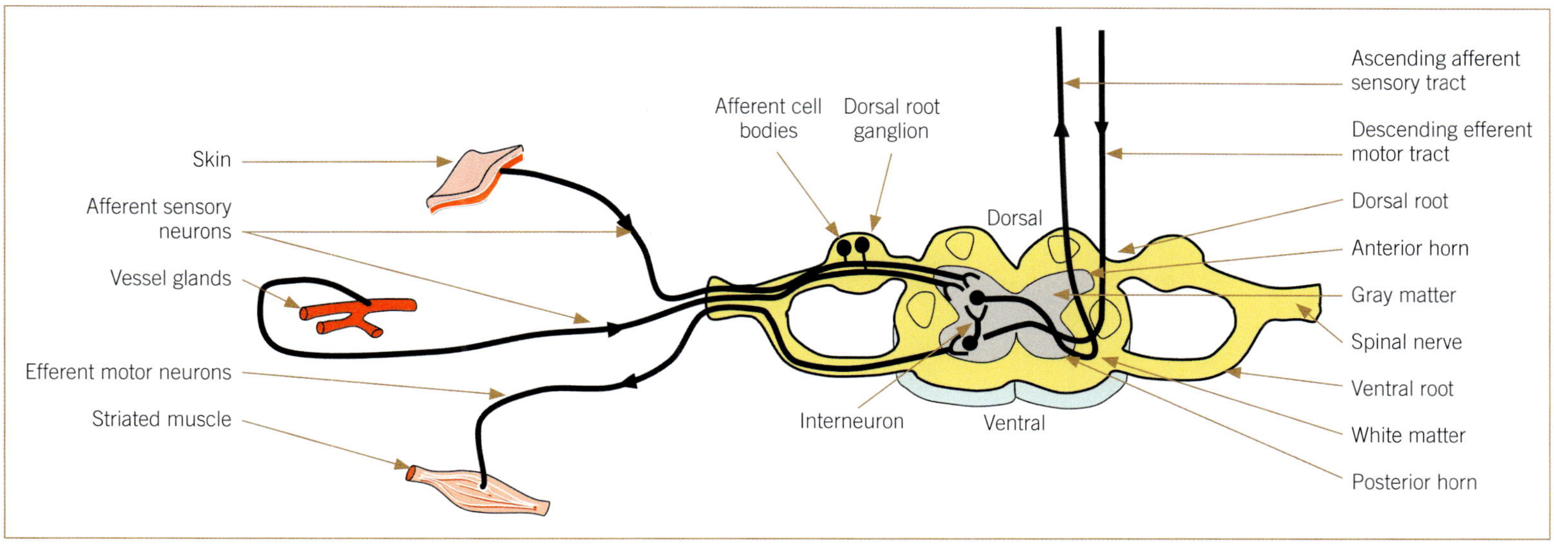

Fig 2-3-5 Section of the spinal column. Sensory primary afferent neurons enter the spinal nerve to pass through the dorsal root into the anterior horn of the central gray matter. They may either connect with interneurons to a spinal reflex circuit or connect to ascending sensory pathways for processing in higher centers. A spinal reflex involves the primary sensory afferent neuron synapsing with an intermediate neuron that synapses with an efferent neuron that passes out of the posterior horn through the ventral root to the muscle.

skeletal muscles, smooth muscle, cardiac muscle, and glands. Function can be reflex, with localized spinal reflexes limited to lower levels or processed from higher levels in the midbrain or cortex (Figs 2-3-4, 2-3-5, and 2-3-6).

Spinal nerves, somatic and visceral afferents, and efferents

There are 31 pairs of spinal nerves, each with a dorsal root and a ventral root. Each spinal nerve contains somatic and visceral afferent sensory neurons and efferent motor neurons. Sensory neurons enter the dorsal root and have their cell bodies in the dorsal root ganglions. Efferent neurons leave through the ventral root to the muscles and viscera (Figs 2-3-4 and 2-3-5).

Somatic afferent neurons

Somatic afferent sensory neurons are sensory neurons that conduct impulses initiated in receptors of the skin, skeletal muscles, tendons, and joints. Peripheral sensation of touch, temperature, pressure, and pain is enabled by sensory afferents called exteroceptors. Receptors in the skeletal muscles, tendons, and joints provide information about body position and movement and are called proprioceptors. These include muscle spindles and Golgi tendon organs. Somatic afferent neurons are unipolar neurons that enter the spinal cord / brain stem through the dorsal root and their cell bodies are located in the dorsal root ganglia. Sensory information from the teeth joints and masticatory muscles is relayed via sensory primary afferent neurons into the sensory roots of the trigeminal nerve (V) into the main sensory nucleus and spinal tract nucleus.

Somatic efferent neurons

Somatic efferent neurons are motor neurons that conduct impulses from the spinal cord or brain stem to skeletal muscles. These neurons are multipolar with cell bodies located in the gray matter of the spinal cord or brain stem. Somatic efferent neurons leave the spinal cord or brain stem through the ventral root of spinal nerves or motor brain stem roots (Figs 2-3-4 and 2-3-5).

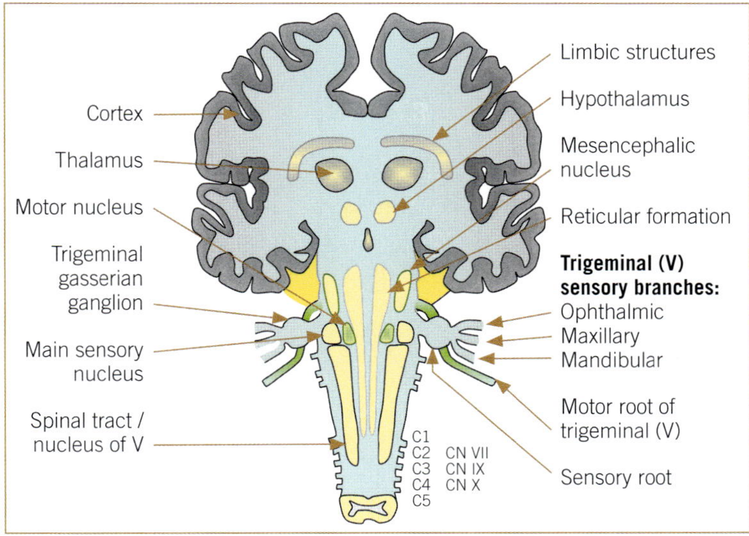

Fig 2-3-6 Illustration of the brain and brain stem showing centers related to sensory and motor neural pathways and the branches of the trigeminal sensory and motor roots (Redrawn from Okeson[1]).

Reflexes

Reflexes are neural responses to internal and external stimuli that are automatic, rapid, and independent of conscious control. They are active in the maintenance of rapid functions and homeostasis. They may be simply composed of monosynaptic pathways or more complex with multiple internuncial neurons or interneurons (Fig 2-3-5).

Simple reflex arc

A simple reflex arc is composed of a receptor that responds to a sensory stimulus, which then passes through its sensory afferent neuron with a single cell body in the dorsal root ganglion. The afferent neuron synapses with an internuncial neuron in the spinal cord for processing or for immediate synapsing with a motor efferent neuron. The motor neuron carries action potentials to the effectors in a muscle or gland for the desired response (Fig 2-3-5).[1,2,4,6,12-14]

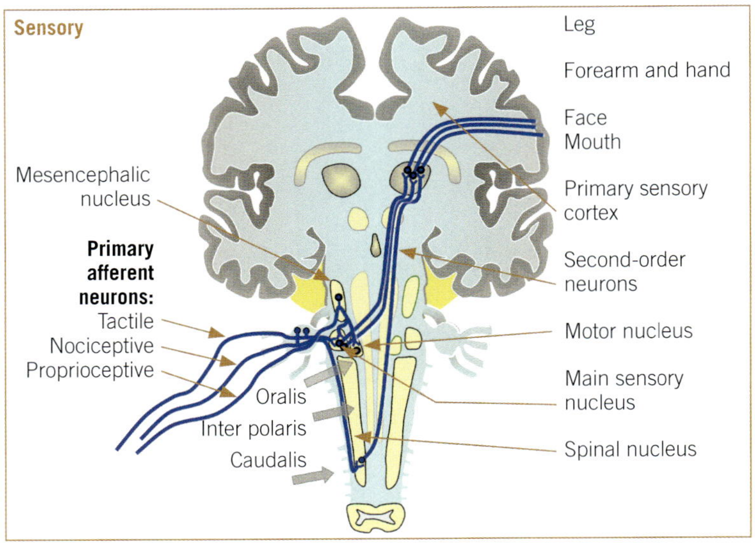

Fig 2-3-7 Primary afferent neurons (PANs) from tactile, nociceptive, and proprioceptive receptors pass to respective centers. Proprioceptive PANs pass to the mesencephalic nucleus to second-order neurons that pass to main sensory nuclei synapses to further internuncial neurons that pass up to the thalamus and sensory cortex. Tactile PANs pass to second-order neurons in the main sensory nucleus. Nociceptive PANs pass to the lower caudal level of the spinal tract nucleus caudalis to synapse with second-order neurons that pass cranially for central processing. (Redrawn from Okeson.[1])

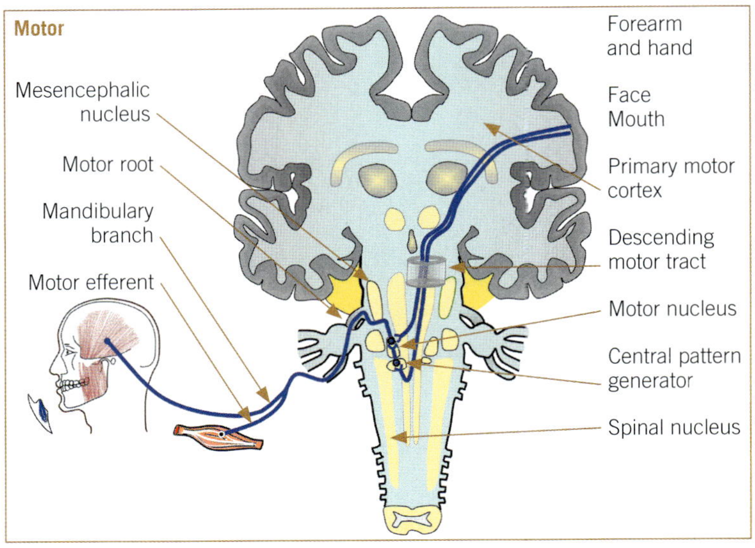

Fig 2-3-8 Motor descending efferent neural pathways. Motor commands pass from the cortex through the descending motor tract to the motor nucleus, the masticatory central pattern generators, and out through the motor branch of the trigeminal nerve (V). (Redrawn from Okeson[1] and other sources.)

The brain stem and its functions

The brainstem is the lower part of the brain, continuous with the spinal cord, and contains parts of the midbrain, the pons, and part of the medulla. It has three major components and functions.

1. It houses ascending and descending sensory and motor neural pathways.
2. It contains major cranial nerve roots and neural pathways.
3. It integrates function and regulatory control of the cardiovascular system, respiration, pain sensitivity, alertness, and consciousness. It contains central pattern generators (CPGs) that include the masticatory and swallowing pattern generators (Figs 2-3-5, 2-3-6, and 2-3-7).[1,2,4,6,15,16]

Ascending and descending neural pathways and tracts

The brain stem functions as the conduit of information between the body and the cerebrum and cerebellum. It contains pathways and tracts for ascending afferent sensory and descending efferent motor neurons. Ascending afferent sensory information from the orofacial region and the trigeminal nerve passes through the main sensory nucleus and the spinothalamic tract. Ascending sensory pathways include the spinothalamic tract for pain and temperature and the dorsal column for the sensations of touch, proprioception, and pressure (Fig 2-3-7).[1-6]

The brain stem provides motor and sensory innervation to the face and neck through the cranial nerves. It contains the main motor and sensory roots and pathways of the trigeminal nerve (V) and other cranial nerves (III to XII) for innervations of orofacial structures and other cervico-cranial structures.

Regulation of vital functions

The brain stem contains the reticular formation extending from the top of the spinal cord to the medulla, pons, midbrain, and hypothalamus. It contains the cardiac and respiratory regulatory centers and is active in the regulation of consciousness, alertness, and sleep. The brain stem contains neural fields of CPGs involved with rhythmic functions that are able to function automatically, independent of voluntary control. The masticatory CPG is located adjacent to the motor center (Fig 2-3-8).

Central pattern generators

CPGs are neural networks that can produce rhythmic patterned outputs without sensory or central input. These are responsible for automatic functions such as walking, breathing, swallowing, and mastication. They may involve the integrated contraction of many muscles with highly complex interactions of facilitation and inhibition of all the muscle groups through the afferent, efferent, and internuncial neurons, and their interactions.

Masticatory pattern generator

The masticatory CPG controls mastication by facilitating an intrinsic rhythmic neural pattern modified by the interaction of sensory feedback from the mouth, muscles, and joints. The pattern is affected by the physical characteristics of food, and varies with age. The CPG consists of a complex of neurons situated in the pons and medulla. It receives inputs from higher centers of the brain, especially from the inferio-lateral region of the sensorimotor cortex and from sensory receptors. The CPG includes a core group of neurons with intrinsic signaling properties, as well as a range of other neurons that receive inputs from oral and muscle spindle afferents. The CPG also modulates reflex circuits in addition to controlling motor neurons supplying the jaw, tongue, and facial muscles.[15-18]

Swallowing pattern generators

Swallowing involves the coordinated contraction of more than 25 pairs of muscles in the oropharynx, larynx, and esophagus, which are active during an oropharyngeal phase, followed by the primary esophageal peristalsis. Swallowing depends on a CPG located in the medulla oblongata, which involves several brain stem motor nuclei and two main groups of interneurons: a dorsal swallowing group (DSG) in the nucleus tractus solitarius and a ventral swallowing group (VSG) located in the ventrolateral medulla. Neurons in the DSG are responsible for the generation of the swallowing pattern. The VSG neurons relay commands to the various motor neuronal pools. As in other CPGs, the functioning of

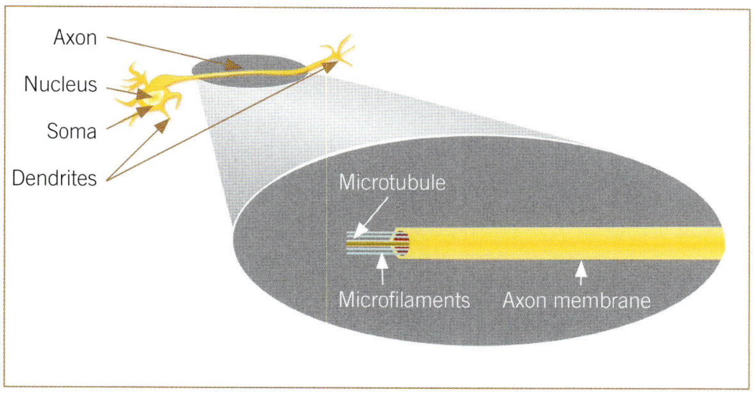

Fig 2-3-9 An unmediated nerve or neuron consists of a cell body, axon, and dendrites. The cell body contains the soma and nucleus. The axon transmits the nerve impulse and can vary in length from a few millimeters up to a meter. A thickening between the cell body and the axon is the axon hillock, which can generate the initiating change in voltage to start a nerve impulse. Dendrites extend from the cell body and the end of the axon. The axon is lined by the axon membrane and contains microtubules and microfilaments.

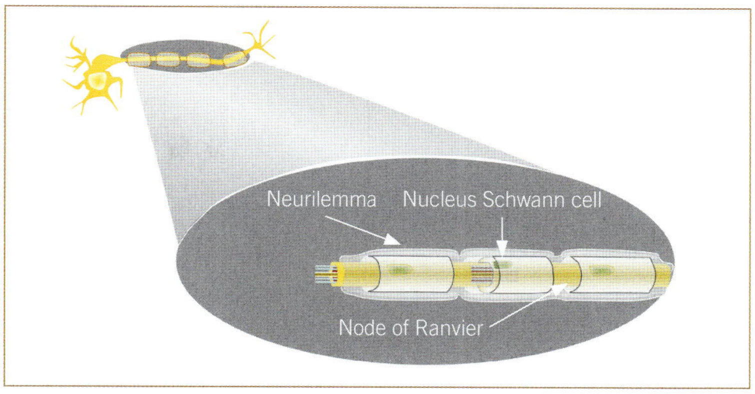

Fig 2-3-10 The majority of nerves in the peripheral nervous system and the white matter of the central nervous system are myelinated. Their axons are lined by regularly spaced insulating sheaths of myelin in Schwann cells. Between the myelin sheaths, the axon is unlined in areas called the nodes of Ranvier. The myelinated nerve is encased by a membrane called the neurilemma.

the central network can be modulated by peripheral and central inputs, so that the swallowing pattern is adapted to the size of the bolus.[1-6,11,12]

Hypothalamus

The hypothalamus is situated below the thalamus and above the brain stem. It is related to metabolic processes and control of the autonomic nervous system, the secretion of hormones, control of body temperature, hunger, thirst, fatigue, anger, circadian cycles, fight-or-flight reflex, and sexual desire. The hypothalamus secretes corticotropin-releasing hormone (CRH) in response to stress that passes to the pituitary gland, which in turn secretes adrenocorticotropic hormone (ACTH) that causes the adrenal gland to secrete cortisol (stress hormone) for the fight-or-flight response.

Cerebellum

The cerebellum plays a significant role in the integration of sensory perception, motor control, and coordination of posture and balance. It integrates proprioceptive information on body position for processing in the cerebral motor cortex and is involved in the control of motor learning, equilibrium, balance, and fine movement. It is also instrumental in the cognitive functions of attention, language, and the sensory processing of sound involved in language and music perception.

Cerebrum

The cerebrum contains the cerebral cortex, medullary body, and basal ganglia.

The cerebrum is involved in cognitive and voluntary processing, and has specific right and left brain functions, with specific areas of motor and sensory processing. Current neuromagnetic resonance imaging and other developing technologies are continuously mapping new areas of neural activity specific to thought, memory, emotion, and psychosocial behavior.

The complex peripheral sensory pathways to the midbrain and thalamus pass to the cerebral cortex for perceptual and cognitive processing. The complex interaction of neural pathways, plastic coordination, and interacting regions facilitate the multifaceted processes of behavior, social interaction, intellect, speech, and all aspects of human activity.

Conscious and voluntary motor functions are directed by the cortex from the primary motor cortex and motor areas in the frontal lobe. Upper motor neurons send axons via internuncial neurons down through the midbrain and spinal column to synapse with the peripheral motor neurons at their neuromuscular junctions.

Afferent and efferent neurons enter and leave the spinal column through the roots of the 31 spinal nerves and the brain stem through the 12 cranial nerve roots. The trigeminal (V) cranial root has three thick sensory roots and a motor root at the upper part of the midbrain (Fig 2-3-6).

Neurotransmission

Nerve anatomy, neurons

The nervous system consists of billions of nerve cells or neurons and neuroglial cells. Specialized receptors create neuronal responses to sensations including touch, pressure, sound, light, and taste. Nerves conduct impulses, and communicate with each other and with other types of cells, such as muscle cells.

The nucleus of a neuron is located in the cell body. Dendrites and axons extend out from the cell bodies varying in length and diameter. Dendrites conduct impulses toward the cell body and axons conduct impulses away from the cell body.

Nerves consist of axons, cell bodies, nerve endings, and dendrites. They may be myelinated or unmyelinated. Nervous transmission occurs when a neuron ending is stimulated by a synapse through a chemical neurotransmitter, changes in voltage, postsynaptic excitatory potential, or by sensory receptors. Axons are surrounded by a membrane called the neurilemma (Figs 2-3-5, 2-3-9, and 2-3-10).

Nerve cell membrane

The nerve cell membrane is hydrophobic and limits diffusion of charged molecules or ions creating a potential difference across its surface known as a membrane potential (Fig 2-3-11). Potential or potential difference may be regarded as synonyms for voltage. The membrane potential is measured and expressed as voltage.

Membrane potential

Electrical potential is the potential energy per unit of charge that is associated with a static electric field. It is measured in volts and the difference in electrical potential between two points is known as the volt-

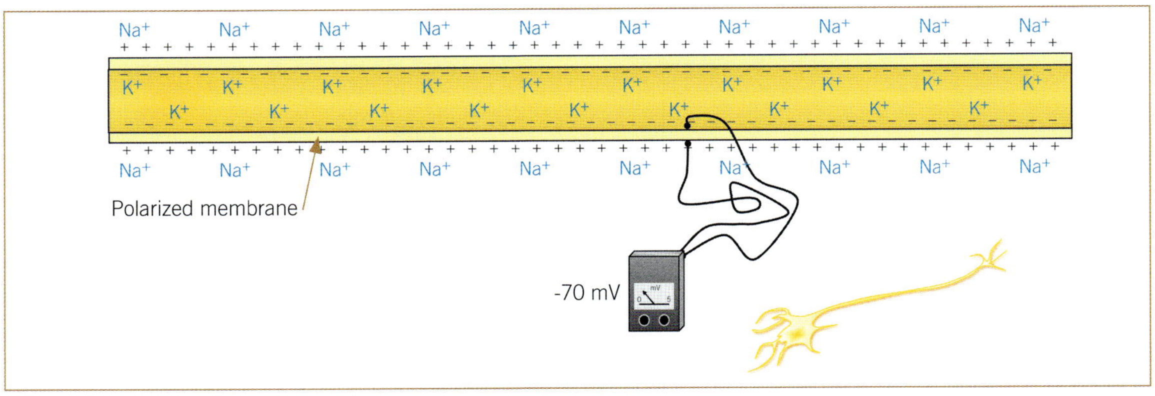

Fig 2-3-11 Unmyelinated nerve axon resting membrane potential. Membranes are polarized and exhibit a resting membrane potential. This is due to an unequal distribution of ions (positively charged K^+ and Na^+ cations) on either side of the nerve cell membrane. This electrical potential is approximately -70 mV (with the inside of the membrane negative with respect to the outside). This is the resting membrane potential occurring when a membrane is not being stimulated or conducting impulses.

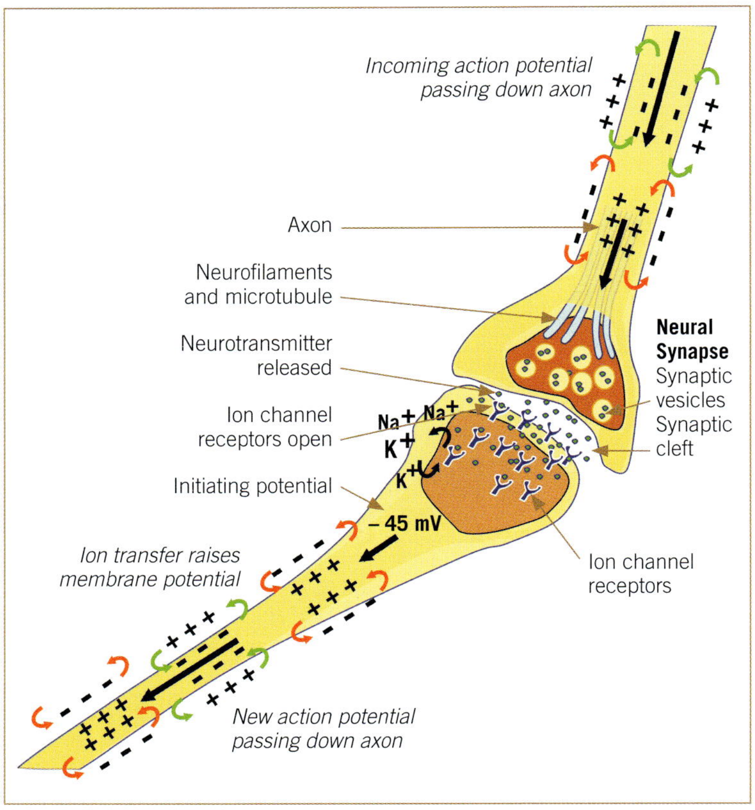

Fig 2-3-12 Neural synapse. Incoming action potential stimulates synaptic vesicles to release neurotransmitters. These cross the synaptic cleft and bind to receptors that are ion channels. This binding opens the ion channels and sodium and potassium ion interchange occurs across the synaptic membrane, raising the membrane potential in the axon hillock. This may (alone or in conjunction with surrounding dendrites) be sufficient to raise the axon hillock potential to -45 mV, sufficient to initiate a new action potential to pass down the nerve axon.

age. The difference in concentration of charged sodium (Na^+) and potassium (K^+) ions on either side of a nerve cell membrane create a potential difference or membrane potential between the inner and outer sides of the membrane.

Membrane resting potential

The equilibrium membrane voltage under normal, unstimulated conditions is called the resting potential (approximately -70 mV) (Fig 2-3-11) At rest, the membrane is more permeable to K^+ than to other ions, with the resting potential close to the K^+ equilibrium potential. In the middle of an action potential, the Na^+ permeability dominates so that the voltage is raised to +30 mV, close to the sodium equilibrium voltage.

Cell walls are impermeable or semi-permeable. Mechanisms in the cell wall control the passage of ions across cell membranes. Na^+ and K^+ ions and their transfer across cellular membranes have several biological functions. They facilitate the propagation of electrical signals as nerve impulses and their conduction along nerves and muscle fibers. In addition, they are instrumental in the transfer of energy, glucose, cell nutrients, and the regulation of cell volume.

Ion channels and passive transport

Neural and muscle membranes contain ion channels that regulate ion passage from the inside to the outside of the nerve or muscle fiber. These are protein pores in the membrane and are specific for particular ions. Sodium and potassium channels are specific to each of these ions. Channels open and close to allow ion transfer by passive transport, which is determined by the membrane voltage and ion concentrations on either side of the membrane (Figs 2-3-11 to 2-3-14).

Ion channel initiation

The "ion channels" involved in the action potential are voltage-sensitive. These will open and close in response to changes in voltage across the membrane. Other types are initiated by chemical, temperature, pressure, and light changes. Ligand-gated channels are another class of channel that open and close in response to the binding of complex molecules (ligands) such as neurotransmitters. Those of sensory neurons are activated by sensory stimuli such as light, temperature, light touch, and pressure.

Ion channels, gates

The electrical signals within biological organisms are most commonly driven by Na^+ and K^+, monovalent cations, passing from one side of a membrane to another through specific gates or channels of complex protein molecules. These allow ionic influx and outflux according to specific trigger mechanisms. Passage of only a few ions or slight changes in voltage stimulation can open the Na^+ and K^+ gates. For nerve impulse transmission, Na^+ and K^+ ions pass from one side of the axon neuron membrane to the other through respective protein Na^+ or K^+ channels or gates. Muscle cell walls (sarcolemma) also transmit impulses into the muscle fiber by the same process of ionic interchange through ion channels. Membrane polarization and depolarization stimulates calcium ion release, which in turn initiates the mechanism of muscle contraction.

Cell wall polarization and depolarization

Throughout the nervous system, the relative Na^+ and K^+ transcellular concentration interactions and transfer are fundamental to the mech-

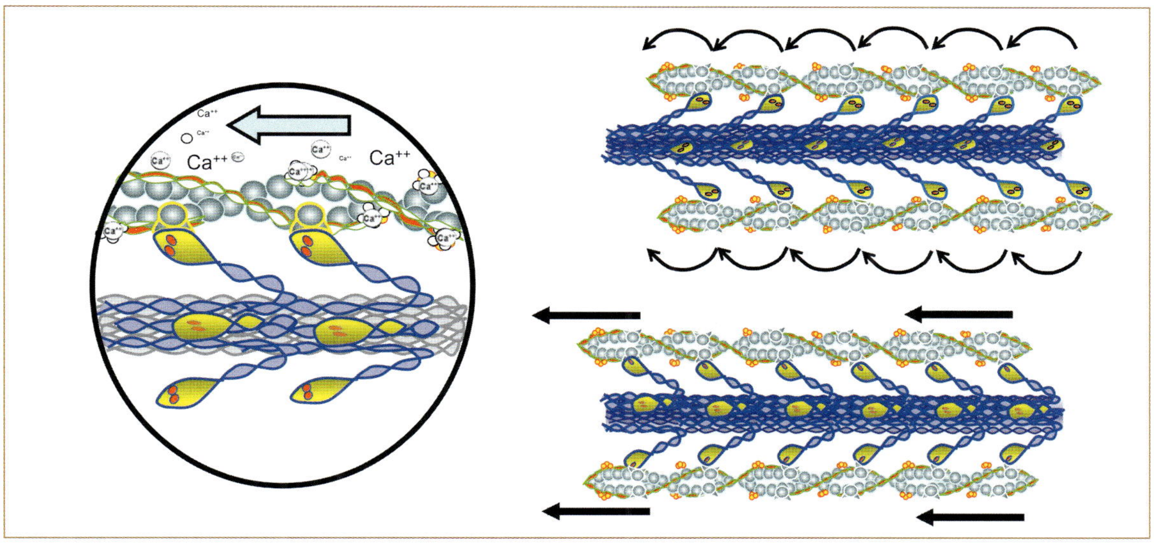

Fig 2-3-25 Myosin heads swivel around their hinges, pulling the attached actin heads around 4 to 7 nm down their long axis as the filaments slide against each other. Sliding filament mechanism: the myosin heads bind to the myosin binding sites in the actin molecules once they are deactivated by the effect of calcium on troponin and tropomyosin. The heads then rotate around their hinges and pull the attached myosin down the long axis.

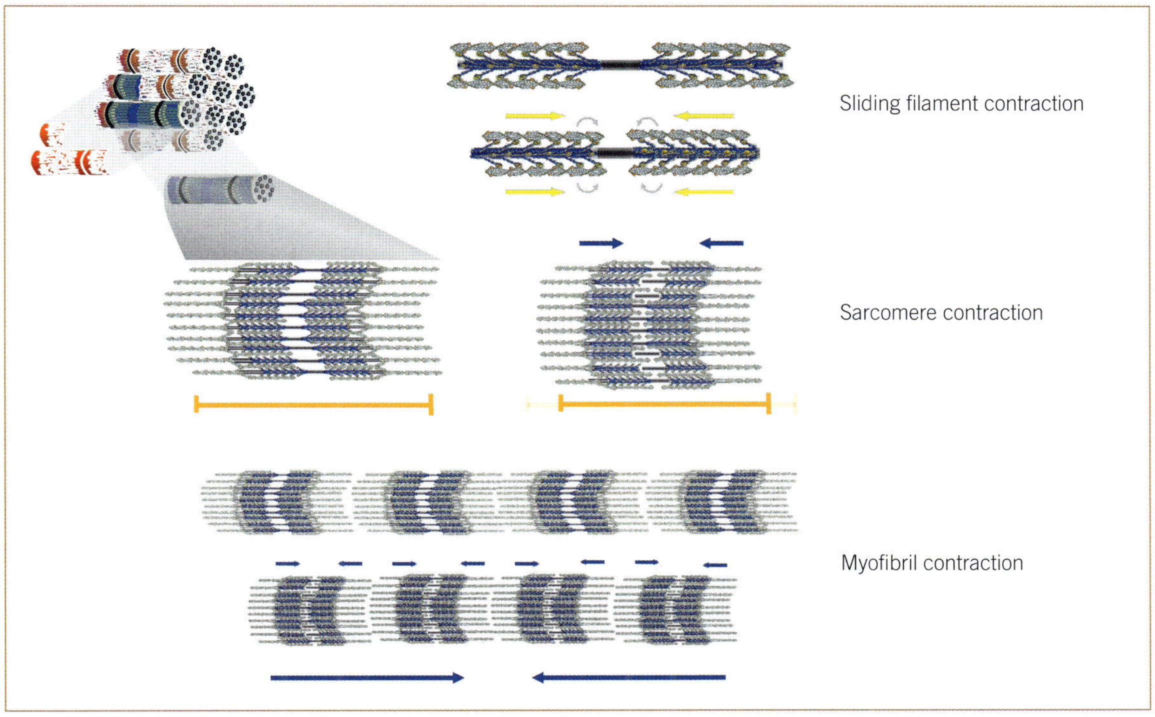

Fig 2-3-26 Myofibrils contain sarcomeres denoted by dark Z-lines. Between the Z-lines the thin myofibrils are arranged in parallel. Thin fibers (light blue) and thick fibers (dark blue). As the central thick fibers pull the surrounding thin fibers towards the middle M-line, the sarcomere contracts. Contraction of the row of continuous sarcomeres results in the contraction of the myofibril.

and uses the energy to move into the "cocked back" relation. Each skeletal muscle myosin head moves around 7 nm on a stroke, with variations of smaller and larger movements dependent on the specific myosin isoform.

This continues as long as ATP is available and calcium is present on the thin filament.

While the above stages are occurring, calcium is actively pumped back into the sarcoplasmic reticulum powered by ATP. The active pumping of calcium ions into the sarcoplasmic reticulum creates a deficiency in the fluid around the myofibrils. This causes the removal of calcium ions from the troponin. Thus, the tropomyosin-troponin complex again covers and blocks the binding sites on the actin filaments. The myosin ceases binding to the thin filament, and the contractions cease.[28-33]

Muscle fiber action potentials

Muscle action potentials are provoked by the arrival of a pre-synaptic neuronal action potential at the neuromuscular junction. The action potential in a normal skeletal muscle cell is similar to the action potential in neurons. Action potentials result from the depolarization of the cell membrane of the muscle fiber, the sarcolemma, which opens ligand-sensitive sodium channels. These subsequently become deactivated and the membrane is repolarized through the outward current of potassium ions. The resting potential prior to the action potential is -90 mV. The muscle action potential lasts roughly 2 to 4 ms, the absolute refractory period is roughly 1 to 3 ms, and the conduction velocity along the muscle fiber is roughly 5 m/s. The muscle membrane action potential passing through the transverse tubules in the sarcoplasmic reticulum releases calcium ions that free the tropomyosin and allow the muscle to contract (Figs 2-3-27 and 2-3-28).[34]

Summary of muscle activation and contraction

Stimulation of the sarcoplasm by electrical and chemical efferent axons causes muscle membrane sarcolemma depolarization and repolariza-

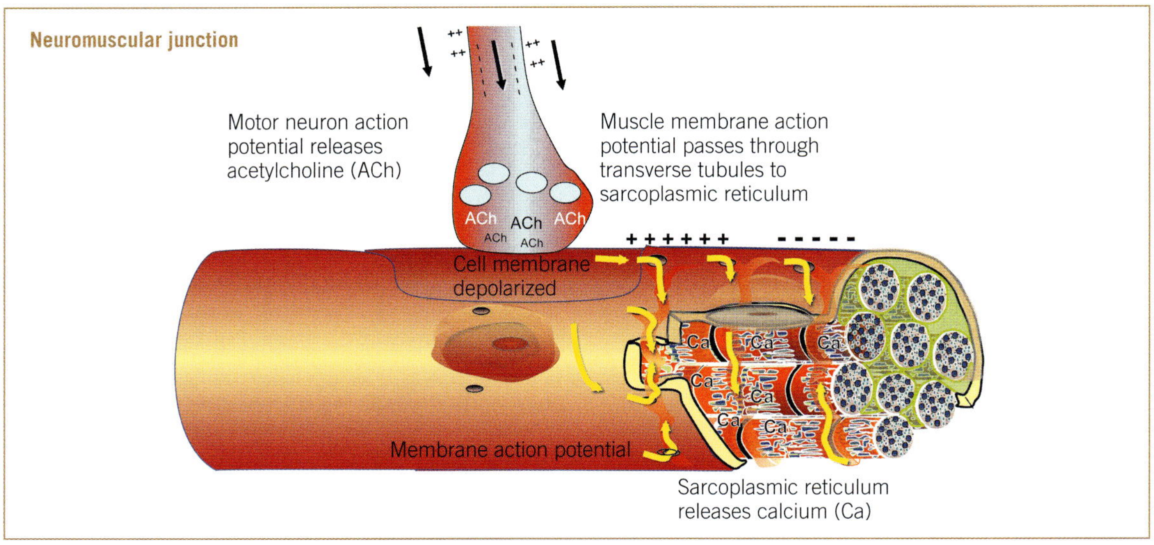

Fig 2-3-27 An action potential passes down the motor neuron to the synapse with the muscle cell membrane (sarcolemma). Acetylcholine is released and causes the depolarization of the muscle cell membrane. The resulting action potential passes through transverse tubules in the membrane wall to the sarcoplasmic reticulum, where this causes the release of calcium ions.

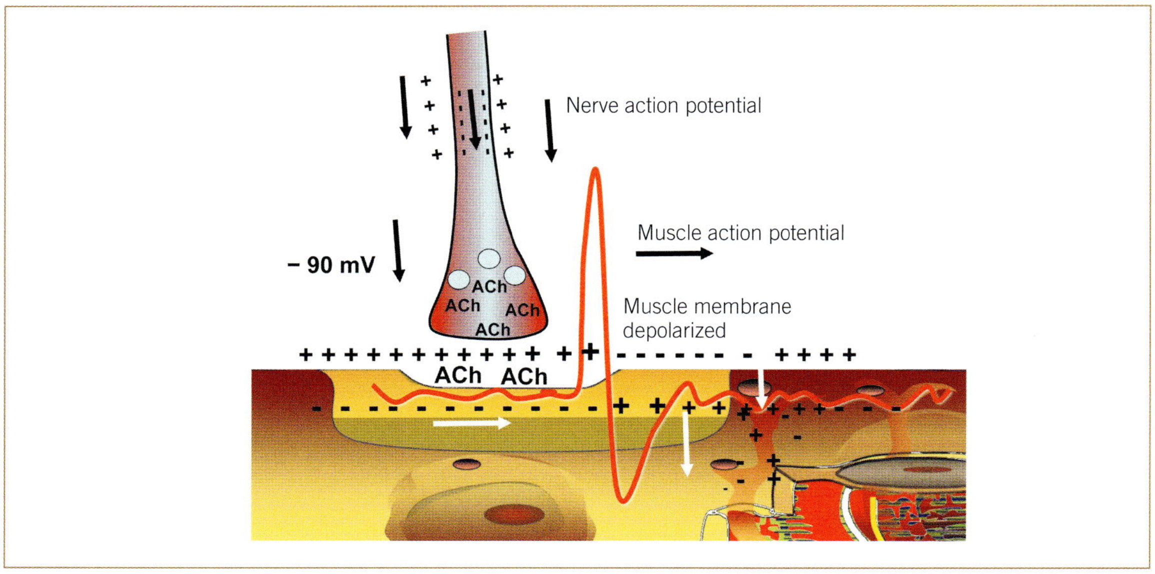

Fig 2-3-28 An action potential generated in muscle fiber occurs on depolarization of the membrane for 2 to 4 ms with the depolarization of the cell membrane. This opens ligand sensitive sodium channels. These then become deactivated and the membrane is repolarized through the outward passage of potassium ions. The resting potential prior to the action potential is typically -90 mV, slightly more negative than in neurons. The muscle action potential lasts roughly 2 to 4 ms, the absolute refractory period is roughly 1 to 3 ms, and the conduction velocity along the muscle is roughly 5 ms. The action potential releases calcium ions that free up the tropomyosin and allow the muscle to contract. Muscle action potentials are provoked by the arrival of a pre-synaptic neuronal action potential at the neuromuscular junction.

tion, releasing calcium ions in the sarcoplasm. This stimulates the interaction of myosin heads with actin, activating the myosin power stroke and sliding of actin filaments. This then causes sarcomere and myofibril contraction, and the generation of muscle force (Figs 2-3-26 to 2-3-29).

Muscle contraction

Voluntary muscle contraction occurs as a result of conscious effort originating in the cerebral cortex. Electrical impulses (action potentials) are transmitted through neural pathways to efferent motor neurons that innervate muscle fibers. In the case of some reflexes, the signal to contract can originate in the spinal cord through a spinal reflex feedback loop. Other actions such as locomotion, breathing, and chewing have a reflex aspect to them. The contractions can be initiated consciously or unconsciously and are continued through unconscious reflex, with proprioceptive feedback.

Proprioception

Proprioception is the sense of the relative positions of neighboring parts of the body. This is unlike the six exteroceptive senses of sight, taste, smell, touch, hearing, and balance by which the outside world is perceived, and the interoceptive senses, that perceive pain and the stretching of internal organs. Proprioception is a third sensory modality that provides feedback purely on the status of the body internally. It is the sense that indicates whether the body is moving with the required effort, as well as where the various parts of the body are located in relation to each other.

The proprioceptive sense is composed of impulses from sensory afferent neurons in the middle ear and stretch and positioning receptors located in the muscles, joints, and the joint-supporting ligaments. There are specific nerve receptors for this form of perception, named proprioceptors. Muscle spindles and tendon organs are the proprioceptive mechanisms in the muscles and tendons; Ruffini endings and Vater-Pacini corpuscles are found in the temporomandibular joints.[35-38]

Muscle spindles

Muscle spindles are found between the muscle fiber bundles. Muscle spindles are sensory mechanisms containing intrafusal muscle fibers distributed throughout the muscles and provide sensory feedback information to the central nervous system regarding the state of tension of the muscle. The masticatory elevators contain relatively high concentrations of muscle spindles. High concentrations are found in the deep masseter, in the vertical temporalis component, and medially in the medial pterygoid. Muscle spindles are not reported in the depressor muscles.[35,38-41]

The number of swallows recorded per day during eating was reported as 146. For 146 swallows at 30 kg of force for 522 ms, the swallowing total was 2,299 kg/s per day. The total force-time activity for chewing and swallowing amounts to 7,800 kg/s per day. The number of swallows recorded at night is approximately 120, thus the swallowing force generated at night can be approximately 5,806 kg/s per night.[13]

The mechanism for swallowing is coordinated by the swallowing center in the medulla and the pons. The reflex is initiated by touch receptors in the pharynx as a bolus of food is pushed to the back of the mouth by the tongue.[20] Swallowing involves a complex mechanism using both skeletal muscle (tongue) and smooth muscles of the pharynx and esophagus. The autonomic nervous system coordinates this process in the pharyngeal and esophageal phases (Fig 2-5-6).

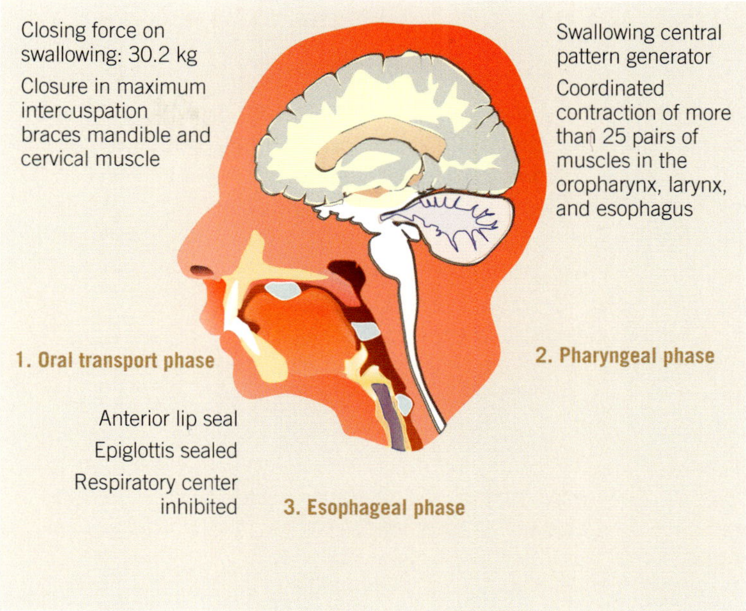

Fig 2-5-6 Swallowing is a complex vital activity that involves coordination of multiple muscles with a central pattern generator in the medulla and pons that coordinates the three stages: 1) oral transport; 2) pharyngeal; and 3) esophageal. Anterior lip, nasopharyngeal, and epiglottis seals must be coordinated to facilitate the swallow and avoid food entering the nasal cavity or trachea.[20] High occlusal forces are applied on closure in MI for mandibular bracing during deglutition.[7,13]

Phases

Normal swallowing consists of three phases following oral preparation:

1. Oral transport
2. Pharyngeal
3. Esophageal

Oral transport phase

The bolus is first moved to the back of the tongue. Next, the anterior tongue rises to the hard palate and retracts in a posterior direction to force the bolus to the oropharynx. The posterior tongue is lifted by the styloglossus and palatoglossus muscles, raising the soft palate and sealing the nasopharynx preventing nasal aspiration. This phase is voluntary and involves the trigeminal (V), facial (VII), and hypoglossal (XII) nerves.

Pharyngeal phase

In this phase, the bolus is advanced from the pharynx to the esophagus through peristalsis. The soft palate is elevated to the posterior nasopharyngeal wall through the action of the levator veli palatini. The palatopharyngeal folds on each side of the pharynx are brought close together through the superior constrictor muscles, so that only a small bolus can pass. Then, the larynx and hyoid are elevated and pulled forward to the epiglottis to relax the cricopharyngeus muscle. This passively shuts off its entrance and the vocal cords are pulled close together. This phase is controlled reflexively and involves cranial nerves V, X (vagus), XI (accessory), and XII (hypoglossal). The respiratory center of the medulla is directly inhibited by the swallowing center for the very brief time that it takes to swallow. This is known as deglutition apnea.

Esophageal phase

The upper esophageal sphincter relaxes to let food past, after which various striated constrictor muscles of the pharynx, as well as peristalsis and relaxation of the lower esophageal sphincter, sequentially push the bolus of food through the esophagus into the stomach (Fig 2-5-6).

Occlusal parafunction, bruxism

Occlusal parafunction and bruxism describe the non-functional activity of clenching and grinding of the teeth. There remains a degree of semantic confusion over the terms "occlusal parafunction" and "bruxism." "Occlusal parafunction" was used as a general term to describe the phenomena of grinding and clenching.[21] "Bruxism" was used more in a clinical restorative context in relation to more severe grinding and clenching, and their destructive effects on the dentition. Mild transient harmless episodes of occasional occlusal parafunction are common and widespread, while the term bruxism has, in the past, described a more persistent, severe, and pernicious form of occlusal parafunction, causing progressive tooth wear and destruction in the dentition.[21-27] The more recent literature on bruxism and temporomandibular disorders (TMDS) now uses the term "bruxism" as the blanket term for parafunctional grinding and clenching.[28-35] Current terminology uses mild, moderate, and severe bruxism to cover the whole range of occlusal parafunction. This includes grinding and clenching and awake bruxism and sleep bruxism – all of which are considered to be separate entities.[29,30] This text will use the terms severe, moderate, and mild bruxism. Occlusal parafunction will also be used as a general synonymous term.

Duration, intensity, and periodicity

Occlusal parafunction/bruxism is a behavioral activity involving the nonfunctional clenching and grinding of the teeth. Up to 90% of a normal population may grind or clench at some time during mild transient episodes. Of a young adult population sample, 91.5% had one or more tooth sites with a significant wear facet.[22,29] Duration, intensity, and periodicity can vary greatly between individuals. Bruxism may be awake bruxism (formerly diurnal bruxism) or sleep bruxism (formerly nocturnal bruxism). Both of these are considered to have differing characteristics and etiologies.[23-27] As previously mentioned, there is some semantic overlap in the usage of the terms bruxism and occlusal parafunction, and both are generally subconscious activities. The etiology is not well understood. Current belief is that bruxism is mainly regulated centrally and not peripherally.[24,27] The primary determinant is behavioral, with emotional and physical stress, and psychosocial factors implicated as risk factors.[25-29] Post-traumatic stress disorder has been cited as triggering more long-term activity.[28]

Awake bruxism

Wake-time parafunction is considered to be mostly associated with clenching rather than grinding. The incidence of awake bruxism is very difficult to measure. Sleep bruxism is more often associated with grinding.[27] Emotional stress can play a role in the etiology of awake tooth clenching.[23] However clenching and grinding can both occur during awake bruxism and during sleep bruxism.[29]

Sleep bruxism (parasomnia)

Sleep bruxism is described by the American Sleep Disorders Association as a stereotyped movement disorder, characterized by grinding or clenching of the teeth during sleep,[30] or as a parasomnia and an oral parafunctional activity during sleep, characterized by either jaw clenching or repetitive phasic jaw muscle activity that produces tooth grinding.[30,31] A parasomnia is a sleep disorder. Sleep bruxism is studied using a polysomnograph in a sleep laboratory that records brain EEG, eye movements, muscle activity (EMG), heart rhythm (ECG), and breathing function or respiratory effort during sleep.

Sleep bruxism exhibits rhythmic jaw muscle activity that can take three forms: phasic (52.5%); tonic (11.4%); and mixed (36.1%).[29]

Sleep bruxism, a "sleep related movement disorder," is further described as secondary to sleep-related microarousals occurring 8 to 14 times per hour with rhythmic masticatory muscle activity peaking in the minutes before rapid eye movement (REM) related to a sleep transition stage.[31]

Sleep cycles, micrarousals, cyclic alternating patterns

A sleep cycle consists of non-REM and REM stages of 90 to 110 min of sleep. One night of sleep is composed of three to five of these cycles. Non-REM sleep has separate stages N1 and N2, and deep sleep of stage N3. Most sleep bruxing episodes are observed in light non-REM sleep, while 10% occur in REM sleep associated with sleep arousal.[31,32]

Microarousals occur during sleep and are defined as 3 to 10 s abrupt shifts in electroencephalography (EEG) activity with a rise in heart rate and muscle tone (EEG arousals). Arousals tend to recur 8 to 15 times per hour of sleep in young healthy subjects. Sleep bruxing has been observed to occur in relation to recurrent arousal within a cyclic alternating pattern (CAP). A CAP repeats every 20 to 60 s during non-REM sleep. Most sleep bruxing (SB) episodes occur in clusters in relation to CAPs. CAP-related arousal is described as a natural process that acts as a sensor for maintaining body homeostasis and as a protection sentinel during sleep.[31]

The origin of most SB episodes follows the following sequence:

- A rise in sympathetic cardiac activity
- A rise in the frequency of EEG activity
- Heart rate tachycardia
- Increased jaw-opener muscle activity, probably for mandible protrusion and airway opening
- An associated increase in the amplitude of respiratory ventilation
- Observable EMG incidents scored as SB-rhythmic masticatory muscle activity (RMMA) with or without tooth grinding (TG).

EMG patterns related to SB have been called RMMA. In normal subjects, RMMA occurs about once an hour during sleep in comparison with 2 to 12 times per hour in SB patients.[31] In approximately half of the SB-RMMA episodes, swallowing activity was observed. No swallowing was observed for several minutes before RMMA-TG episodes.[31]

Individual bruxers with significant tooth wear may be unaware of this activity. Occasionally, a spouse may report grinding noises at night. The natural history of sleep bruxism varies and can be cyclic, progressive, or self-limiting. The incidence in different age groups has been described as high from the teens to the forties, and as decreasing with advancing age.[31-35]

Forces generated by bruxism may be considerable and have been measured in the range from 70 to 400 kg. No single etiological component has been identified in severe bruxers, either in their psychological profile or environmental scenarios. Active periods of occlusal parafunction may be diagnosed by the presence of shiny wear facets in enamel, porcelain, or metal and opposing wear facets aligned in particular mandibular excursions.

So-called occlusal disorders have, in the past, been considered to constitute a significant etiological component,[36,39] however this is no longer considered to be the case.[37,40-42] While occlusal elements such as occlusal interferences or steep vertical overlap may not be the direct cause of occlusal parafunction, they constitute the sites of high stress concentration on which this activity occurs. High stress concentrations on these and other sites of excursive grinding or clenching can cause significant wear and damage to the teeth, their restorations, and supporting structures.

Incidence of bruxism

Determining the incidence of occlusal parafunction is confounded by difficulties in diagnosis. The most common method used in studies diagnosing bruxism is by asking the subject if they clench or grind by way of an interview or questionnaire. This "self-reported" method is notoriously inaccurate. Sleep laboratories with polysomnography are the most accurate environments to study SB. Spouse or family member reporting and wear facets are also used as measures of incidence. Bruxism may be mild, moderate, or severe in intensity and duration over specific periods and may fluctuate over time. It is difficult to objectively distinguish between mild, moderate, and severe activity.

Different values for studies on incidence depend on the method of observation, population, and type of bruxism studied. Ranges fluctuate wildly, with extremes of 6% to 91% for overall populations in varying countries and cultures.[29,33-38] Variables of clenching, grinding, gender, and age have been studied. A comprehensive review of 34 cross-sectional general population studies based on questionnaires and interviews[29] shows the majority (25/34) to be in the 3 to 20% incidence range for wake clenching (WkCl) and sleep grinding (SlGr). Seven out of 34 were in the 20 to 45% incidence range. Out of 10 longitudinal studies, the mean SlGr and WkCl incidence was between 19 and 25%. Wake clenching incidence was greater than sleep grinding. Incidence in children is high, becomes reduced through teens and adulthood, and is reduced at more advanced ages. Incidence values from studies based on occlusal wear facets are much higher than from questionnaires and interviews. Mean incidence in 11 studies using questionnaire and interviews with TMD patients was 25% for SlGr, 46% for WkCl, and 44% for WkCl + SlGr for combined age groups. Incidence in studies based on occlusal wear ranged from 47 to 100%. The average incidence of wear from 12 studies was 71%.[29]

The incidence of mild transient episodes of clenching and grinding in the general population is likely to be far higher than indicated by questionnaire studies, with transient grinding and clenching proving to be a normal adaptive feature. No difference was seen between gender, and incidence decreased with age.[28]

Etiology

Three etiological theories for the origins of bruxism have been described:

1. Peripherlal morphologic (occlusal)
2. Psychologic
3. Psychosocial[29]

Occlusal theories have been all but abandoned due to claims of insufficient evidence and flawed studies.[36-39] Experimental occlusal interference studies have shown equivocal results. Some studies showed short-term muscle and joint symptoms and some showed increased clenching and parafunction.[39,42] Others do not show these effects.[40-42] While these probably do not cause long-term parafunction, the significance in terms of new single contacts in new restorations and their potential damage to the restoration or supporting structures remain a concern in oral rehabilitation.[39-42] The origin of bruxism has been stated to be multifactorial with central, as yet undefined, processes be-

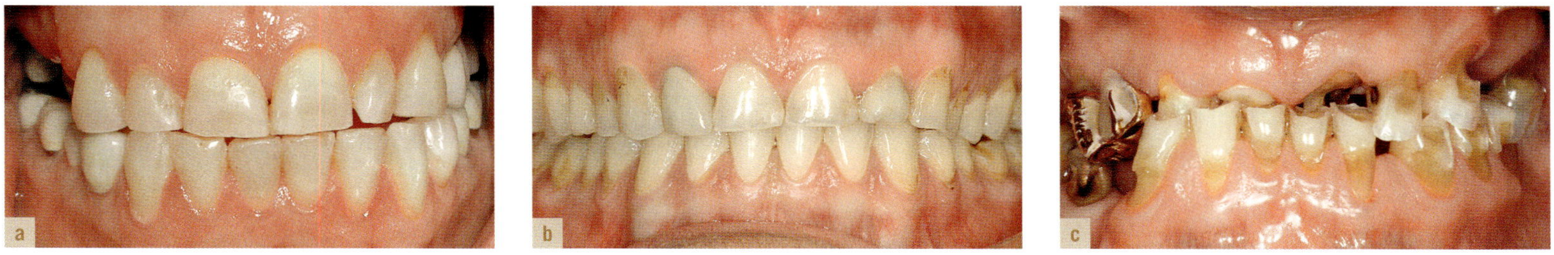

Fig 2-5-7 Categories of occlusal wear: a Mild includes wear facets with incipient loss of crown height. b Moderate includes loss of 1/3 to ½ of crown height. c Severe describes wear resulting in loss of more than ½ of crown height.

ing primarily responsible. Disturbances in the central dopaminergic system have been implicated, with circadian rhythm influences and neurotransmitters under investigation.[24,31]

Stress, behavior, psychosocial factors, TMDs, and bruxism

The interrelation between bruxism, TMDs, and psychosocial (axis II) determinants is not well understood. The term "psychosocial" as a determinant in TMDs is loosely used and can include stress, anticipation of stress, fear, anxiety, and the full psychosocial gamut of behavioral, emotional, and psychological states and conditions.[21,43] Psychosocial disorders are considered in the TMD axis II classification and TMD research diagnostic criteria.[43]

Psychological and psychosocial factors, with stress, anxiety, depression, and somatization are implicated in causing pain modulation affecting muscle and joint pain in TMDs. Stress is also implicated in causing muscle tension and is also cited as a risk factor more in relation to awake bruxism than sleep bruxism.[23-27]

However, the etiological contribution of these factors to awake bruxism and sleep bruxism is yet to be clarified. Cause and effect have not been proven, and association is commonly demonstrated but confounded by the incidence of severe wear cases not being unequivocally linked to chronic stress, personality stereotypes, or TMD symptoms.

Stress

Stress is a part of normal life. Different people react differently to potentially stressful conditions and situations. Stress is a severe medical problem contributing to two-thirds of medical visits, heart disease, mental disorders, and other diseases.[43-46] Stress is the emotional and physical strain caused by the response to pressure from the outside world. Common stress reactions include tension, irritability, inability to concentrate, anxiety, fear, and a variety of physical symptoms that include headache and a fast heartbeat.

While many feel stress plays a significant role in occlusal parafunction, difficulties in measuring and quantifying stress, and bruxism have led scientific purists to cast doubt on the existence of a direct cause and effect relationship.[29,31]. Stress is currently designated as a risk factor in bruxism.

The grinding and clenching of bruxism is strongly implicated in producing local muscle and joint tissue damage, which sets off a cascade of events involving peripheral and central sensitization that cause muscle and joint pain.[21,28,29]

Psychological stress has also been found to exacerbate sleep bruxism and/or daytime clenching.[46]

Adverse effects of bruxism

The forces of occlusal parafunction can be extremely destructive. They can have deleterious effects on the teeth, dental restorations, implants, the supporting structures the muscles, and the temporomandibular joints.[47-56]

Effects of bruxism on the teeth

Occlusal wear classification

Wear of the teeth by parafunctional grinding can range from mild to severe wear. Various classifications have been proposed that describe the degrees of progressive loss of surface tooth substance.[47,48] A simple classification is proposed here of mild, moderate, and severe, which reflects the overall loss of crown height. Mild includes wear facets with incipient loss of crown height. Moderate includes loss of $^1/_3$ to $^1/_2$ of crown height. Severe describes wear resulting in loss of more than $^1/_2$ of crown height (Fig 2-5-7).

In more severe occlusal attrition cases, the bone may not be adversely affected, but may be thickened and widened and is described as buttressing. Initially, wear of the enamel, cracks in the teeth, and cervical abfractions are observed. As occlusal wear continues more rapidly in the dentin, it may occur together with erosion of the dentin affected by dietary elements, such as acidic drinks or foods.[51]

Erosion and attrition

Occlusal tooth wear is described as occurring by a combination of attrition, usually from occlusal parafunction, and by erosion. Abrasion is also included as a potential component of tooth wear. The relative contributions are difficult to ascertain clinically and are contested academically.[52]

Rate of wear

In a systematic review, the predicted percentage of adults presenting with severe tooth wear increased from 3% at the age of 20 years to 17% at the age of 70 years. The overall percentages of extensive wear varied from 1.4 to 5.7% for occlusal and from 3.9 to 24% for cervical wear.[49]

The teeth may become worn down to the gingival level and the dental pulp may become exposed. In cases of steep vertical overlap (class II division 2), the overlapping teeth will be worn initially. In cases of flatter guiding inclines, such as class III, anterior and posterior teeth will become worn simultaneously. It is not clear whether specific grinding patterns may be predominantly anterior or lateral. Severe wear and successive fractures and prosthetic complications are pathognomonic for heavy bruxers.

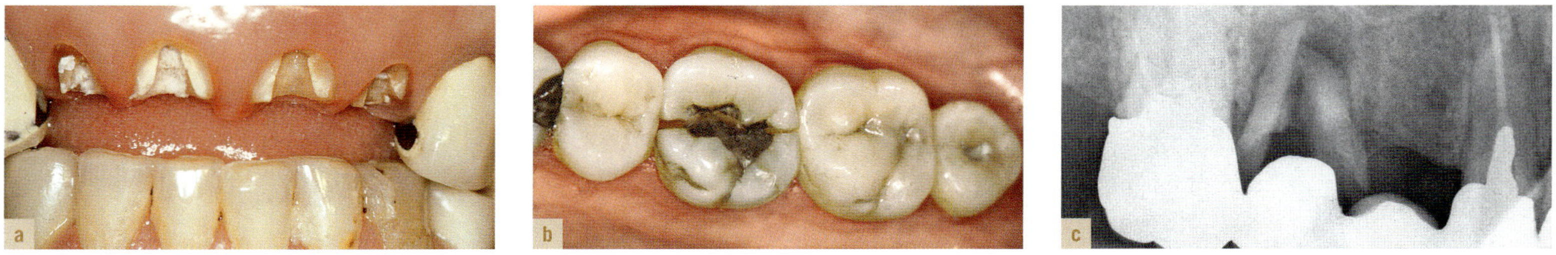

Fig 2-5-8 Fracture of root-treated **a** teeth, **b** crowns, and **c** roots.

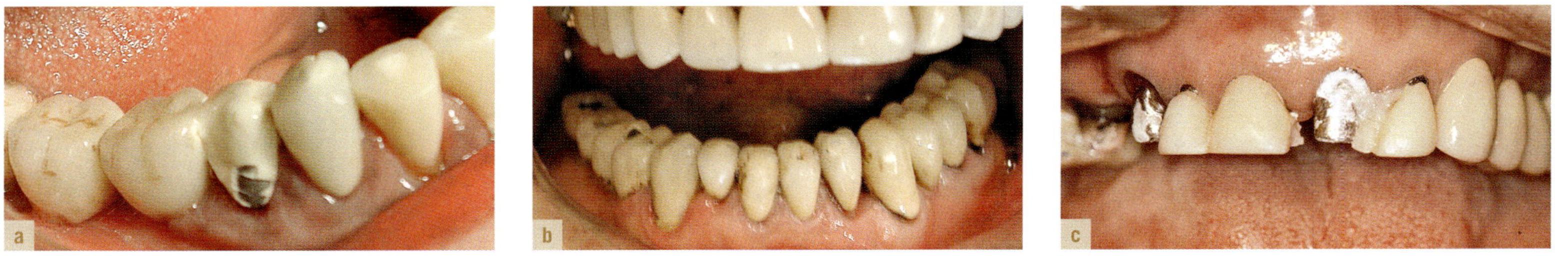

Fig 2-5-9a to c Fracture of porcelain and acrylic resin veneers in fixed restorations.

Direction of parafunctional grinding

Some authors maintain that severe wear in bruxers can be in an anterior direction or protrusive, or can be in a lateral direction, from side to side.[53] In some cases, there appears to be more wear of the anterior teeth and in others there is more wear of the posterior teeth. Whether this is a function of a distinctive protrusive habit as opposed to a specific lateral habit or whether this is simply a function of the vertical overlap is not clear. Lateral grinding nocturnally on occlusal appliances recurred consistently with lateral facets and was seen in 80% of observed cases.[54]

Effect of occlusal parafunction on dental restorations

Restoration of the teeth with tooth- or implant-supported restorations in heavy bruxers is particularly problematic and unpredictable. In such cases, the incidence and probability of occlusal wear, superstructure fracture, root fracture, decementation, secondary caries, abutment screw loosening, or implant or implant component fracture are particularly high. Restoring the dentition at a particular occlusal vertical dimension or with a particular occlusal scheme will not necessarily prevent the continuation of occlusal parafunction and its potentially destructive effects. Mechanical failures of this nature are extremely common and problematic and significantly reduce the prognosis of the restored dentition and its supporting structures. The use of occlusal appliances such as night guards will not stop the parafunction, but will reduce the destructive effects (Fig 2-5-7 to Fig 2-5-10).[54-56]

Effect of occlusal parafunction on the supporting structures of the teeth

Occlusal trauma

High parafunctional occlusal loads are transmitted by the occluding teeth to the periodontal and alveolar supporting structures. Normal occlusal loading in mastication and swallowing, in the absence of periodontal inflammation, stimulate periodontal and alveolar turnover and remodeling of the bone, maintaining a steady state of periodontal and alveolar health. Intermittent and occasional high masticatory loads may cause microtrauma that is followed by repair and maintenance of health. Prolonged, continued occlusal parafunctional loading can cause damage to the supporting structures.

Wolff's Law, Frost mechanostat model, remodeling, modeling, resorption, apposition

Wolff's Law of 1892 proposed that bone achieves maximum mechanical efficiency with minimum mass, and that bone structure adapts in response to a changing mechanical environment. Trabecular orientation is aligned with the principal stresses and bone density is highest in areas of the highest shear (bending) stress.[57]

A model of bone response to varying loading levels was presented by Frost.[57] This defines a range of physiologic load within which normal turnover, named "remodeling," maintains the gross morphology in response to normal functional loading. This was based on a long-bone model (Fig 2-5-11).[57,58] A distinction is made between remodeling (physiologic load), modeling (mild overload), and fracture (pathologic overload). Modeling occurs in the mild overload range, in which modeling occurs as a change in form. This may be additive, as a hypertrophic increase in bone volume, or may result in a decrease in volume. This model was applied originally to the long bones. A direct analogy to bone at the tooth and implant level has been made [59] However, loss of alveolar bone around a tooth or an implant is generally due to local loading or overload and/or a consequence of the bacterial inflammatory process. Maintenance of maxillary and mandibular form is a consequence of the dynamic interaction of the masticatory muscles, dental occlusion, and its osseous and skeletal supporting structures (see Box 2-5-1).

Occlusal trauma, occlusal traumatism

Occlusal trauma is described as the injury to the attachment apparatus as a result of excessive occlusal force. Occlusal trauma is the tissue injury, and not the occlusal force. *The Glossary of Prosthodontic Terms*

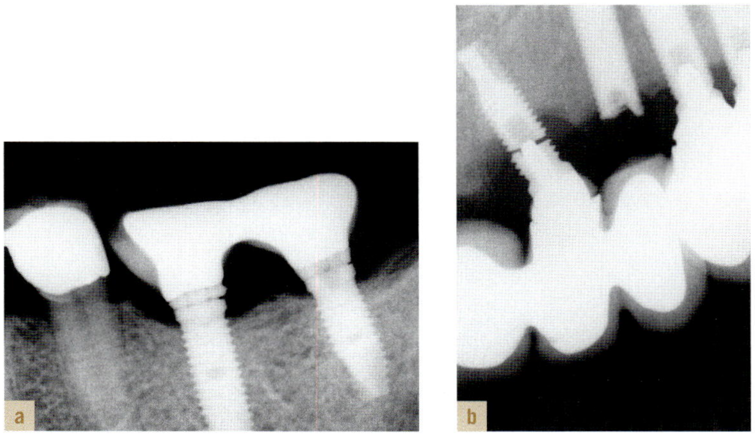

Fig 2-5-10a and b Damage to implants: screw loosening, abutment screw fracture, implant fracture, and loss of alveolar bone.

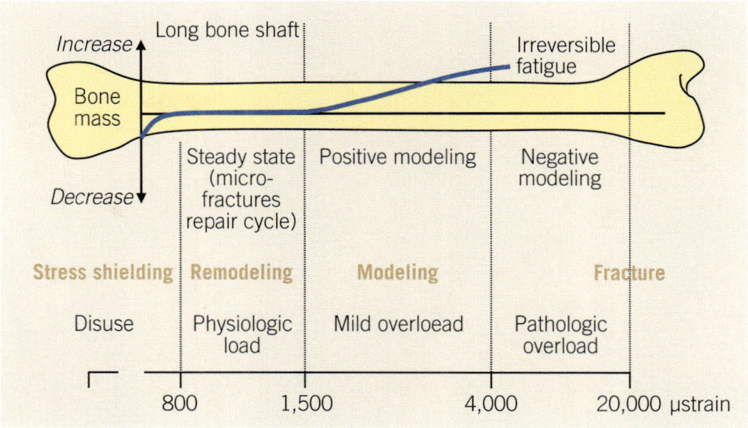

Fig 2-5-11 Frost's mechanostat model from the Utah paradigm of bone physiology. Bone response to increasing levels of loading.[57,58]

Box 2-5-1 Remodeling, modeling, resorption

Remodeling
Remodeling is the process that maintains the bone in a stable steady state. When bone is remodeled it undergoes both new formation and resorption without a net change in shape or size.

Modeling
Bone modeling is the sum of the activities of the endosteum and periosteum of bone producing a net change in bone form. This may be additive and hypertrophic, with increased bone volume, or reductive, with reduced bone volume.

Resorption
The process of losing substance. Bone resorption is the process by which osteoclasts break down bone by acidic demineralization and degradation of the organic matrix.

defines occlusal trauma as "trauma to the periodontium from functional or parafunctional forces causing damage to the attachment apparatus of the periodontium by exceeding its adaptive and reparative capacities. It may be self-limiting or progressive."[60] A distinction is made between primary and secondary occlusal trauma. This definition does not include damage to the crowns and roots of the teeth, prosthetic and single restorations, or implants that are commonly compromised by occlusal parafunction (Figs 2-5-7 to 2-5-10).

The lesion of trauma

A lesion of trauma is described as resulting from continuous "traumatic" pressure to a tooth. At the compression site, increased vascularity, vascular thrombosis, and disorganization of cells and collagen fibers occurs, with necrosis of periodontal tissues (hyaline degeneration) at the bone front. Adjacent osteoclast activity resorption is followed by osteoclastic resorption at the bone front.[61-64] The net result is resorption on the compression side. On cessation of the applied force, the lesion of resorption undergoes repair and results in a widened periodontal membrane. The cervical attachment of the periodontal ligament (PDL) to the neck of the tooth is not lost and there is no apical loss of attachment (Figs 2-5-12 to Fig 2-5-15). An activated orthodontic wire is sufficient to cause this resorption on the pressure side, with deposition on the tension side. Alternating occlusal parafunctional forces acting for prolonged periods on a tooth in opposing directions have been named "jiggling forces." By a cyclic sequence of resorption and repair, bone PDL space is widened by such jiggling forces and the tooth becomes mobile.[65-67]

Primary and secondary occlusal trauma

A distinction has historically been made between primary and secondary trauma.

Primary occlusal trauma

Primary occlusal trauma is defined as "the effects induced by abnormal or excessive occlusal forces acting on teeth with normal periodontal support."[60] This is occasionally observed when a tooth or teeth are mobile and a radiographic widening of the periodontal space is apparent with no probing or attachment loss. Cessation of the traumatic force will cause repair, narrowing of the periodontal space, and a cessation of mobility (Figs 2-5-16 and Fig 2-5-18).

Secondary occlusal trauma

Secondary occlusal trauma is defined as "the effects induced by occlusal force (normal or abnormal) acting on teeth with decreased periodontal support [60] (Fig 2-5-17).These effects may include an initial widening of the PDL spaces followed by increased and often increasing mobility (Fig 2-5-19).[67-76] Fremitus may be detected as buccal movement of the maxillary teeth on closure into maximum intercuspation (Fig 2-5-20). In situations where occlusal pressure is unidirectional, when the alveolar bone support is reduced and the restraining forces of the soft tissue are inadequate, teeth may migrate. This is observed in the maxillary anterior teeth as flaring and migration, and as tipping and tilting of the posterior teeth.[68-71] When forces are multidirectional, the trauma to the supporting structures will more readily result in a widening of the PDL and increased mobility.

Increased and increasing mobility

Mobility may be increased or increasing (Fig 2-5-19). Increased mobility occurs when there is mobility of a tooth or teeth, usually with widening of the PDL space, where the mobility is self-limiting. This has been described as a physiologic adaptation to loading and is often reversible. In situations where the mobility is not self-limiting and is observed to be increasing, there exists an increased possibility of eventual tooth loss. Increasing mobility more often than not occurs following bone loss from

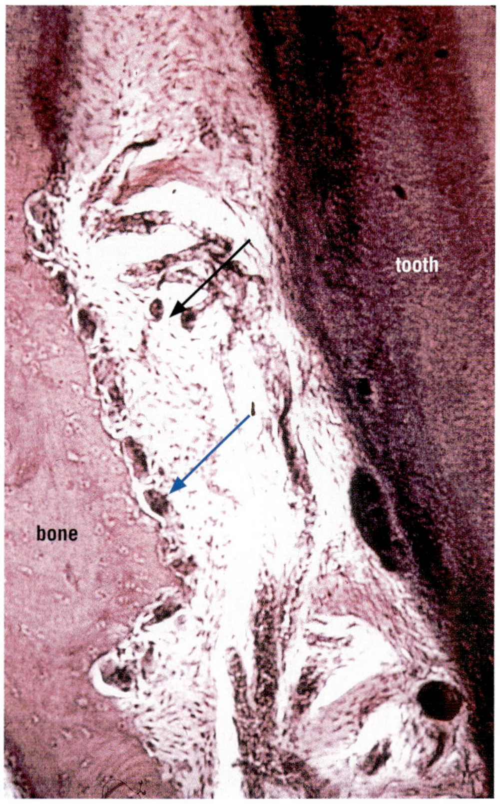

Fig 2-5-12 Lesion of occlusal trauma with widened and disorganized periodontal membrane (black arrow) and frontal resorption (compression site), showing osteoclastic front (blue arrow). (Image courtesy of Professor DW Cohen.)

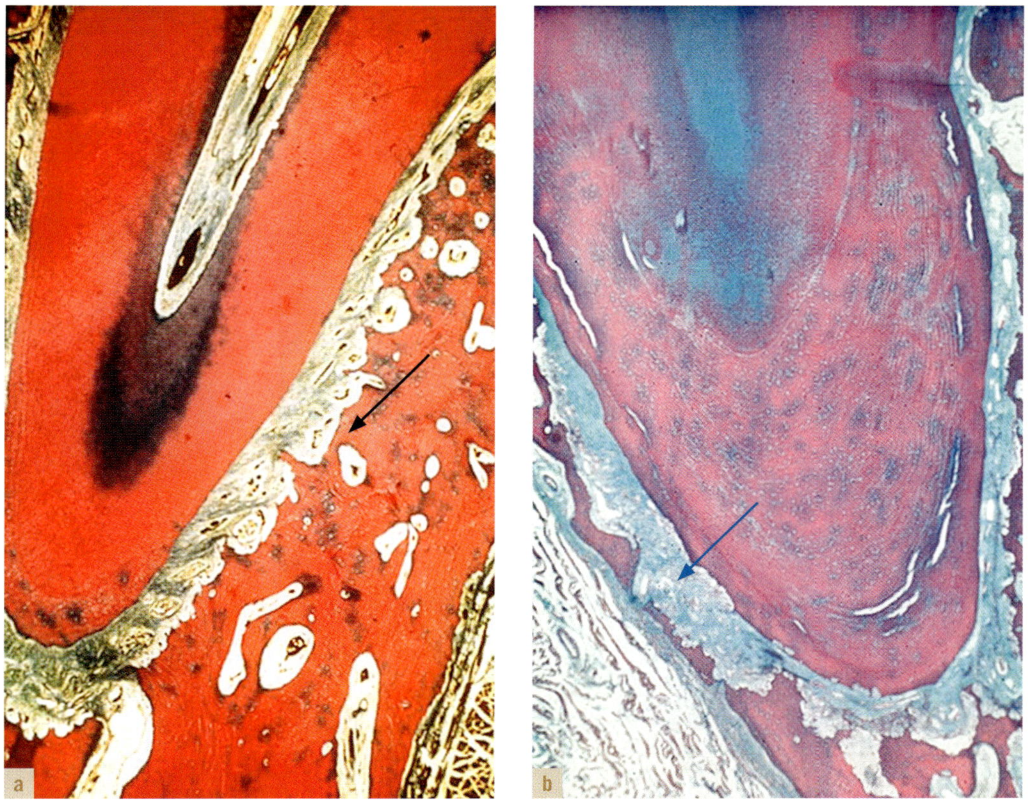

Fig 2-5-13a and b Lesion of occlusal trauma. Widening of the periodontal spaces, frontal resorption, and resorption lacunae in the apical region. (Images courtesy of Professor E Rozenberg.)

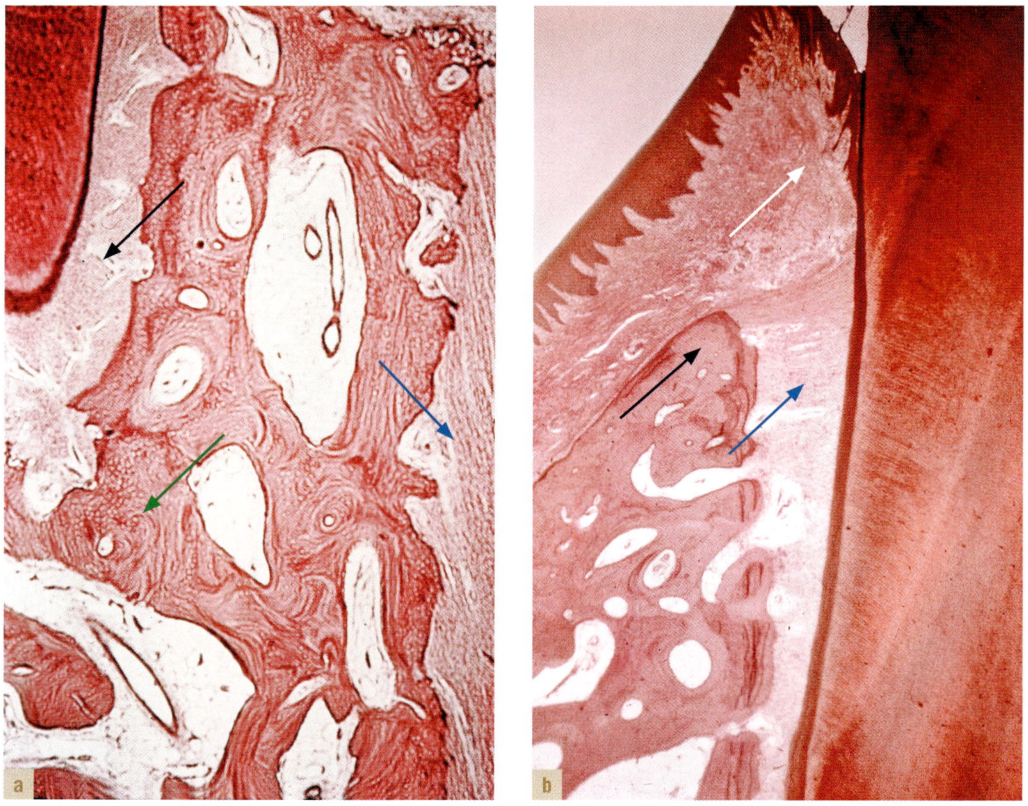

Fig 2-5-14a Apical area, compressed and disorganized periodontal ligament (black arrow), with widened stretched ligament under tension (blue arrow); green arrow: secondary osteons. b Cervical crestal area with widened periodontal ligment (blue arrow) and stretched fibers without loss of attachment (white arrow); black arrow: alveolar crest (Images courtesy of Professor DW Cohen.)

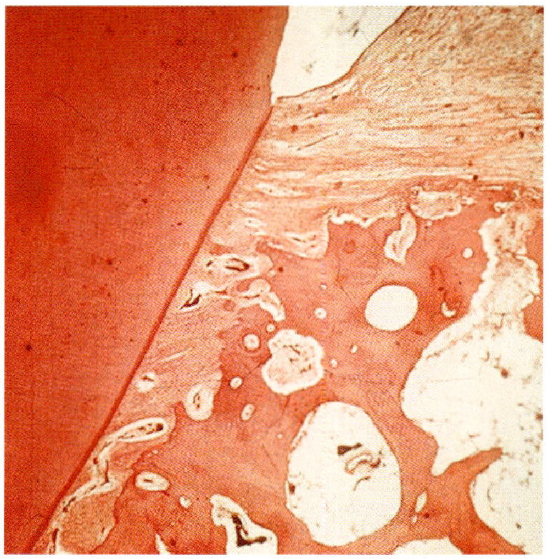

Fig 2-5-15 Widened periodontal ligament, horizontal fibers, and bone front resorption at the crest (Image courtesy of Professor E Rozenberg.)

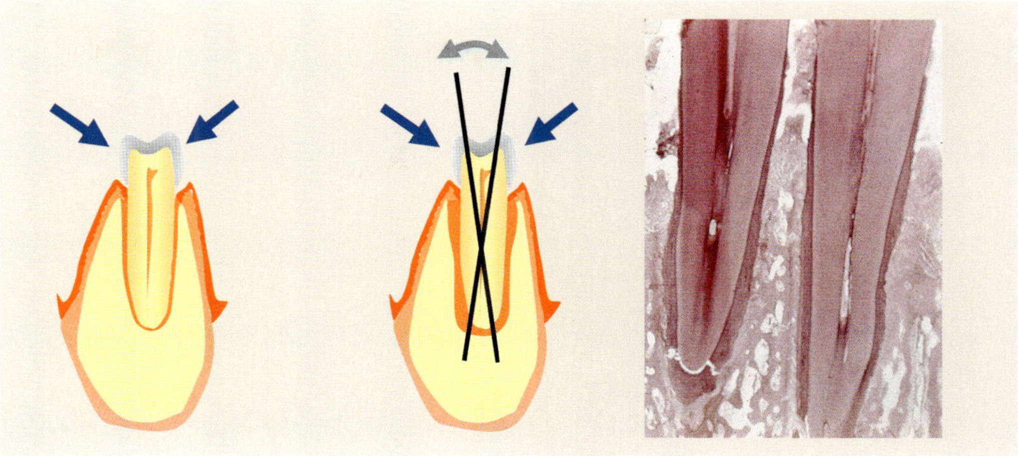

Fig 2-5-16 Primary occlusal trauma is defined as excessive occlusal forces acting on teeth with normal periodontal support.[60] This is clinically seen as widening of the periodontal membrane and increased or increasing mobility. There is no loss of cervical periodontal attachment. The mobility and widened PDL are reversible once abnormal forces are removed. (Histology courtesy of Professor E Rozenberg).

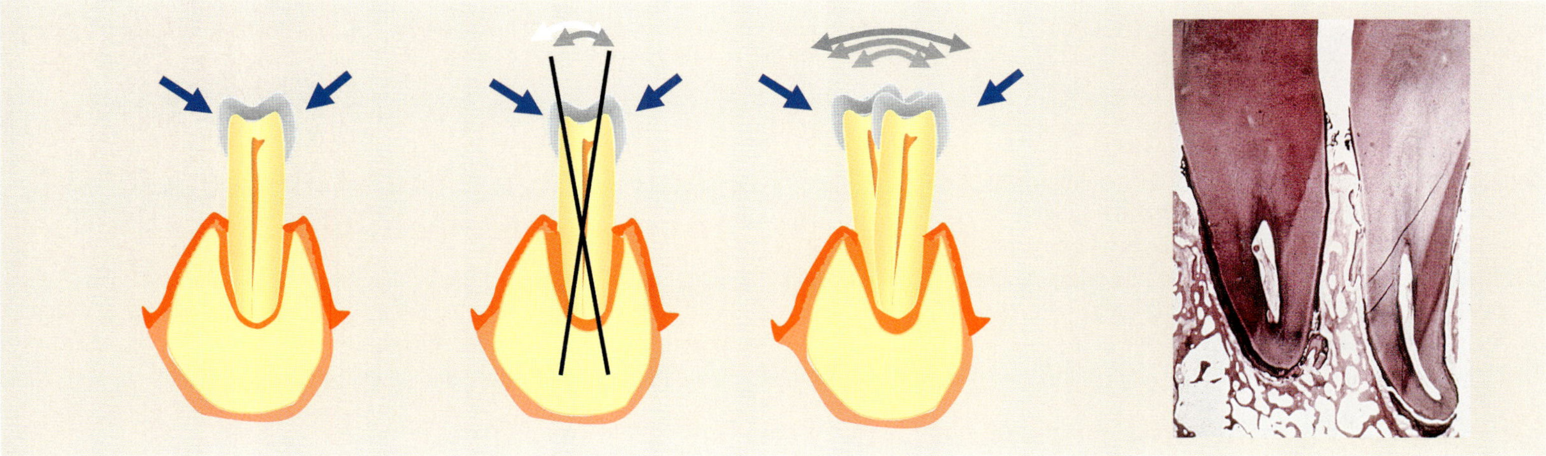

Fig 2-5-17 Secondary occlusal trauma is defined as normal occlusal forces acting on teeth with reduced periodontal support. This may manifest clinically with or without widening of the periodontal membrane. Increased or increasing mobility and fremitus on closure and excursion.[60] (Histology courtesy of Professor DW Cohen.)

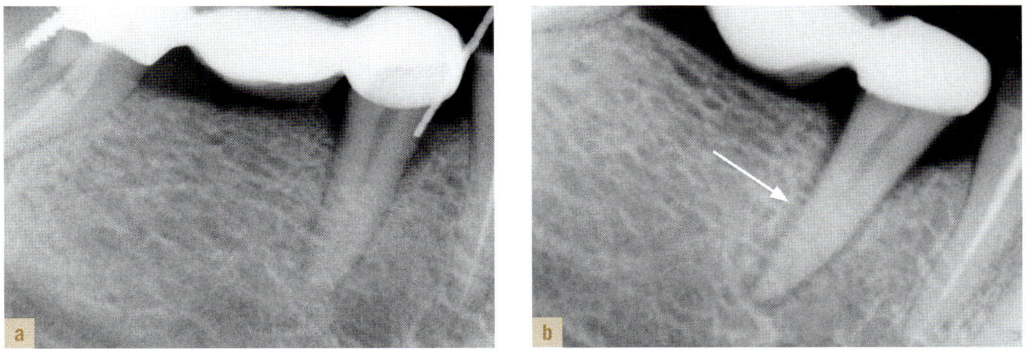

Fig 2-5-18a and b Mandibular right second premolar with primary occlusal traumatism with widened PDL (arrow). Periodontal probing of 3 mm. Distal abutment had been decemented for some time. Patient was a heavy bruxer.

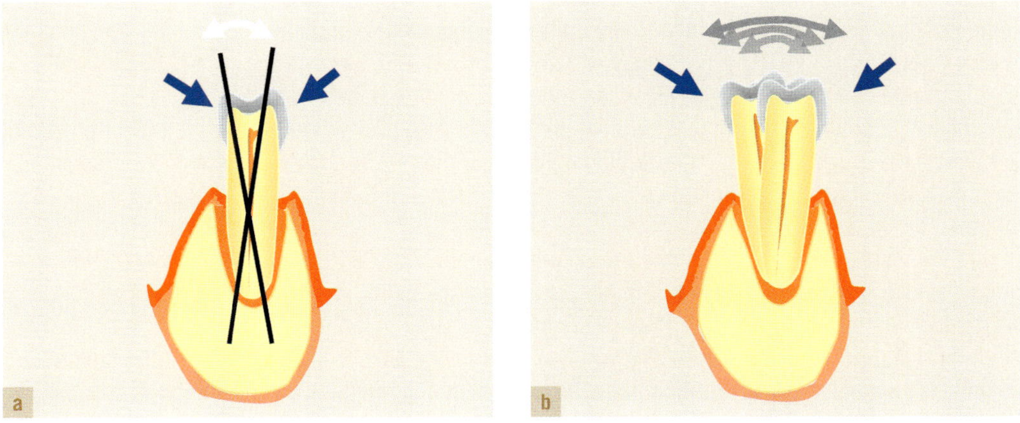

Fig 2-5-19a Increased mobility is tooth mobility that occurs within a circumscribed range that is greater than normal tooth mobility but does not change over time. b Increasing mobility is tooth mobility that increases over time. The PDL widens continuously as the tooth becomes progressively more mobile (right).[67-76]

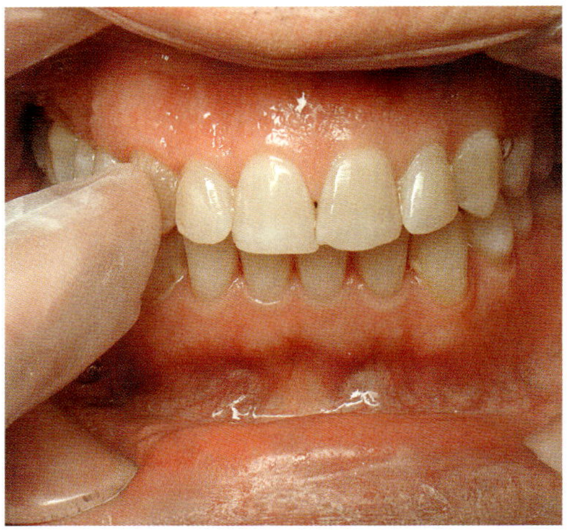

Fig 2-5-20 Fremitus: in cases of secondary traumatism, mobility may be felt on the buccal aspect of the maxillary teeth on closure into maximum intercuspation.

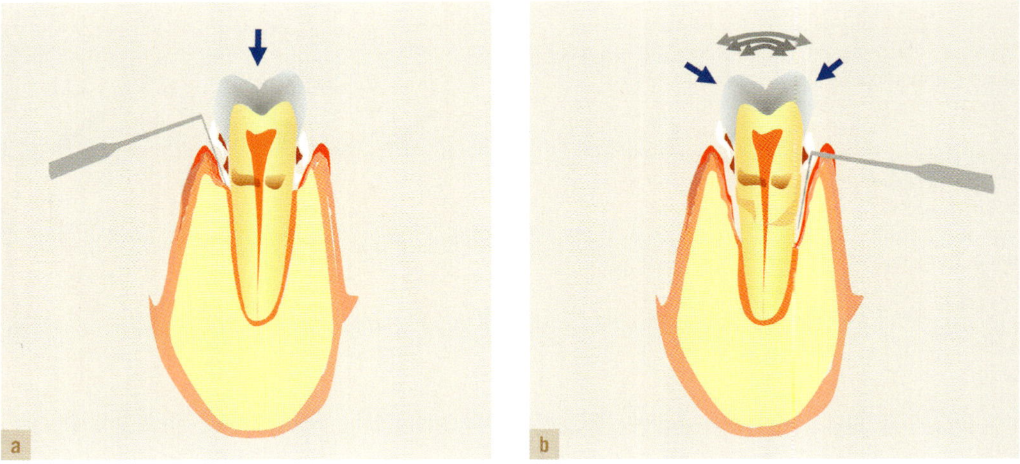

Fig 2-5-21a Combined occlusal trauma and periodontitis (co-destruction). Chronic plaque-induced inflammatory periodontitis results in loss of attachment and infrabony lesions. b Superimposed lesion of trauma from chronic jiggling and parafunctional occlusal forces together with progressively increasing mobility may cause more bone and attachment loss than that occurring from periodontitis alone.[74-82]

periodontitis and often requires splinting of the teeth. In the absence of marginal periodontal inflammation, both situations do not lead to loss of cervical attachment.[67-73] In a review on tooth mobility and periodontal disease, it was concluded that progressively increasing tooth mobility may be regarded as a contributing factor in progressive periodontitis.[68]

Occlusal trauma and periodontitis (co-destruction)

The role of occlusion in the progression of periodontal disease remains a controversial subject. When a lesion of occlusal trauma and a lesion of marginal periodontitis are superimposed, an increased potential exists for greater attachment loss as compared to periodontitis alone. This has been named co-destruction (Fig 2-5-21).[74,75] This has been shown to occur in beagle dog models, where bone loss and attachment loss with ligature-induced periodontitis, combined with jiggling forces were greater than for ligature-induced periodontitis alone.[76,77] This was not shown to occur in an equivalent squirrel monkey study.[78]

The effect of jiggling forces, superimposed on a condition of established plaque-associated periodontal disease, is still not properly understood. In beagle dog studies, traumatic jiggling forces were able to produce a progressively increasing mobility that resulted in a progression of plaque-associated lesions.[76,77] On the other hand, an equivalent experiment in squirrel monkeys concluded that the traumatic forces resulted in an "increased" tooth mobility but not in larger loss of attachment than that caused by subgingival plaque formation.[78] Human studies have found that teeth with initial occlusal discrepancies had significantly deeper initial probing depths, greater mobility, and a worse prognosis than teeth without initial occlusal discrepancies.[79] Treatment of occlusal discrepancies in these studies significantly reduced the progression of periodontal disease.[79,80]

In clinical situations of chronic marginal periodontitis, it is difficult to separate and distinguish between the periodontal and occlusal factors. In the presence of bone loss and active periodontitis with bleeding on probing, subgingival plaque and calculus, occlusal deflective contacts, and increasing mobility, the principal etiological element is likely to be plaque-induced periodontal inflammation with the occlusal trauma playing a subsidiary part. Periodontal and occlusal treatment approaches must be combined.[81,82]

Clinical signs and symptoms of trauma from occlusion

Clinical features from which a diagnosis of occlusal traumatism may be made have been proposed as indicators of trauma from occlusion.[81,82]

Clinical indicators include:

- Mobility
- Tooth migration
- Pain on chewing or percussion
- Fremitus
- Occlusal prematurities/discrepancies
- Wear facets in the presence of other clinical indicators
- Chipped or fractured tooth (teeth)
- Thermal sensitivity

Radiographic indicators include:

- Widened PDL space, disruption of the lamina dura
- Bone loss (furcations; vertical; circumferential)
- Root resorption

Differential diagnosis is necessary to identify other sources that may have caused or coexist with the above indicators.[81,82]

Splinting teeth (and implants)

Splinting mobile teeth provides the splinted unit with combined resistance to displacing forces that is further enhanced by non-collinear splinting in an arc as cross-arch splinting. Splinting mobile teeth with reduced alveolar bone support does not necessarily eliminate their mobility,[73,83,84] but it provides stability to the splinted unit. Improved patient comfort is cited as the most justified indication for splinting mobile teeth.[67,72,82] Splinting is indicated for increasing tooth mobility.[68] Other indications include the prevention of tooth migration, with reduced alveolar support and the stabilization of teeth following orthodontic movement to avoid relapse.[73,82] Parameters of care for chronic periodontitis with advanced loss of periodontal support and splinting strategies have been proposed.[67,85] Splinting multiple abutments in tooth-supported restorations to enhance resistance and retention is contentious, particularly in cases of reduced clinical crown height and increased intercrestal crown space. While some degree of resistance and retention may be enhanced, the effects of large moment arms on

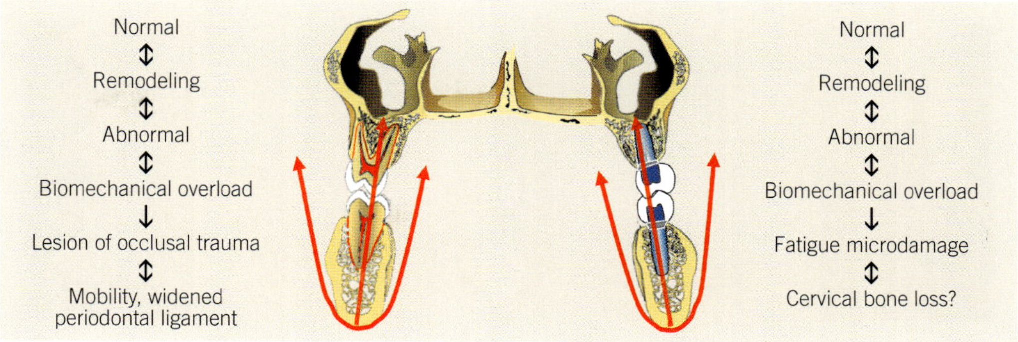

Fig 2-5-22 Normal and abnormal loading responses of teeth and implants. Teeth: normal loading in normal housing maintains intact morphology in a steady state of remodeling. Excessive loading may cause a lesion of trauma at the compression site, primary occlusal trauma with healing, widening of the PDL, reversible increased tooth mobility, and no loss of attachment. Implants: normal loading causes remodeling and steady state. Biomechanical overload may cause an abnormal response of fatigue microdamage with possible irreversible cervical bone loss.[91,92]

long splinted tooth-supported restorations increase the risk of decementation, particularly in terminal abutments. Larger tooth-supported fixed partial dentures had a greater failure rate due to recurrent caries than smaller restorations.[86] Splinting mobile teeth to implants is also contentious. While leaving splinted implants and splinted teeth as separate is most widely recommended,[87] their rigid combination has also been justified depending on the individual clinical determinants. The risk of a 5% incidence of root intrusion with a non-rigid connection must be weighed against considerations of retrievability and component complexity of a rigid tooth-to-implant connection.[88-90]

Normal and abnormal loading of teeth and dental implants

Dental implants are attached to the jawbone via direct bone-to-implant contact at the bone–implant interface. This difference in connection, as compared with the periodontal attachment of teeth in their alveolar housings, manifests in a difference in reaction to normal and abnormal occlusal loading. In addition to a difference in resiliency on normal loading, the histological reaction to abnormal loading between teeth and implants varies (Fig 2-5-22).

Teeth

Normal loading is created by the forces of mastication and swallowing that are part of normal life. Remodeling of the alveolus and periodontal interface maintain normal alveolar anatomy. Transient mild clenching and grinding are also extremely common and may be considered as part of normal loading. These forces serve to maintain the macro- and microstructural integrity and natural turnover of the bones of the facial skeleton and the alveolar housing of the teeth. This is part of normal remodeling of the bone. Abnormal loading may be due to a high and sustained force, repetitive jiggling force, or a small but continuously sustained force. These may result in a lesion of occlusal trauma, tooth mobility, and widening of the PDL in the absence of periodontal inflammation. This process is considered by some to be an adaptive response to overload.

Implants

Loaded dental implants connected to the bone by an osseointegrated bone interface are able to function and respond to normal loading with remodeling of the bone–implant interface. A process of fatigue microdamage with microfracture of bone at the interface and subsequent repair facilitates the process and remodeling. This perpetuates a steady state at the interface. It has been postulated that when loading is increased to the extent that the rate of repair of the microdamage is unable to keep up with the rate of imposed microdamage, a net loss of cervical bone attachment may occur as regressive modeling with irreversible marginal bone loss(Figs 2-5-22 to 2-5-24).[91,92]

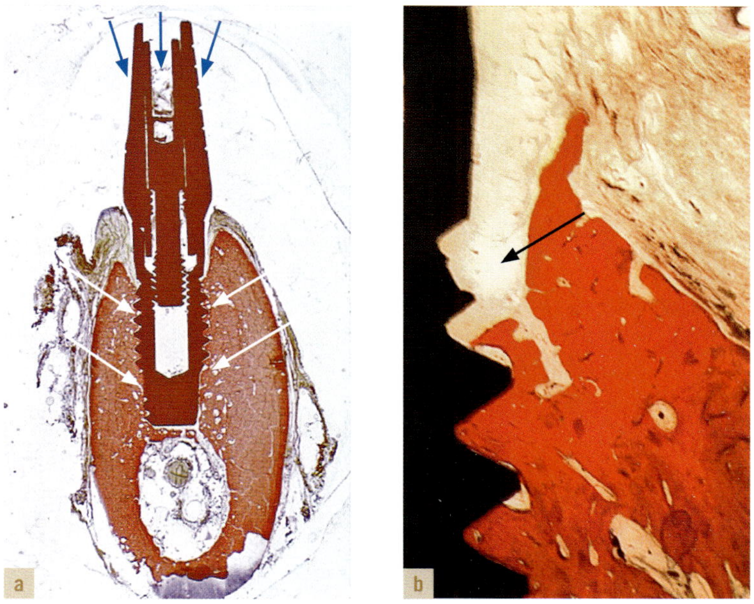

Fig 2-5-23 Fatigue microdamage (FMD) is the mechanism proposed as causing bone loss round implant necks and further bone loss. a FMD and repair maintains marginal bone and the interface (white arrows). b FMD without repair can cause cervical bone loss.[91,92] (Histology courtesy of Professor A Koslovsky.)

Occlusal overload, crestal bone loss, and peri-implantitis

The combined effects of mechanical overload and plaque induced peri-implant inflammation are still under debate.

Peri-implantitis has been variously defined as "a site specific, plaque-induced infection with progressive loss of the bone supporting a functioning implant",[93] and as "an infection with suppuration associated with clinically significant progressive crestal bone loss after the adaptive phase" of osseointegration.[94]

Suppuration is not always apparent clinically. "Peri-implant mucositis and peri-implantitis are infectious diseases. Peri-implant mucositis describes an inflammatory lesion that resides in the mucosa, while peri-implantitis also affects the supporting bone."[95] Peri-implantitis has been simulated in ligature plaque-induced animal models.[96]

Co-destruction has been shown to occur in teeth in the beagle dog.[76,77] This has also been shown to occur in implants in a beagle dog model with the combination of ligature-induced peri-implantitis and occlusal trauma induced by implant restorations in supraocclusion (Fig 2-5-25).[97] This

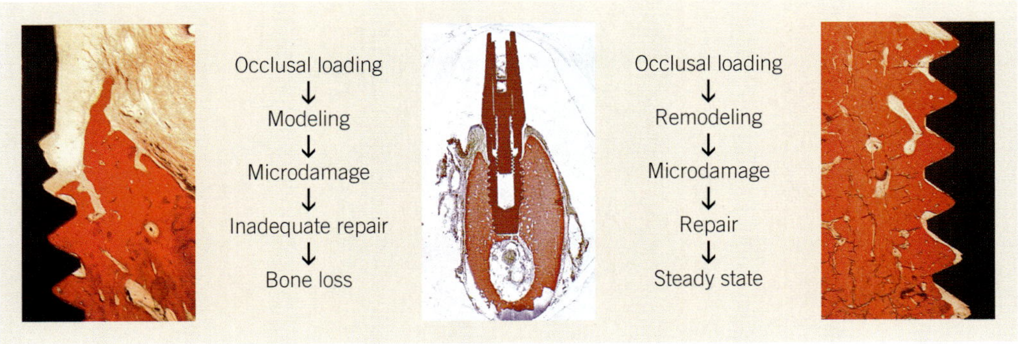

Fig 2-5-24 Remodeling repairs the fatigue microdamage at the implant–abutment interface to maintain a steady state. Modeling and regressive modeling as irreversible cervical bone loss occurs when the rate of repair cannot keep up with the rate of microdamage[91,92] (Histology courtesy of Professor A Koslovsky.)

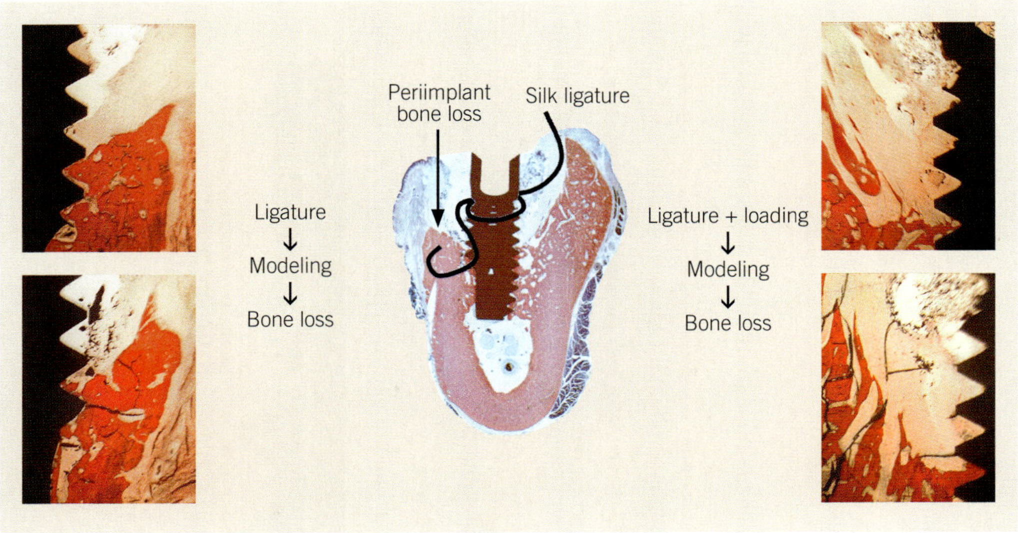

Fig 2-5-25 Co-destruction occurring in a beagle dog model. The cervical bone loss of ligature-induced peri-implantitis and occlusal overload (right) was greater than the cervical bone loss induced by occlusal overload alone (left). (Histology courtesy of Prof A Koslovsky et al.[97])

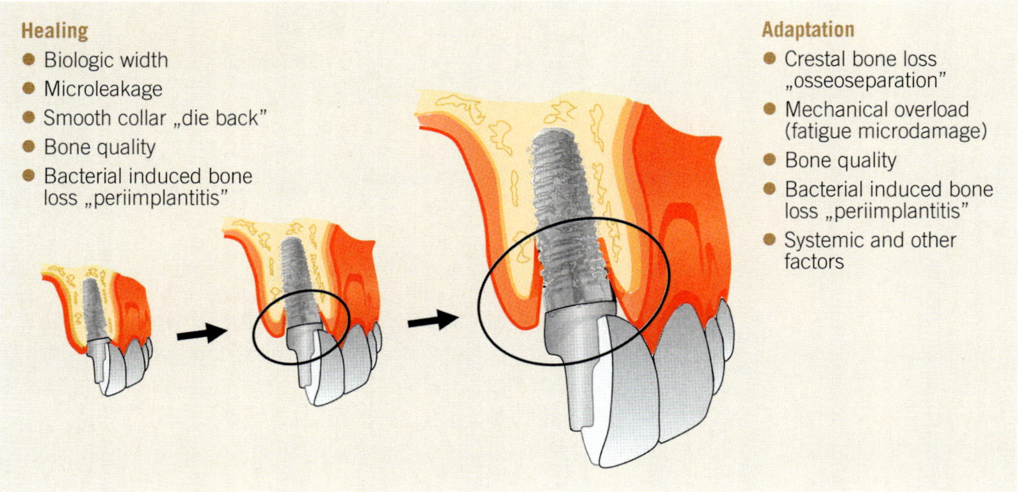

Fig 2-5-26 Postulated progression of crestal bone loss.[94,101,102] The process of bone loss in the "healing" and subsequent "adaptation" period are differentiated.[94,101,102] Crestal bone loss in the late adaptation stage is subject to multiple time-dependent host and local variables

was also seen in a macaca monkey model[98] but not in cynomolgus monkeys[99] nor in another beagle dog study[100] (see Chapter 7).

Postulated mechanisms of implant marginal bone loss

In humans, bone loss occurs in a small number of implants. Alternative terms for peri-implant bone loss have been coined as "osseoseparation" and "osseodisintegration." The term "peri-implantitis" has been considered as an unsuitable term to describe all crestal bone loss.[94,101,102]

When bone loss occurs around implants, it is often difficult to know the exact reason. Two types of bone loss are reported: early and late. Early loss occurs in the healing phase and later bone loss in the subsequent functional adaptive phase.[94,101,102] Initial early cervical bone loss in the range of around 0.5 to 2 mm occurs around most implants following healing and osseointegration after one year (early loss). In a small number of implants further bone loss may occur over varying extended periods of time. This has also been called osseodisintegration.[94,101,102] "Osseosuficiency" is described as the adequate host and implant conditions at the implant host site required to develop and maintain a successful interface.[101] Osseoseparation was described as a condition where host and/or implant factors combine to cause late marginal bone loss, osseodisintegration, and possible eventual implant loss.[101]

Late bone loss in the adaptation period has most commonly been related to plaque-induced inflammatory peri-implantitis and to regressive modeling related to mechanical overload. Several other case-specific, time-dependent, patient, and implant factors are likely to be involved but their relative contribution in each case is often difficult to determine.[94,101]

Contributing factors have been advanced and demonstrated in animal models. Creation of a biologic width during the healing phase caused cervical loss in a beagle dog model.[103] Microleakage from bac-

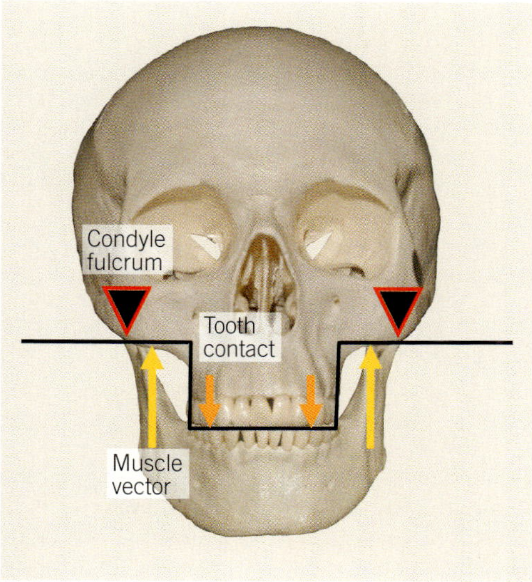

Fig 2-7-20 Closure in the frontal aspect acts as a loaded beam. Yellow arrows: muscle vectors. Orange arrows: tooth contact and resultant occlusal force. Condyle eminence force at condylar fulcrums.

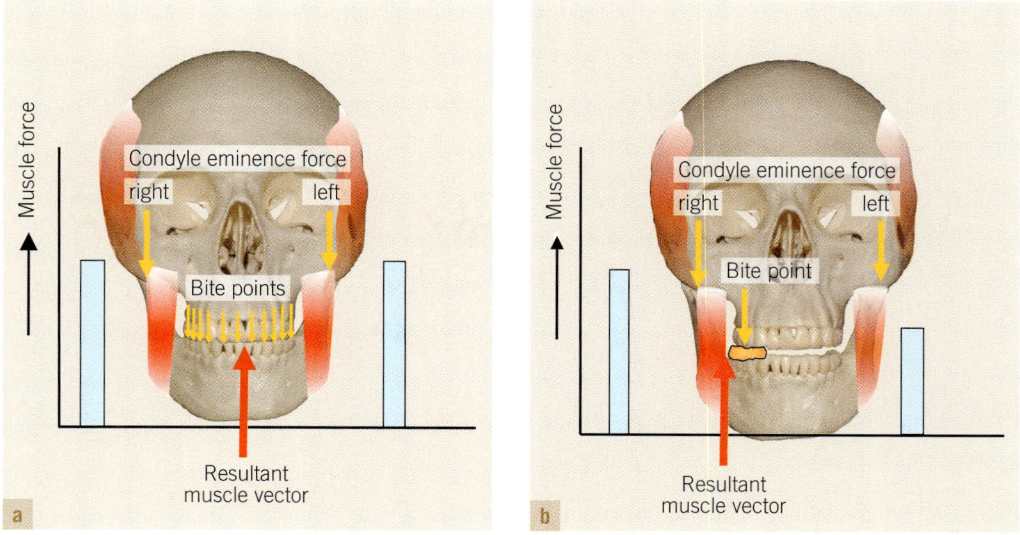

Fig 2-7-21a Symmetrical loading of the system with the total resultant muscle vector in the midline. b Greater loading on one side causes the muscle vector to move towards the side with the greater recruitment and loading.

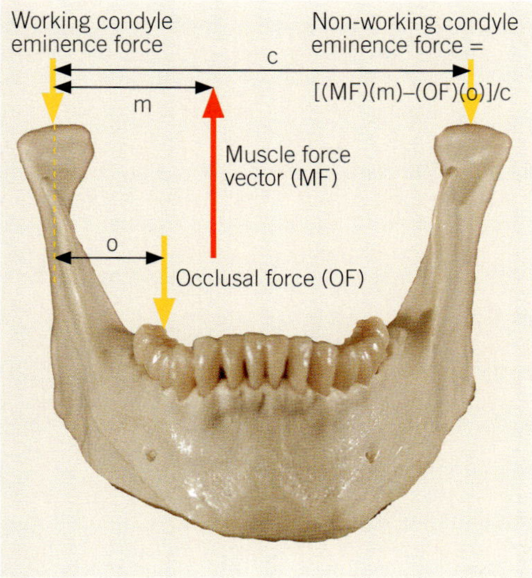

Fig 2-7-22 Frontal moment analysis.[17,19,23,87]

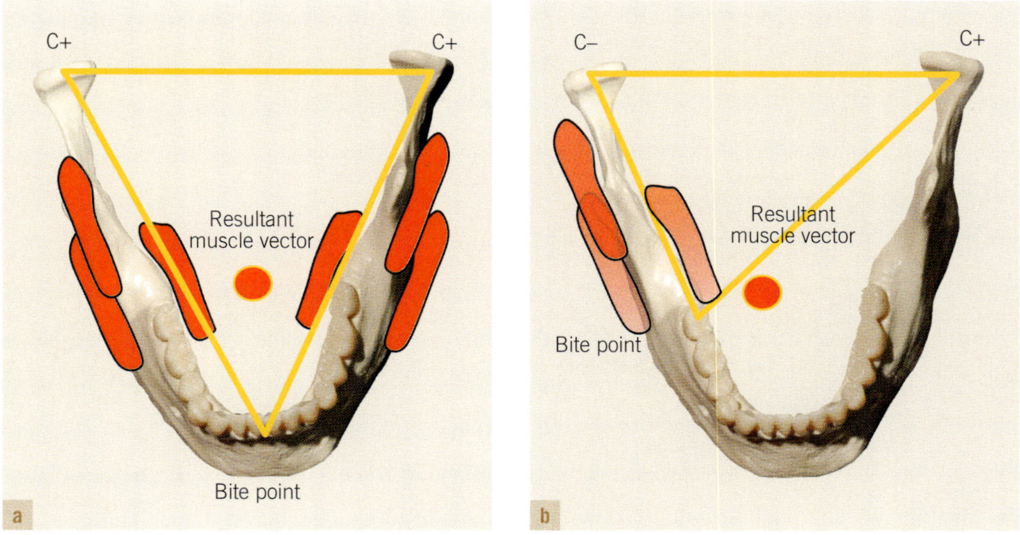

Fig 2-7-23 Triangles of support: condylar compression (C+), condylar unloading (C–). a With the resultant muscle inside the triangle of support, the system is stable and both condyles are under compressive loading. b When the resultant muscle vectort is outside the triangle of support, the posterior bite point acts as a pivot, resulting in decompression of the working condyle and compression of the non-working condyle.

Loading of the TMJs

The question of whether the condyles act as a fulcrum on closure was debated over several years.[14-16,88-90] In part, this debate was influenced by the fact that the TMJs are lined by fibrous connective tissue rather than cartilage that is typical of other load-bearing joints. Current concepts consider that the TMJ is a stress-bearing joint and that it becomes more heavily loaded on incisor biting (Figs 2-7-18 and 2-7-19).[17,23] Differential loading of the working and non-working sides of joints is a function of the relative recruitment of the working and non-working elevator muscles. Thus, working and non-working side condyles may alternatively be placed under more or less compression as the recruitment side varies (Figs 2-7-21 to 2-7-23). The non-working side condyle is considered to be loaded more than the working side condyle during forceful unilateral working side chewing and biting.[23] Compression of the working side disc is greater than that of the non-working side disc.

During the closing stroke of chewing, the working side mandibular corpus is twisted around its long axis. This twisting causes the lower body of the corpus to be everted and the alveolus and teeth to be inverted. During the closing stroke, the lateral aspect of the disc becomes more heavily compressed than the medial aspect.[17]

Condylar compression on forced lateral closure

Several studies have measured superior condylar displacement on different occlusal contact conditions.[91-93]

Clenching on a stabilization maxillary splint and an anterior repositioning splint with MI produced no superior condylar movement. Clenching on a maxillary splint with anterior contact only produced upward condylar movement of 0.44 mm and anterior movement of 0.19 mm.[91]

The condylar position was 0.30 mm more superior and 0.10 mm more anterior during clenching than without clenching on an anterior splint.[92] Condyle position, keyed with an anterior stop, was located an average of 0.45 mm more superior with heavy closing force (clenching) than with light comfortable closing force.[93]

Lateral contacts and working and non-working condylar displacement

Unilateral clenching on the canine caused smaller superior displacement of the non-working side condyle than group function.[94] Controlled clenching on a unilateral canine and group function caused jaw tipping with non-working side TMJ compression. Introduction of simultaneous balancing contacts reduced this tipping.[94] Working side vertical movement was in the range of 0.1 to 0.2mm and non-working side vertical movement in the range of 0.2 to 0.4 mm.[94]

Clenching on the canine caused a cranial movement of the non-working side condyle that was reduced by 0.6 to 0.9 mm by placement of artificial non-working side contacts.[95] It has been postulated by some that these and other studies suggest that non-working contacts may be protective of the non-working TMJ.[91-96]

References

1. Hanken J,Thorogood P. Evolution and development of the vertebrate skull: The role of pattern formation. Trends Ecol Evol 1993;8:9–15.
2. Lieberman D, Mowbray K, Person O. Basicranial influence on overall cranial shape. J Hum Evol 2000;38:291–315.
3. Pickford M. Major stages of the evolution of primate neurocranium. Hum Evol 1988;3:449–460.
4. Leonard WR. Food for thought. Dietary change was a driving change in human evolution. Sci Am 2002;287:106–115.
5. Herring S. The masticatory muscles and the skull: a comparative perspective. Arch Oral Biol 2007;52:296–299.
6. Rossie JB. The phylogenetic significance of anthropoid paranasal sinuses. Anat Rec 2008;291:1554–1563.
7. DuBrul EL. Sicher and DuBrul's Oral Anatomy, ed 8. St Louis: Ishiyaku EuroAmerica, 1988.
8. Sicher H. Oral Anatomy, ed 2. St Louis: CV Mosby, 1952.
9. Marquez S. The paranasal sinuses: the last frontier in craniofacial biology. Anat Rec (Hoboken) 2008;261:1350–1361.
10. Taylor AB. Feeding behavior, diet, and the functional consequences of jaw form in orangutans, with implications for the evolution of Pongo. J Human Evol 2006;50:377–393.
11. Weidenreich F. The brain and its role in the phylogenetic transformation of the human skull. Am Phil Soc 1941;31:321–442.
12. Healy SD, Rowe C. A critique of comparative studies of brain size. Proc Biol Sci 2007;274:453–464.
13 Taylor AB. A comparative analysis of temporomandibular joint morphology in the African apes. J Hum Evol 2005;48:555–574.
14. Gingerich PD. The human mandible: lever or link, or both? Am J Phys Anthropol 1979;51:135–137.
15. Hylander WL, Johnson KR. In vivo bone strain patterns in the craniofacial regions of primates. In: McNeill C (ed). Science and Practice of Occlusion. Chicago: Quintessence Publishing, 1997:165–178.
16. Hylander WL. Functional anatomy and biomechanics of the masticatory apparatus. In: Laskin D, Green CS, Hylander WL (eds). Temporomandibular Disorders: An Evidence-based Approach to Diagnosis and Treatment. Chicago: Quintessence Publishing, 2006:1–34.
17. Hylander WL. Mandibular function and temporomandibular joint loading. In: Carlson DS, McNamara JA, Ribbens KA (eds). Developmental Aspects of Temporomandibular Joint Disorders. Monograph 16. Craniofacial Growth Series. Ann Arbor: University of Michigan, 1985.
18. Hinton RJ, Carlson DS. Temporal changes in human temporomandibular joint size and shape. Am J Phys Anrop 1979;50:325–334.
19. MacDonald JWC, Hannam AG Relationship between occlusal contacts and jaw-closing muscle activity during tooth clenching: Part II. J Prosthet Dent 1984;52:862–867.
20. Van Eijden TM. Three-dimensional anlyses of human bite-force magnitude and movement. Arch Oral Biol 1991;36:535–539.
21. Van Eijden TM. Jaw muscle activity in relation to the direction and point of application of bite force. J Dent Res 1990;69:901–905.
22. The glossary of prosthodontic terms. J Prosthet Dent 2005;94:10–92.
23. Caputo AA, Standlee JJ. Biomechanics in Clinical Dentistry. Chicago: Quintessence Publishing, 1987.
24. Gibbs CH, Mahan PE, Lundeen HC, Brehnan K, Walsh EK, Holbrook WB Occlusal forces during chewing and swallowing as measured by sound transmission. J Prosthet Dent 1981;Oct;46:443–449.
25. Gibbs CH, Mahan PE, Lundeen HC, Brehnan K, Walsh EK, Sinkewiz SL, et al. Occlusal forces during chewing – influences of biting strength and food consistency. J Prosthet Dent 1981;46:561–567.
26. Gibbs CH, Lundeen HC. Jaw movements and forces during chewing and swallowing and their clinical significance. In: Lundeen HC, Gibbs CH (eds). Advances in Occlusion. Boston: John Wright, 1982:23.
27. Nishigawa K, Bando E, Nakano M. Quantitative study of bite force during sleep associated bruxism. J Oral Rehabil 2001;28:485–491.
28. Gibbs CH, Mahan PE, Mauderli A, Lundeen HC, Walsh EK. Limits of human bite strength. J Prosthet Dent 1986;56:226–229.
29. Kiliardis S, Johansson A, Haraldson T, Omar R, Carlsson GE. Craniofacial morphology, occlusal traits, and bite force in persons with advanced occlusal tooth wear. Am J Orthod Dentofacial Orthop 1995;107:286–292.
30. van der Bilt A, Tekamp A, van der Glas H, Abbink J. Bite force and electromyograpy during maximum unilateral and bilateral clenching. Eur J Oral Sci 2008;116:217–222.
31. Nie X. Cranial base in craniofacial development: developmental features, influence on facial growth, anomaly, and molecular basis. Acta Odontol Scand 2005;63:127–135.
32. Davis WE, Templer J, Parsons DS. Anatomy of the paranasal sinuses. Otolaryngol Clin North Am 1996;29:57–74.
33. Enlow DH. The Human Face: An Account of the Postnatal Growth and Development of the Craniofacial Skeleton. New York: Hoeber Medical Division, Harper and Row Publishers, 1968.
34. Witmer LM. Bones, air sacs and natural selection: a new perspective on the function of pneumatic sinuses [abstract]. J Morphol 1997;232:340.
35. Gannon PJ, Doyle WJ, Ganjian E, Ma'rquez S, Gnoy A. Gabrielle HS, et al. Maxillary sinus mucosal blood flow during nasal vs tracheal respiration. Arch Otolaryngol Head Neck Surg 1997;123:1336–1340.
36. Lundberg JO. Nitric oxide and the paranasal sinuses. Anat Rec 2008;291:1479–1484.
37. Lundberg JO, Rinder J, Weitzberg E, Lundberg JM, Alving K. Nasally exhaled nitric oxide in humans originates mainly in the paranasal sinuses. Acta Physiol Scand 1994;152:431–432.
38. Throckorton GS, Throckmorton LS. Quantitative calculations of TMJ reaction forces – I. The importance of magnitude of the jaw muscle forces. J Biomech 1985;18:445–452.
39. Preuschoft H, Witte H, Witzel U. Pneumatized spaces, sinuses and spongy bones in the skulls of primates. Anthropol Anz 2002;60:67–79.
40. Gross MD, Arbel G, Hershkovitz I. Three-dimensiona finite element analysis of the facial skeleton on simulated occlusal loading. J Oral Rehabil 2001;28:684–694.
41. Arbel G, Hershkovitz I, Gross MD. Strain distribution on the skull due to occlusal loading: an anthropological perspective. Homo 2000;51:30–55.
42. Richmond BG, Wright BW, Grosse I, et al. Finite element analysis in functional morphology. Anat Rec A Discov Mol Cell Evol Biol 2005;283:259–274.
43. Marquez S, Laitman JT. 2008. Climatic effects of the nasal complex: a CT imaging, comparative anatomical and morphometric investigation of *Macaca mulatta* and *Macaca fascicularis*. Anat Rec 291:1420–1445.
44. Sicher H, Tandler J. Anatomie Fur Zahnartzte. Berlin: Springer, 1928.
45. Richter W. Der Obergesichtsschadel des menschen als gebisturm, ein statische kunstwerk. Dt Mschr Zahnheilk 1920;38:49–68.
46. Bluntschli H. Ruckirkung des kieferapparates auf den gesamtschadel. Z Zahnarztl Orthopad 1926;18:57–59.
47. Roberts DR, Tattersall I. Skull form and mechanics of mandibular elevation in mammals. Am Mus Novit 1974;2536:1–9.
48. Couly JD. The mechanical adaptation of bones. Princeton NJ: Princeton University Press, 1976.
49. Demes B. The resistance of the primate skull against mechanical stresses. Z Morphol Anthropol 1981;72:47–64.
50. Throckmorton GS, Throckmorton LS. Quantitative calculations of temporomandibular joint reaction forces – I. The importance of the magnitude of the jaw muscle forces. J Biomech 1985;18:445–452.
51. Benninghoff A. Spaltlinien am knochen, ein methoce zur ermittlung der architectu platter knoche. Verh Anat Ges 1925;34:189–206.
52. Tappen NC. A functional analysis of the facial skeleton with split line technique. Am J Phys Anthropol 1953;11;503–532.
53. Tappen NC. A comparative functional analysis of primate skulls by the split-line techniques. Hum Biol 1954;26:220–238.
54. Moss ML, Young RW. A functional approach to craniology. Am J Phys Anthropol 1960;18:281–291.
55. Endo B. Distribution of stress and strain produced in the human face by masticatory forces. J Anthrop Soc Nippon 1965;73:123–135.
56. Endo B. A biomechanical study of the human facial skeleton by means of strain-sensitive lacquer. Okajimas Folia Anat Jpn 1966;42 205–217.
57. Endo B. Analysis of stresses around the orbit due to masseter and temporalis muscles respectively. J Anthrop Soc Nippon 1970;78:251–266.
58. Demes B, Preuschoft H, Wolffe JEA. Stress-strength relationships in the mandibles of hominoids. In: Chivers D, Wood BA, Bilsborough A (eds). Food Acquisition and Processing in Primates. London: Plenum Press, 1984:369–396.
59. Preuschoft HB, Demes M, Meyer M, Bar HF. The biomechanical principles realized in the upper jaw of long snouted primates. In: Else JG, Lee PC (eds). Primate Evolution. Cambridge: Cambridge University Press, 1986:249–264.
60. Preuschoft H, Witzel U. The functional shape of the skull in vertebrates: which forces determine skull morphology in lower primates and ancestral synapsids? Anat Rec 2005;283:402–413.
61. Rak Y. The Australopithecine Face. New York: Academic Press,1983.

62. Demes B. Another look at an old face: biomechanics of the Neanderthal facial skeleton reconsidered. J Hum Evol 1987;16:297–303.
63. Moss ML, Young RW. A functional approach to craniology. Am J Phys Anthrop 1960;18:281–291.
64. Ravosa MJ. Browridge development in Cercipithecidae: A test of two models. Am J Phys Anthrop 1988;76:535–555.
65. Ravosa MJ. Ontogenic perspective on mechanical and nonmechanical models of primate circumorbital morphology. Am J Phys Anthrop1991;85:95–112.
66. Koolstra JH, van Eijden TM, Weijs WA, Naeije M. A three-dimensional mathematical model of the human masticatory system predicting posterior bite forces. J Biomech 1988;21:563–576.
67. Koolstra JH, van Eijden TM. Biomechanical analysis of jaw closing muscles. J Dent Res 1995;74:1564–1570.
68. Misch CE, Bidez MW. Implant-protected occlusion: a biomechanical rationale. Compendium 1994;15:1330, 1332, 1334; quiz 1344.
69. Alexandridis CA, Thanos CE, Caputo AA. Distribution of stress patterns in the human zygomatic arch and bone. J Oral Rehabil 1981;8:495–505.
70. Alexandridis CA, Caputo AA, Thanos CE. Distribution of stresses in the human skull. J Oral Rehabil 1985;12:499–507.
71. Gross MD, Nissan J, Rellu S. Stress distribution around maxillary implants in anatomic photoelastic models of varying geometry. Part I. J Prosthet Dent 2000;85:442–449.
72. Gross MD, Nissan J, Rellu S. Stress distribution around maxillary implants in anatomic photoelastic models of varying geometry. Part II. J Prosthet Dent 2001;85:450–454.
73. Benzing UR, Gall H, Weber H. Biomechanical aspects of two different implant-prosthetic concepts for edentulous maxillae. Int J Oral Maxillofac Implants 1995;10:188–198.
74. Miyasaka J, Tanne K, Tsutsumi S, Sakuda M. Finite element analysis for the biomechanical effects of orthopedic forces on the craniofacial skeleton. Construction of the 3-dimensional finite element model of the craniofacial skeleton. Osaka Daigaku Shigaku Zasshi 1986;31:393–402.
75. Miyasaka J, Tanne K, Yamagata Y, Sakuda M, Tsutsumi S. Finite element analysis for biomechanical effects on craniofacial skeleton. J Dent Res 1987;66:323.
76. Tanne K, Hiraga J, Kakiuchi K, Yamagata Y, Sakuda M. Biomechanical effect of anteriorly directed extraoral forces on the craniofacial complex: a study using the finite element method. Am J Orthod Dentofacial Orthop 1989;95:200–207.
77. Korioth TWP. Simulated physics of the human mandible. In: McNeill C (ed). Science and Practice of Occlusion. Chicago: Quintessence Publishing, 1997:179–186.
78. Korioth TWP, Romily DP, Hannam AG. Three-dimensional finite element stress analysis of the dentate human mandible. Am J Phys Anthrop 1992;88:69–96.
79. Clelland NL, Lee JK, Bimbent OC, Brantley WA. A three-dimensional finite element stress analysis of angled abutments for an implant placed in the anterior maxilla. J Prosthodont 1995;4:95–100.
80. Cattaneo PM, Dalstra M, Melsen B. The transfer of occlusal forces through the maxillary molars: A finite element study. Am J Orthod Dentofacial Orthop 2003;123:367–373.
81. Curtis N, Koreliue K, O'Higgins P. Predicting skull loading: applying multibody dynamics analysis to a macaque skull. Anat Rec (Hoboken) 2008;291:491–501.
82. Lieberman DE, Krovitz GE, Yates FW, Devlin M, St Claire M. Effects of food processing on masticatory strain and craniofacial growth in a retrognathic face. J Hum Evol 2004;46:655–677.
83. Rafferty KL, Herring S, Marshall CD. Biomechanics of the rostrum and the role of facial sutures. J Morphol 2003;257:33–44.
84. Herring SW, Rafferty KL, Liu ZJ, Marshall CD. 2001. Jaw muscles and the skull in mammals: the biomechanics of mastication. Comp Biochem Physiol A Mol Integr Physiol 2001;131:207–219.
85. Zingone A. Shell Structures in Civil and Mechanical Engineering. Theory and Closed Form Analytical Solutions. London: Thomas Telford Publishing, 1997.
86. Ohmori H, Yamamoto K. Shape Optimization of Shell and Spatial Structures for Specified Stress Distribution. Memoirs of the School of Engineering. Nagoya University, 1998;50:1–32.
87. Smith RJ. Mandibular biomechanics and temporomandibular joint function in primates. Am J Phys Anthropol 1978;49:341–376.
88. Greaves WS. The jaw lever system in ungulates: A new model. J Zool Lond 1978;184:271–285.
89. Druzinsky RE, Greaves WS. A model to explain the posterior limit of the bite point in reptiles. J Morphol 1979;160:165–168.
90. Robinson M. The temporomandibular joint: theory of reflex controlled nonlever action of the mandible J Am Dent Assoc 1946;33:1260–1271.
91. Ito T, Gibbs CH, Marguelles-Bonnett R, Lupkiewicz SM, Young HM, Lundeend HC, et al. Loading on the temporomandibular joints with five occlusal conditions. J Prosthet Dent 1986;56:478–484.
92. Teo CS, Wise MD. Comparison of retruded axis articulator mounting with and without applied muscle force. J Oral Rehabil 1981;8:363–376.
93. Lundeen HC. Centric relation records: the effect of muscle action. J Prosthet Dent 1974;31:244–253.
94. Okano N, Baba K, Akishige S, Ohyama T. The influence of altered occlusal guidance on condylar displacement. J Oral Rehabil 2002;29:1091–1098.
95. Seedorf H, Weitendorf H, Scholz A, Kirsch I, Heydecke G. Effect of non-working occlusal contacts on vertical condyle position. J Oral Rehabil 2009;36:435–441.
96. Baba K, Yugami K, Yaka T, Ai M. Impact of balancing side tooth contact on clenching induced mandibular displacements. J Oral Rhabil 2001;28:721–727.

3 Fundamentals of Occlusion

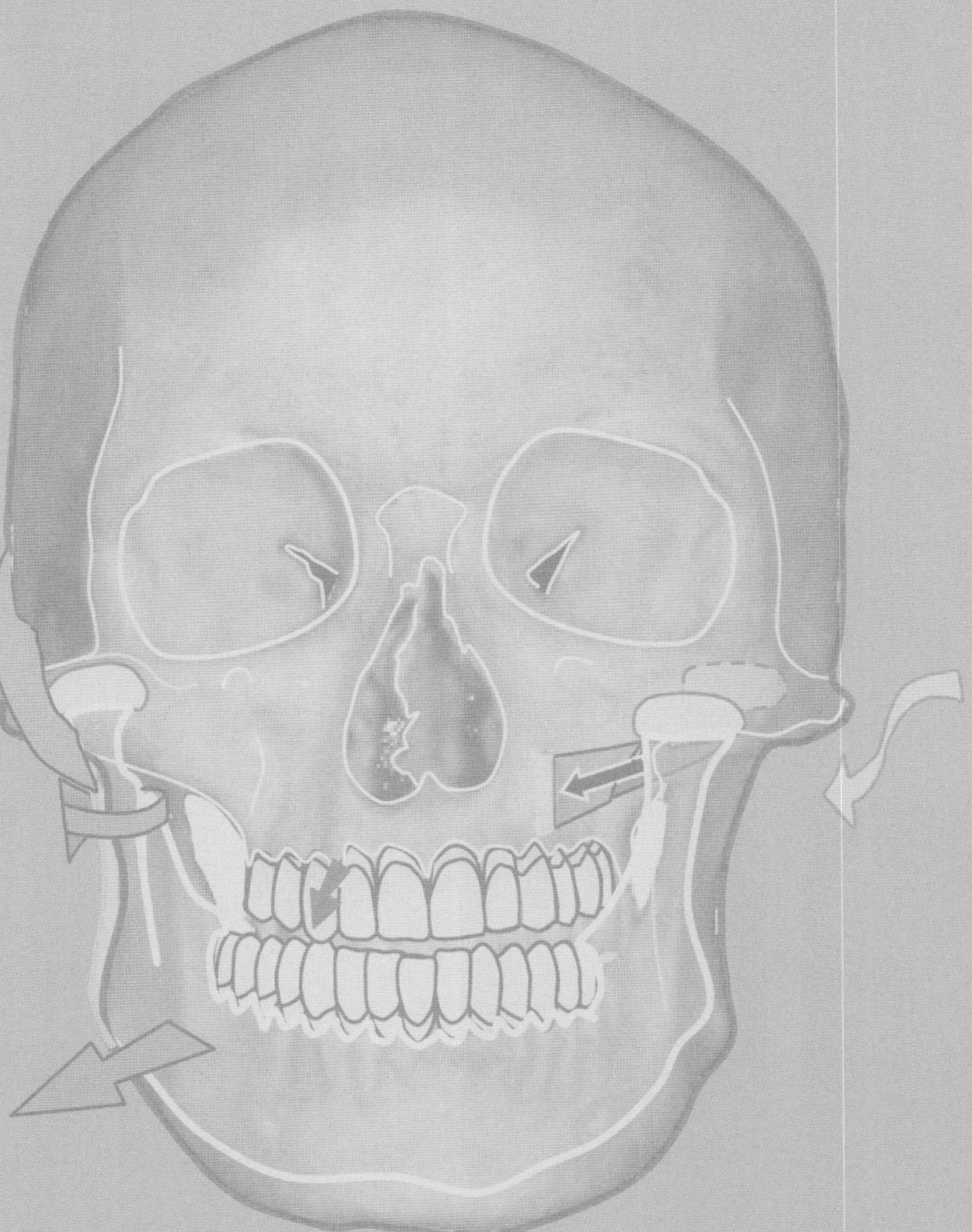

3.1 Functional Anatomy and Dynamics of the Masticatory System

Contents

Structures of the facial skeleton

The skull

The human skull is a complex hollow structure containing the essential functional and perceptual systems and centers of survival (Fig 3-1-1). It constitutes the structural housing for the opposing teeth for mastication and trituration of food for swallowing and digestion. The upper two-thirds are hollow complex shell structures comprised of thin membranous bone, with outer aspects containing the origins of the masticatory muscles for insertion into the opposing mandible.[1-4]

Maxilla

The maxilla consists of thin membranous bone housing the posterior maxillary teeth and the premaxilla housing the anterior maxillary teeth (Fig 3-1-2). The maxillary sinus borders the nasal cavity medially, the floor of the orbit superiorly, and the lateral wall merging with the zygomatic process.[2-8]

The principal load-bearing region is at the base of the zygomatic process above the first and second maxillary molars. This is seen in most mammals and particularly in carnivores, with the big cats for instance having a single crushing molar behind the carnassial situated under the base of the zygomatic arch. Forces are dissipated up the thin lateral walls of the maxilla towards the zygomatic and frontal processes. The inferior border of the maxilla constitutes the vaulted structure of the membranous hard palate that merges peripherally with the alveolar housing of the maxillary teeth.

The maxillary molars and premolars are aligned in their alveolar housings with very thin cortical buccal plates of bone on the facial aspect. The buccal roots are aligned with the outer maxillary wall and lateral aspect of the zygomatic root, while the maxillary roots are more inclined towards the lateral ascending walls of the palatal vault. The volume of trabecular bone above the molar roots varies, with more trabeculation closer to the roots, and generally has low bone density.

The anterior maxillary teeth are bound superiorly by the floor of the nasal cavity. The amount of alveolar bone above the apices varies. Buccal walls are generally thin. Lingually, the alveolar plates merge with the hard palate.

Mandible

The mandible is a solid bone of varying trabecular density surrounded by a thicker cortical shell (Fig 3-1-3). The mandible is derived from Meckel's cartilage from the fifth branchial arch. The teeth are aligned in a continuous arch with the molars more solidly embedded in the surrounding bone. Trabeculation is more concentrated immediately around the roots and becomes less dense with increasingly larger trabecular spaces at the lower border around and below the mandibular nerve. The anterior incisors, canines, and premolars are surrounded by more dense bone and have, as in the maxillary teeth, very thin buccal plates.

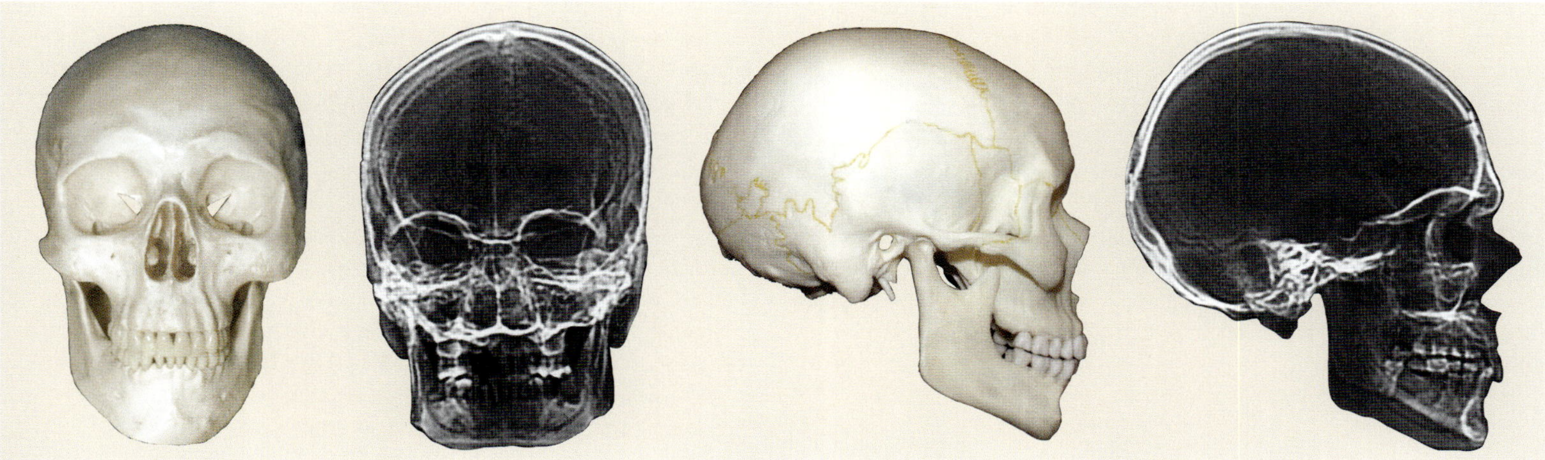

Fig 3-1-1 Frontal and sagittal views of the skull.

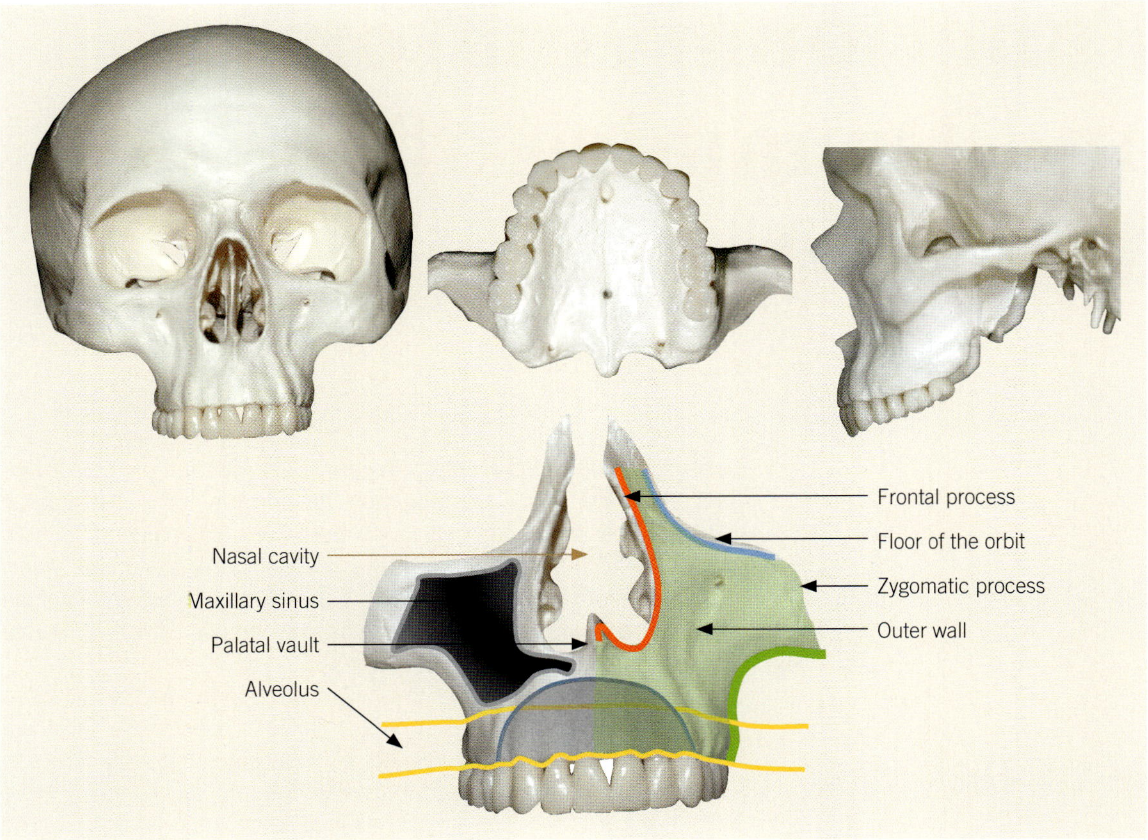

Fig 3-1-2 Frontal, occlusal, and lateral views of the maxilla.

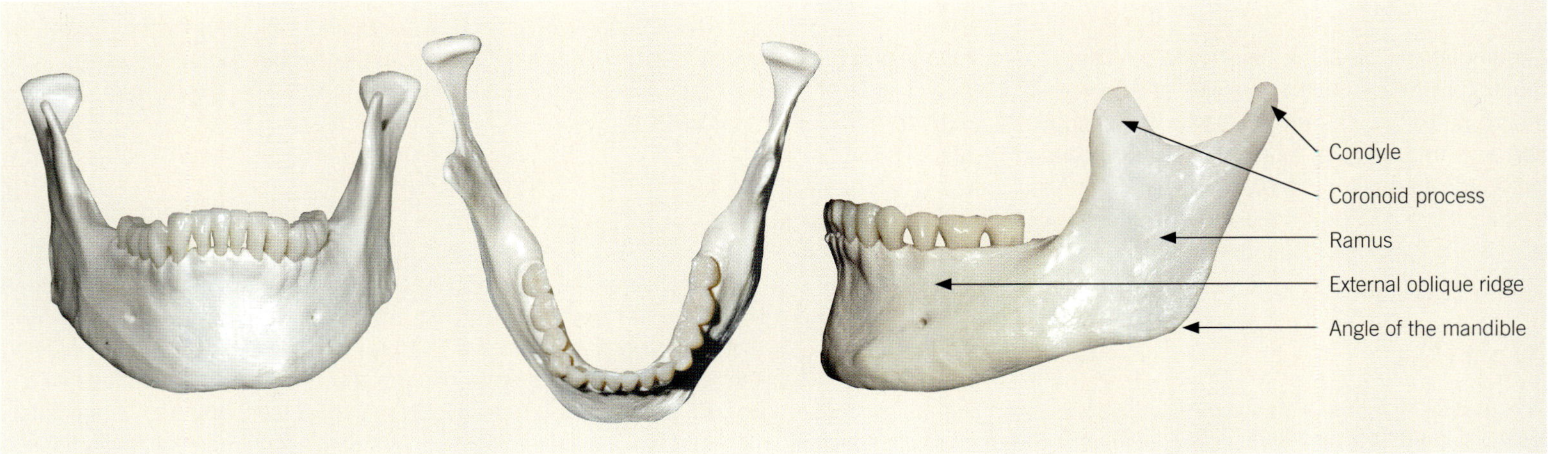

Fig 3-1-3 Frontal, occlusal, and sagittal views of the mandible.

Muscle attachments

Two main muscle groups that are attached to the mandible are the muscles of mastication and the suprahyoid muscles. The masticatory muscles act by connection to the cranium and the suprahyoids by connection to the hyoid bone. The mandible contains the attachments of the elevator masseter and medial pterygoid sling at the angle, the medial pterygoid at the coronoid process, and the protruding lateral pterygoid at the condylar neck. Depressor muscles are attached by the anterior belly of the anterior digastric at the genial tubercles. Other depressor muscle attachment is to the genial tubercles, and glossal tongue muscles attach to the genial tubercles and mylohyoid ridges. Suprahyoid muscles include the digastrics, mylohyoid, geniohyoid, and stylohyoid. Infrahyoid muscles that counter-stabilize the hyoid bone constitute the sternohyoid, omohyoid, sternothyroid, and thyrohyoid muscles.

Occlusion of the maxillary and mandibular teeth

The elevator muscles close the mandible into a maximal intercuspal occlusal relation with the maxilla (Fig 3-1-4). This is a stable relation that allows significant generation of occlusal forces necessary for mastication and deglutition. The posterior teeth support most of the occlusal load with the principal line of action passing through the first molar region near the root of the zygoma. The anterior teeth bear less of the occlusal load in maximum intercuspation (MI). The temporomandibular joint (TMJ) allows a full range of closing and opening movement and is not a classical load-bearing joint. Functionally, the occlusion may be considered to consist essentially of the support of the posterior segment of molars and premolars, an anterior segment comprising the incisors and canines, and the distally related TMJs (Figs 3-1-5 and 3-1-6).

The teeth intercuspate in a maximal intercuspal relation that ensures the stability of the intra-arch and interarch relations maintaining the complex of teeth periodontium, alveolus, basal bony housing, tongue, cheeks, and lips in a state of dynamic equilibrium.

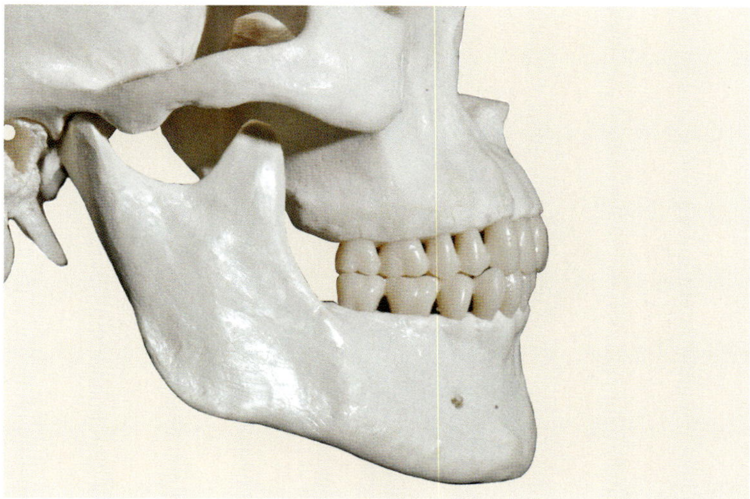

Fig 3-1-4 Sagittal view of the teeth in occlusion.

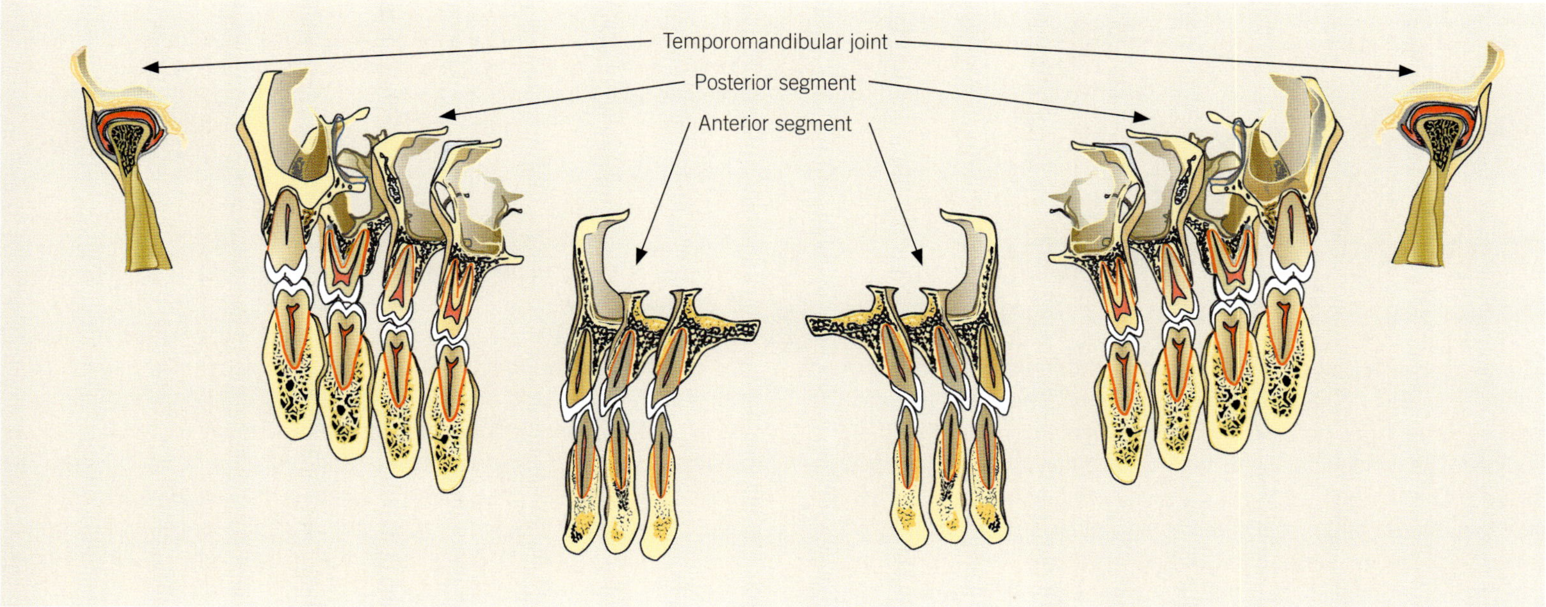

Fig 3-1-5 The load-bearing components of the occlusion. The posterior segment, the anterior segment, and the temporomandibular joints.

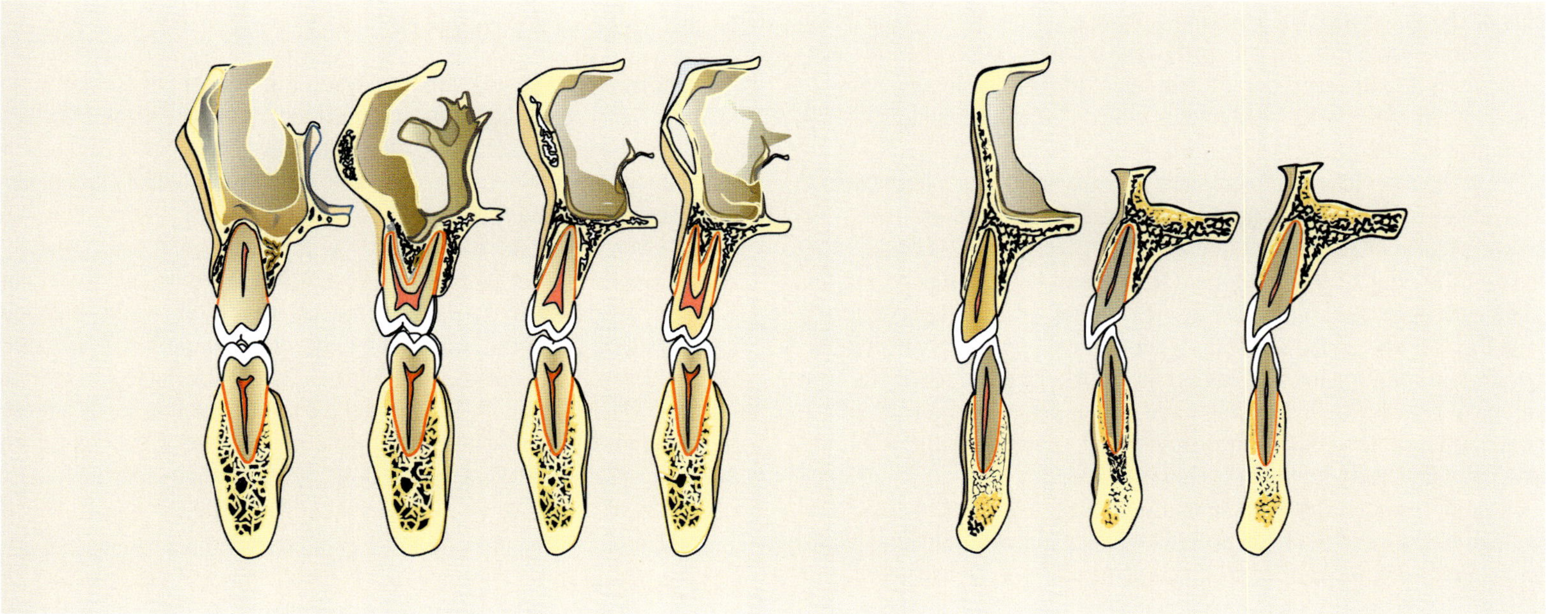

Fig 3-1-6 The supporting anatomy of the teeth in maximum intercuspal relation.

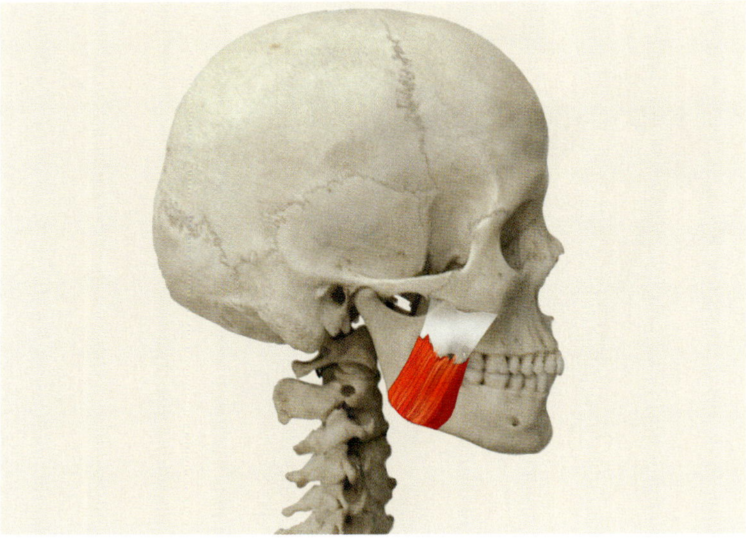

Fig 3-1-7 Masseter. The strongest closing muscle has its origin at the zygomatic arch and insertion at the angle of the lower border of the mandible.

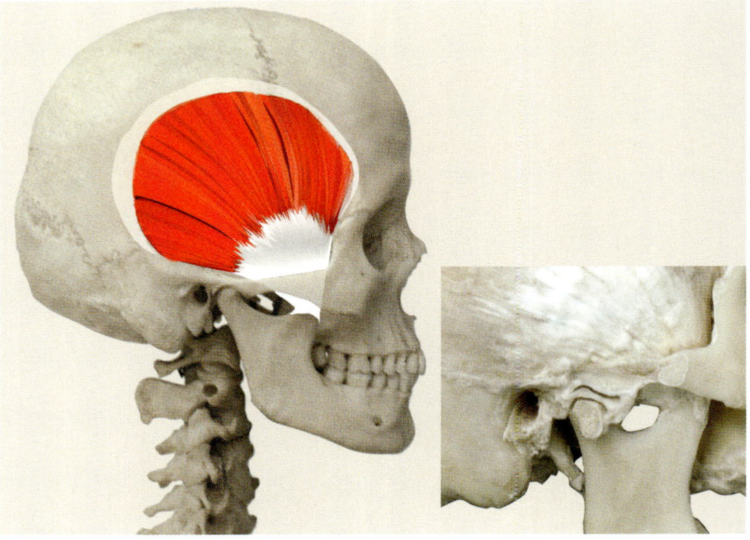

Fig 3-1-8 Temporalis. Closing and positioning muscle. Origin is at the infratemporal line of the cranium. Attachment is at the coronoid process and anterior ramus. Contains anterior, middle, and posterior functional sections. The anterior vertical section elevates. The middle oblique section elevates backwards. The posterior horizontal section retrudes the mandible.

Muscles of mastication

Attachments and insertion

Muscles move bodies to which they are attached by voluntary or reflex contraction. Muscles are generally connected at one end to a solid non-moving part in their "origin" and to the part that is moved by their "insertion." The connection to the origin or insertion is usually by tendinous tissue or fascia. The muscles of mastication work in complex synchrony to effect the full range of potential mandibular movement. While illustrated in the following sections as single muscles, they work in unison for specific voluntary, subconscious, or reflex activities involved in function and parafunctional mandibular movements.

Masseter

The masseter muscle is one of the principal elevator and closing muscles of the mandible. The rectangular-shaped muscle has its origin at the inferior aspect of the temporal and anterior portion of the zygomatic arch and its insertion at the angle of the mandible, extending to the ascending posterior border of the ramus and the posterior lower border of the mandible.[3]

It has a superficial intermediate and deep arrangement of fibers.[3,9] This is a very strong muscle and acts as the principal elevating and power closure muscle of the mandible and can generate considerable forces. The orientation of the main fiber mass is in a superior and anterior oblique direction (Fig 3-1-7). The line of action passes obliquely past the first and second molars. Fiber orientation can vary with different muscle components. The fibers of the posterior deep part run almost vertically downward, in contrast to the remainder of the muscle, whose fibers are directed roughly downward and posterior. Superficial and intermediate fiber orientation is also varied.[9-12]

A study using surface electrodes demonstrated that the superficial masseter was more active in an incisal bite position.[12] For varying bite force direction, the system chooses a single pattern of muscle activation.[9]

Temporalis

The temporalis muscle acts as a mandibular elevator and positioner. This is a fan shaped muscle with its origin connecting to a semi-lunar infratemporal line covering parietal, temporal, frontal, and sphenoid surfaces of the cranium. Many fibers also originate in an aponeuorsis of the temporal fascia. The muscle converges through the space between the zygomatic arch and the lateral skull wall where it attaches to the coronoid process and down the anterior border of the mandibular ramus. The muscle is usually described as consisting of three functional units: anterior, middle, and posterior. The anterior fibers are oriented vertically, the middle oblique and the posterior horizontal. The main fiber body is vertically orientated in the anterior aspect. The temporalis is structured more for positioning than for generating power. The anterior aspect elevates, while the middle and posterior bodies retrude (Figs 3-1-8 and 3-1-13).

The temporalis is covered anteromedially with a fibrous fascia connecting the zygoma to the anterior temporal line. This is a strong tendinous connection and acts as a counter to the downward pull of the mandible on the zygomatic arch.[12-14]

Medial pterygoid

The medial pterygoid is a strong elevator muscle slightly weaker than the masseter. The medial pterygoid muscle originates from the pterygoid fovea, the medial aspect of the lateral pterygoid plate, and has a tendinous attachment to the pyramidal palatine and the maxillary tuberosity. The insertion is at the medial surface of the angle of the mandible. The line of action is superior and oblique, similar to that of the masseter.

The medial or internal pterygoid is a square-shaped bulky elevator muscle synergistic with the adjacent masseter with some of the insertion fibers merging under the body of the angle of the mandible. Their combined elevator action has been described as the masseter and medial pterygoid elevator sling.[14-16] In spite of the medial relation of the attachment and insertion the medial pterygoid had no lateral synergistic interaction with the lateral pterygoid (Figs 3-1-9 and 3-1-10).

Digastric

The digastric muscles are the main depresser or opening muscles of the mandible. The digastric consists of two bellies joined in the middle by a tendon that is related to the hyoid bone by a fibrous sling. The posterior attachment of the posterior belly connects to the mastoid notch at the mastoid process. The anterior aspect of the anterior belly connects

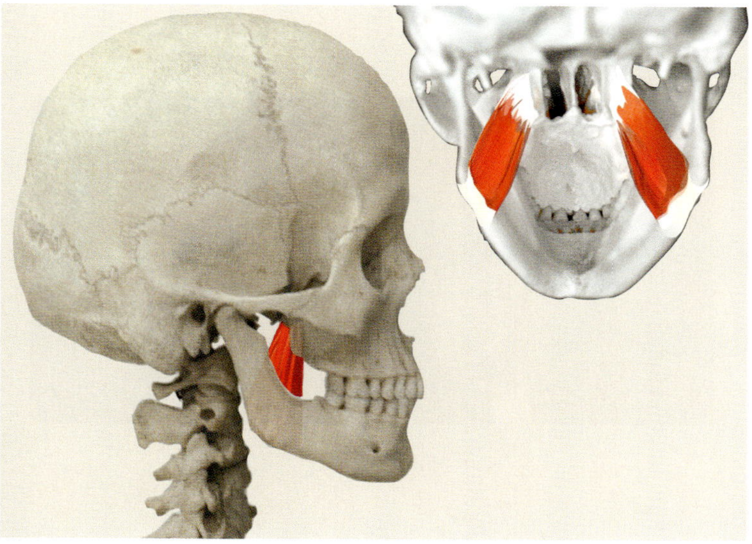

Fig 3-1-9 Medial pterygoid. Closing muscle. Origin is at the medial aspect of the lateral pterygoid plate. Insertion is at the lower medial border of the angle of the mandible.

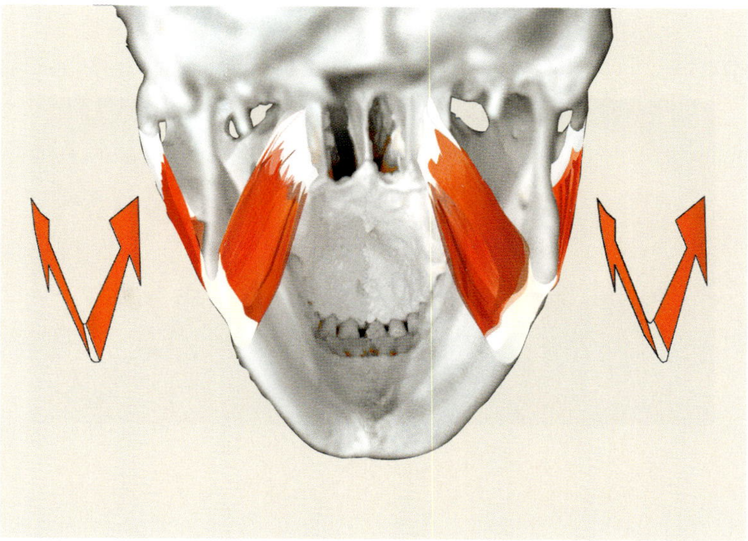

Fig 3-1-10 Masseter/medial pterygoid sling. Muscles act unilaterally or bilaterally as a sling closing the mandible from the lower posterior border towards the maxilla and cranium.

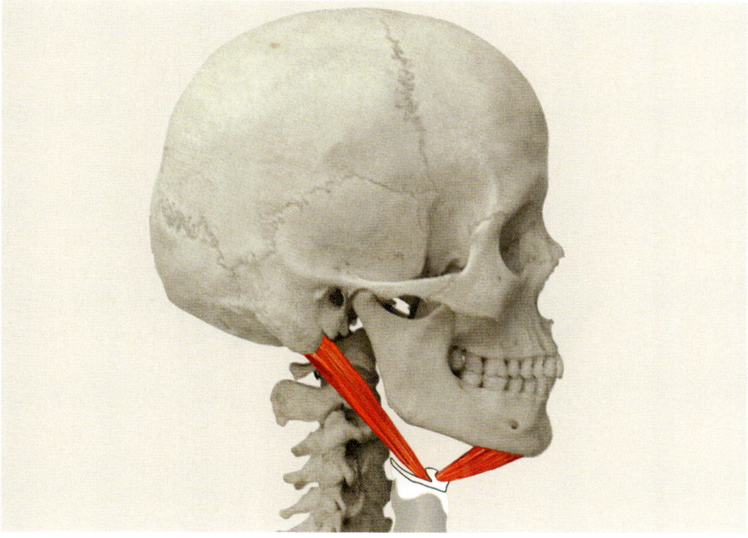

Fig 3-1-11 Digastric. Origin of the posterior belly is at the mastoid notch. Insertion of the anterior belly is at the lower anterior border of the mandible. Inferior sling from the hyoid bone acts as a pulley.

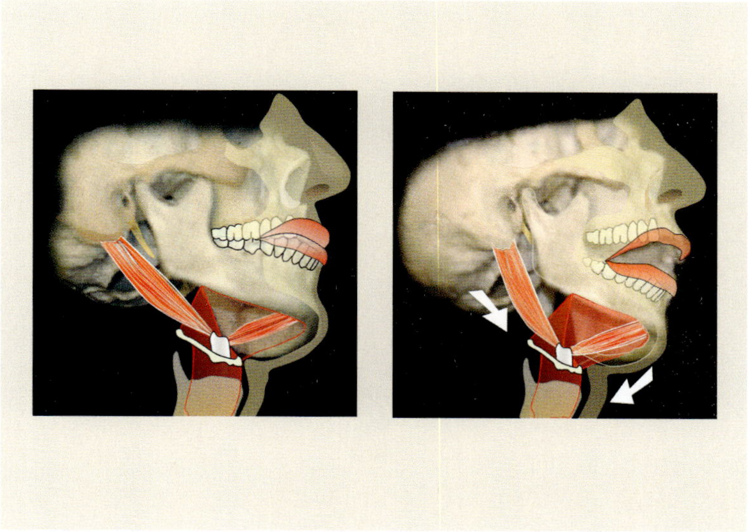

Fig 3-1-12 Opening contraction of anterior and posterior digastric against the hyoid sling and contraction of the infrahyoids opens the mandible.

to the digastric notch at the anterior inferior border of the mandible close to the midline (Figs 3-1-11 and 3-1-12). Contraction of the two digastric bodies against the hyoid pulley sling is countered by the synergistic contraction of the infrahyoid muscles. The posterior body is innervated by the facial nerve and the anterior is innervated by the mandibular nerve.

Mandibular closure and opening

Mandibular closure is carried out by the masseter, medial pterygoid, and temporalis muscles in synchrony. Voluntary closure elevates the mandible directly into its stable intercuspal relation of MI. The anterior temporal acts as a positioner directing final closure into intercuspation. The masseter is the most powerful of the closing muscles. Forceful closure occurs with varying degrees of force synchrony between all the elevator muscles (Figs 3-1-13 and 3-1-14).[15-18]

Lateral pterygoid

The lateral pterygoid consists of two heads: a larger inferior head and a smaller superior head.[19] The larger inferior head originates from the lateral aspect of the lateral pterygoid plate. Fibers pass horizontally backwards and laterally to insert into the anterior aspect of the condylar neck and capsule (Figs 3-1-15 to 3-1-18).[3,19-22]

The smaller superior head originates from the roof of the infra temporal fossa of the greater wing of the sphenoid and inserts into the anterior aspect of the condylar neck and with some fibers to the anterior aspects of the articular disc and joint capsule.[3,19-22]

The superior and inferior heads have been ascribed differing functions but can act together. Their relative functions are still contentious and studies on their roles are dependent on experimental variables in needle electrode studies.[19]

Fibers of the superior and lateral heads converge onto a small insertion site on the condylar fovea, capsule, and disc from the broad origin at the roof of the infratemporal fossa and lateral pterygoid plate. Fiber orientation varies from both upper to lower and medial to lateral. This

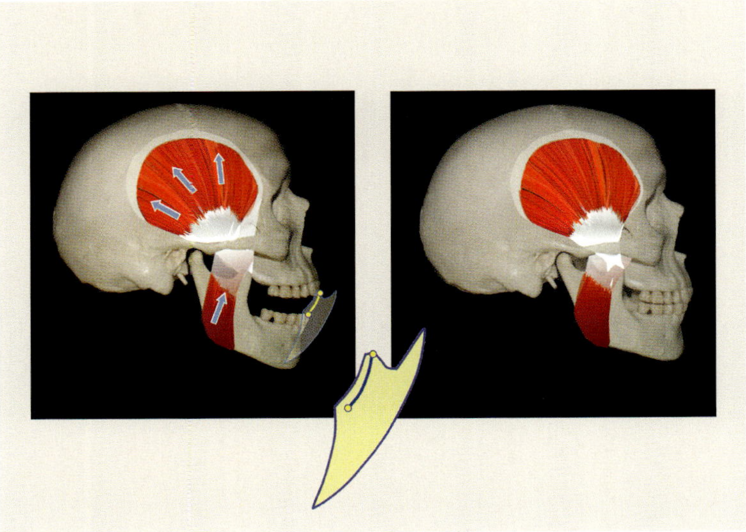

Fig 3-1-13 Mandibular closure is carried out by contraction of elevator muscles. The lines of action of masseter and anterior, middle, and posterior temporal are shown by the arrows.

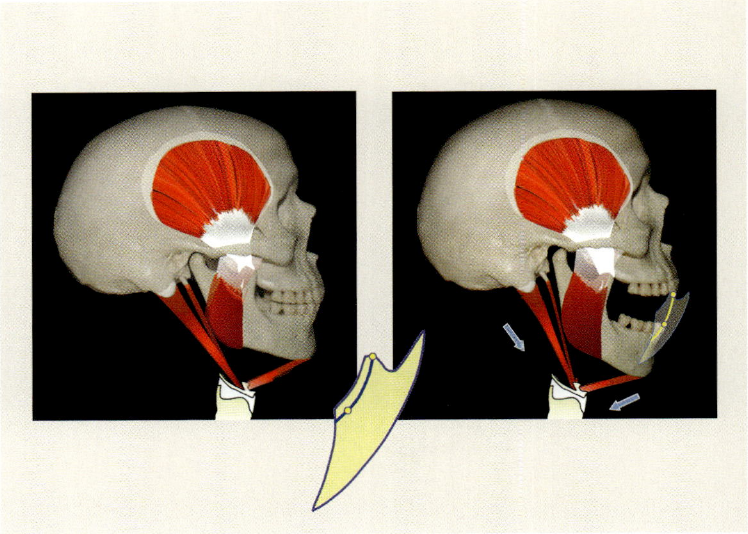

Fig 3-1-14 Mandibular opening or depression is carried out by the anterior and posterior bellies of the digastric in harmony with the infrahyoid cervical muscles stabilizing the hyoid bone and the digastric connection in the hyoid sling.

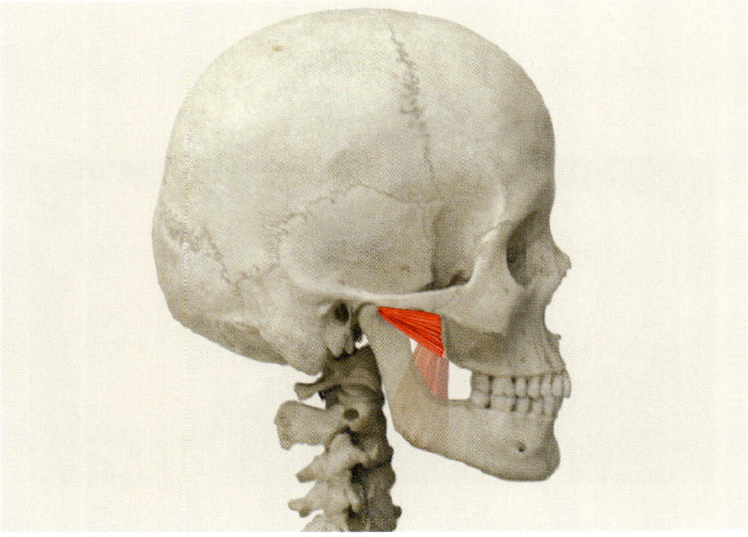

Fig 3-1-15 The lateral pterygoid muscle is located superior to the medial pterygoid.

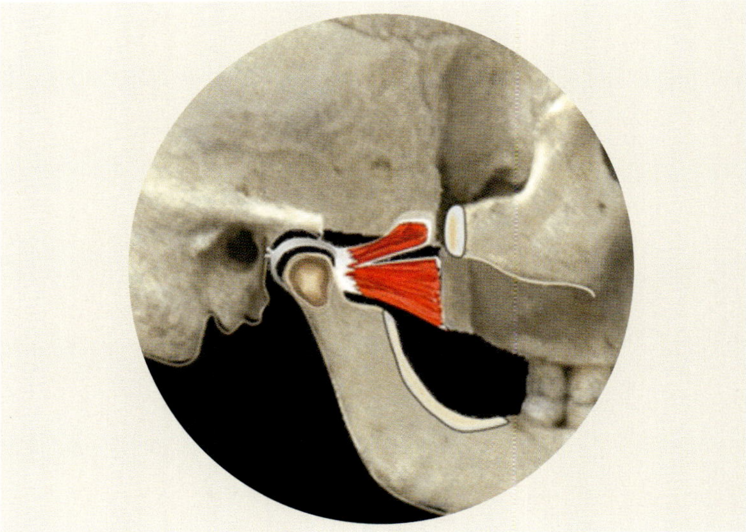

Fig 3-1-16 The lateral pterygoid has a superior and an inferior head. The larger inferior head has its origin at the lateral aspect of the lateral pterygoid plate and its insertion at neck of the condyle. The origin of the superior head is at the infratemporal surface of the greater wing of the sphenoid and the insertion at the anterior aspect of the temporomandibular disc, the capsule, and the condylar neck.

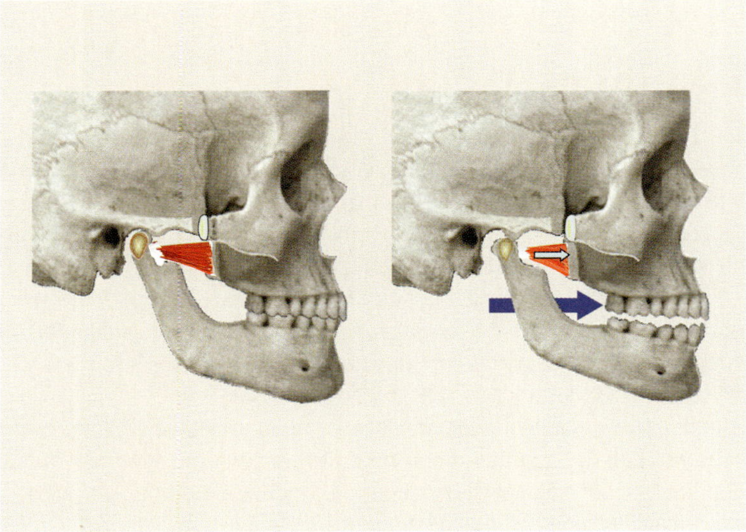

Fig 3-1-17 Lateral view. Simultaneous contraction of inferior heads of the left and right lateral pterygoids pulls the condyles forward in a protrusive movement.

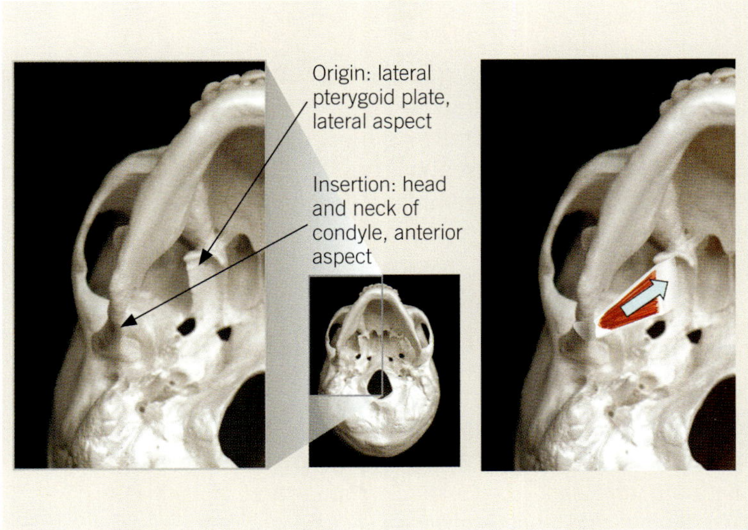

Fig 3-1-18 Inferior view of skull showing the relation between the condyle neck and the lateral pterygoid plate and origins and insertions of the inferior head of the lateral pterygoid.

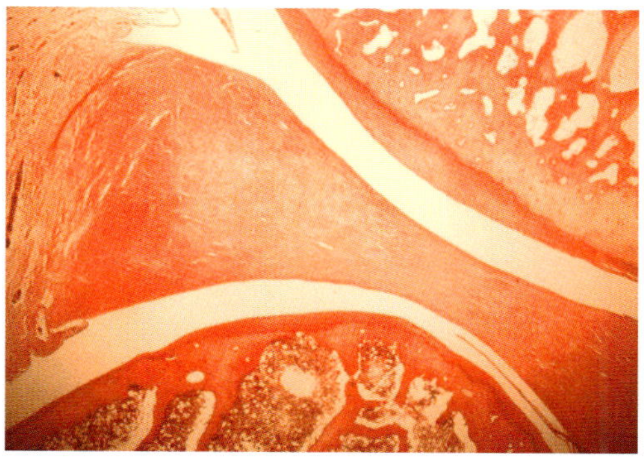

Fig 3-1-29 Histological section of disc and opposing functional surfaces of the condyle and eminence. Thin intermediate zone of disc. Thick posterior band of disc posteriorly with attachment to the retrodiscal tissues. Disc widens anteriorly to the thicker anterior band. (Image courtesy of Professor N Mohl.)

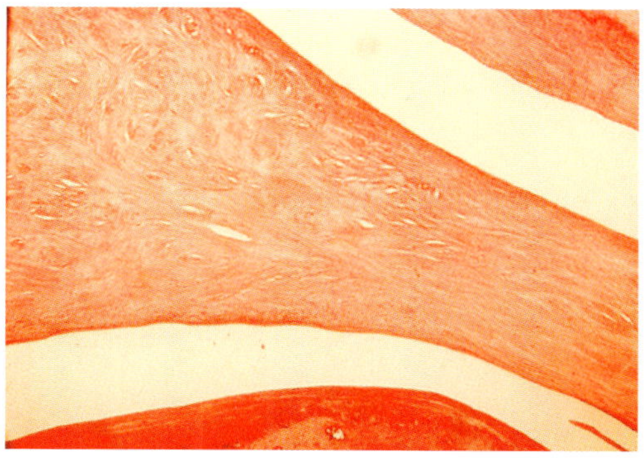

Fig 3-1-30 Close-up of the avascular fibrous intermediate zone of the disc. (Image courtesy of Professor N Mohl.)

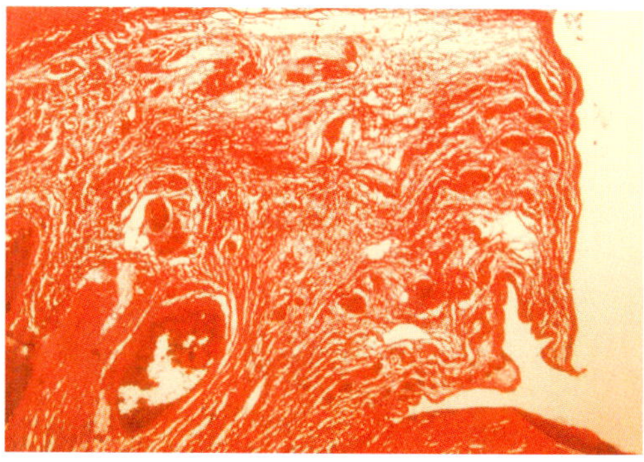

Fig 3-1-31 Retrodiscal tissue of the bilaminar zone. (Image courtesy of Professor N Mohl.)

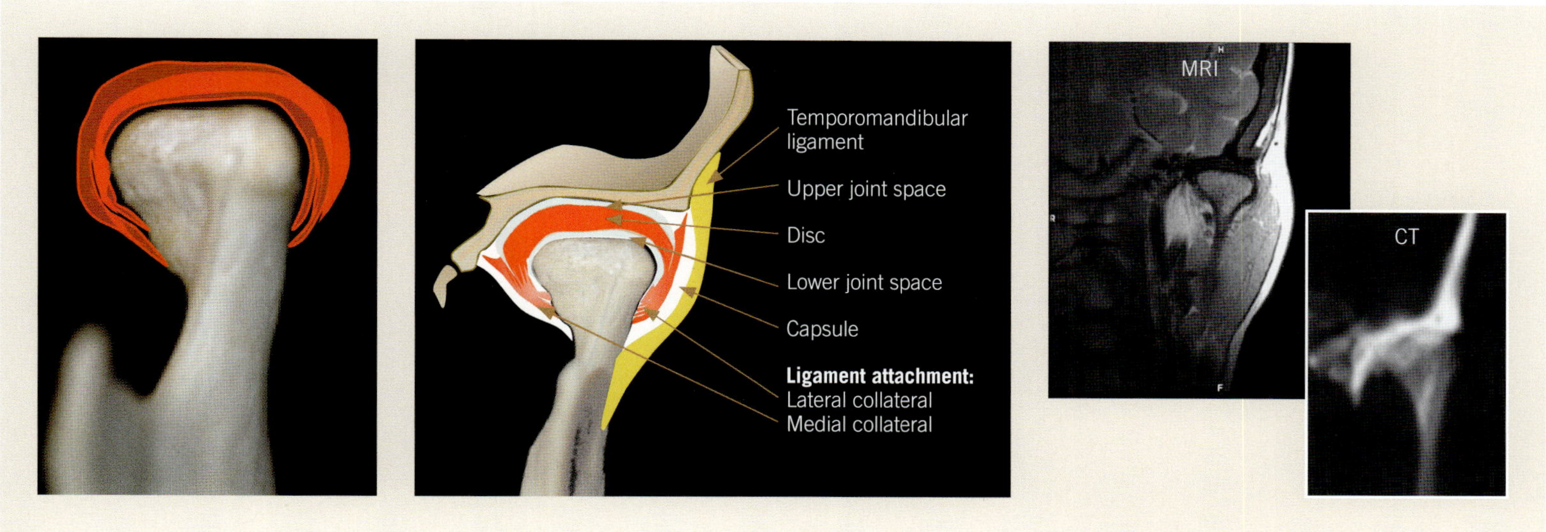

Fig 3-1-32 Condyle relation in frontal section. The disc is attached with collateral ligaments to medial and lateral aspects of the condyle neck. The disc can slide forwards and backwards over the head of the condyle.

Fig 3-1-33 Condyle relation in maximum intercuspation. The upper head of the lateral pterygoid contracts (black arrow) together with the other elevator muscles and pulls the condyle and disc in their functional relation against the eminence. Blue arrow: temporalis contraction.

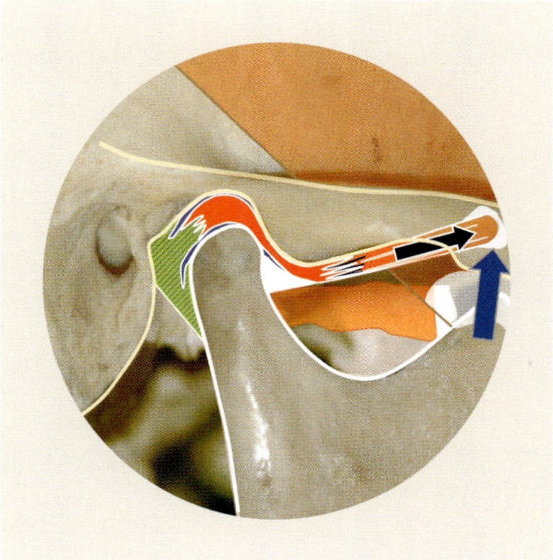

Fig 3-1-34 Condyle relation in maximum intercuspation. Functional anterior superior aspect of the condyle contacts the distal incline of the eminence with the thin intermediate section of the disc interposed (arrows).

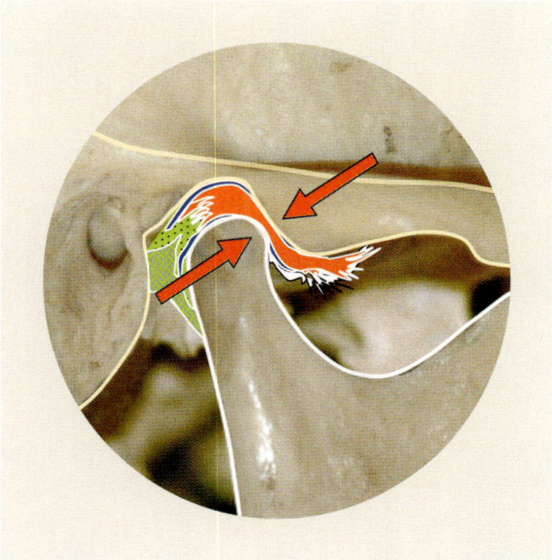

tact around which the condyles can rotate. The condyles are connected to the temporal by the capsular attachment and restrained at the lateral aspect by the temporomandibular ligaments as they rotate against the opposing inclines of the eminences (Fig 3-1-35).

Condylar relation in protrusion, condylar guidance

The mandible is protruded by simultaneous contraction of the lower bodies of the right and left lateral pterygoids pulling the condyles downwards and forwards against the inclines of the articular eminences (Fig

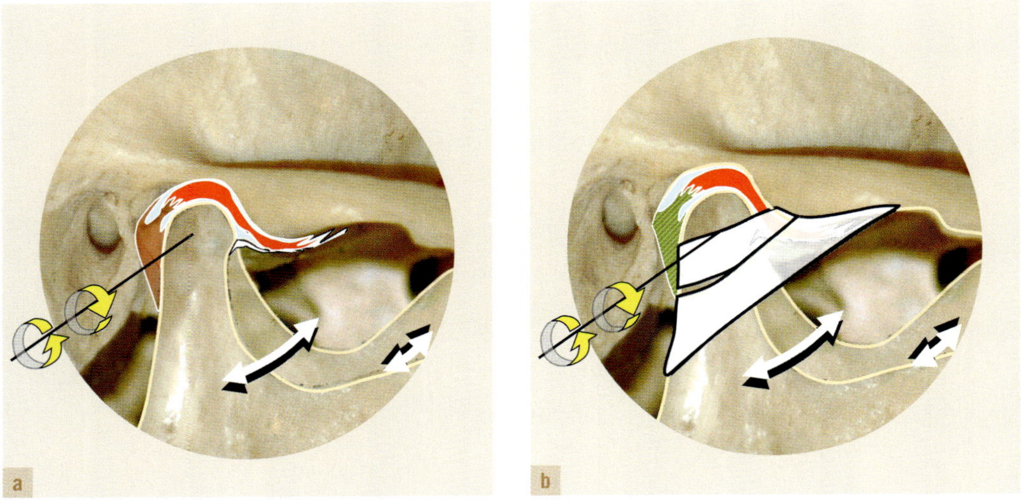

Fig 3-1-35a Condyle relation in centric relation. Condyle rotates open and closed around its terminal transverse horizontal axis of rotation. b The stretched temporomandibular ligament on the lateral aspect restrains the condyle preventing distal movement.

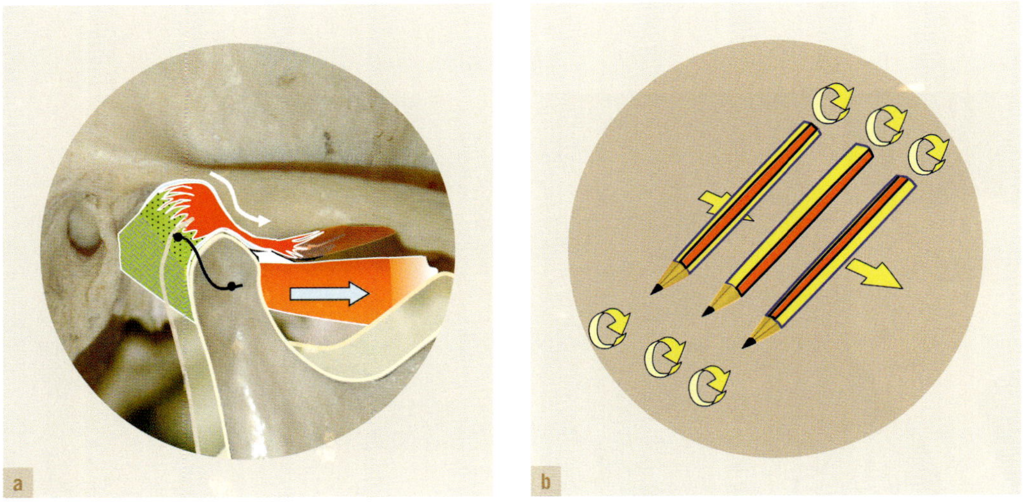

Fig 3-1-36a On protrusion the lower body of the lateral pterygoid pulls the condyle and disc forwards, down the guiding incline of the articular eminence. Condylar guidance: The mandible moves by translation. b Translation: A pencil rolling on a flat surface moves bodily by translation and simultaneously rotates round its long axis.

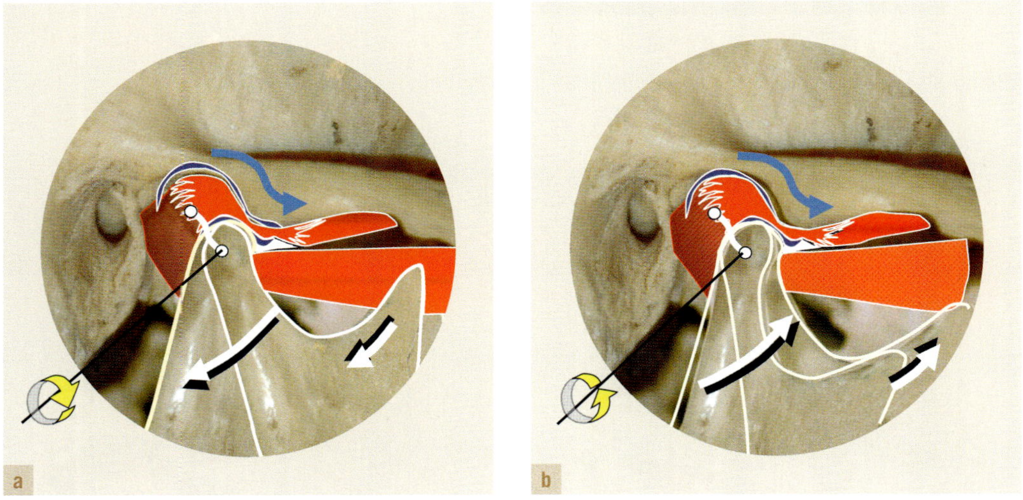

Fig 3-1-37 The condyle moves bodily down the eminence by translation. It can simultaneously open and close around its transverse horizontal hinge axis during the translatory movement. a Protrusion and simultaneous opening. b Protrusion and simultaneous closure.

3-1-19). The condyles and discs move bodily down the guiding inclines of the eminences facilitated by the upper synovial joints spaces. This is termed the "condylar guidance" (Fig 3-1-36a).

In the class I occlusion, the anterior teeth guide the mandible anteriorly, with the lower incisors pulled forward and down the guiding palatal inclines of the maxillary incisors. This protrusive incisal guidance requires the condyles to rotate open slightly around their horizontal axis of rotation facilitated by the lower joint spaces (Fig 3-1-37).

The disc moves passively with the condyle. On protrusion, the elastic superior fibers of the superior lamina of the posterior laminar zone become stretched. During closure, the more ligamentous inferior lamina passively limits forward rotation of the disc on the condyle serving as a restraining ligament.[36-38]

Translation and rotation

The upper and lower synovial joint spaces above and below the disc allow independent bodily movement or "translation" of the condyle down the eminence and simultaneous rotation around the transverse horizontal axis in the lower compartment (Fig 3-1-37). The condyle and disc move down the eminence facilitated by the superior joint space.[37,38] Translation is the bodily movement of an object. Simultaneous translation and rotation is seen as a pencil rolls along a flat surface (Fig 3-1-36b).

In this way, the mandible can be protruded while simultaneously opening and closing around its moving horizontal axis. The mandible can in this way follow a varying protrusive incisal guidance that may be either steep or flat, or the mandible may be opened and protruded

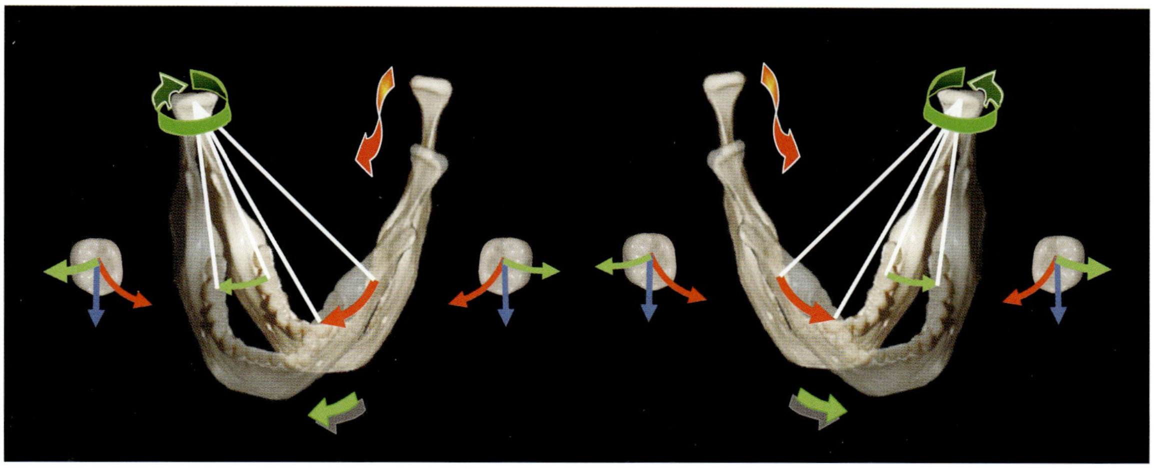

Fig 3-2-27 Right and left lateral border movements. The mandible rotates around the vertical axis of the working side condyle. The green line indicates the path of movement of the working side mandibular first molar. The red line indicates the path of movement of the non-working side first molar. The blue line shows the protrusive path of movement.

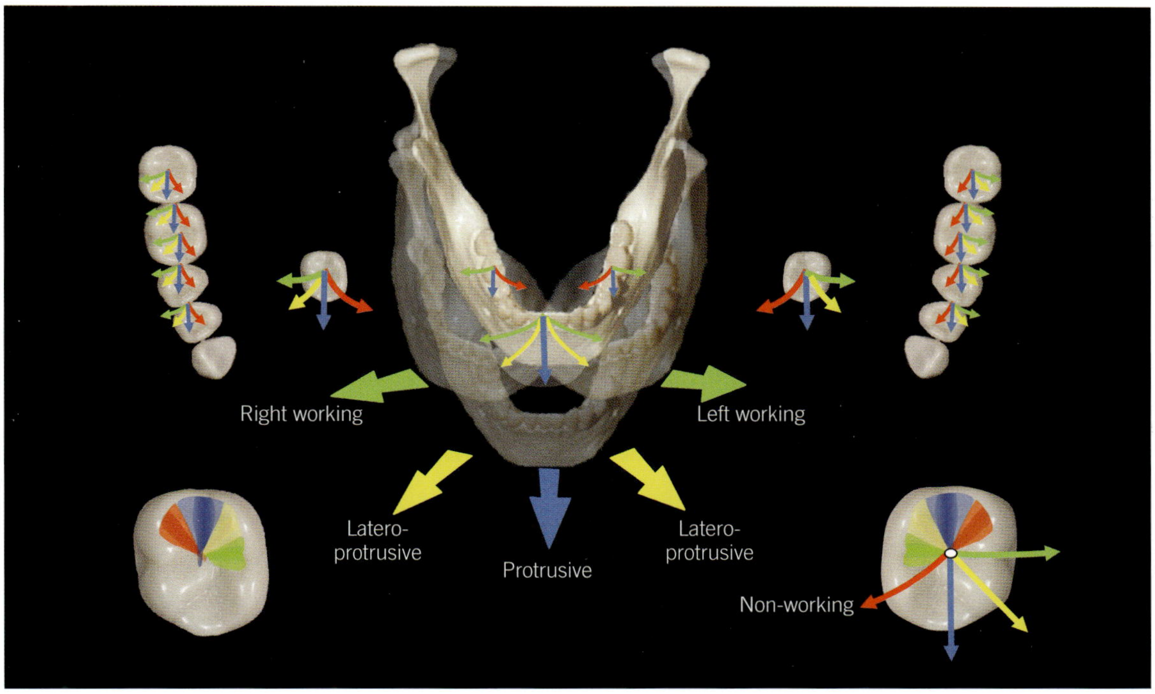

Fig 3-2-28 Paths of movement of mandibular fossae (marginal ridges and incisor midpoint): working, green; non-working, red; protrusive, blue; and lateroprotrusive, yellow. Shaded areas in mandibular first molars show potential contact areas of opposing maxillary mesiopalatal supporting cusps.

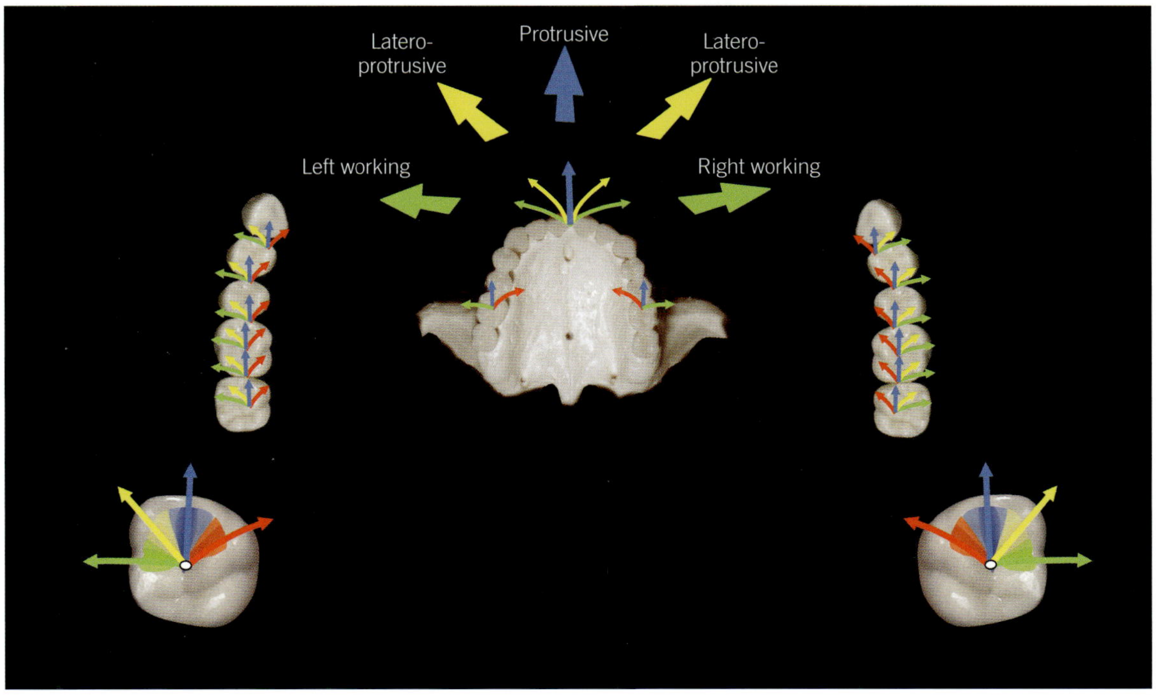

Fig 3-2-29 Paths of movement of mandibular buccal supporting cusps and incisor midpoint relative to the maxilla: working, green; non-working, red; protrusive, blue; and lateroprotrusive, yellow. Shaded areas of maxillary first molars show potential contact areas of opposing mandibular mesiobuccal supporting cusps.

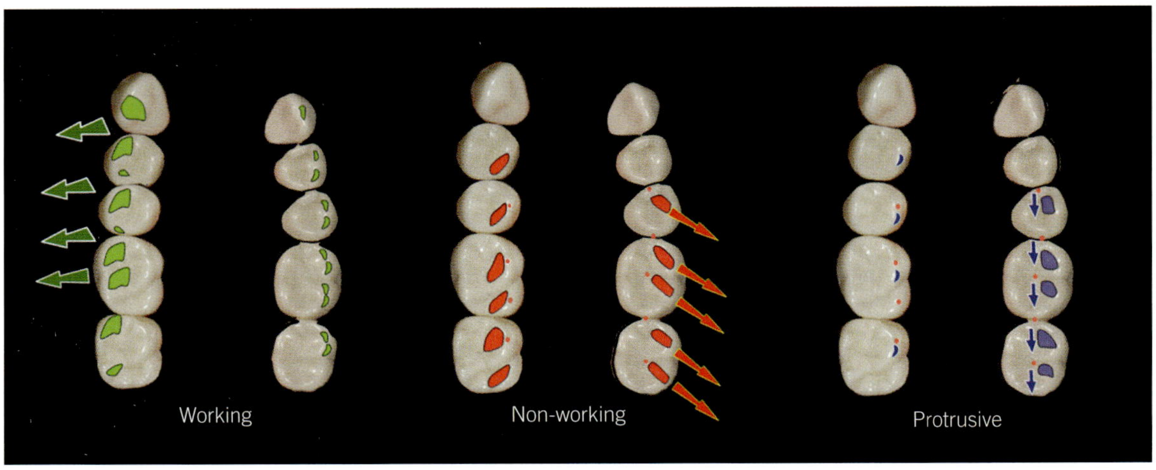

Fig 3-2-30 Potential working, non-working, and protrusive contacts. Arrows indicate movement of mandibular cusps relative to the opposing maxillary teeth.

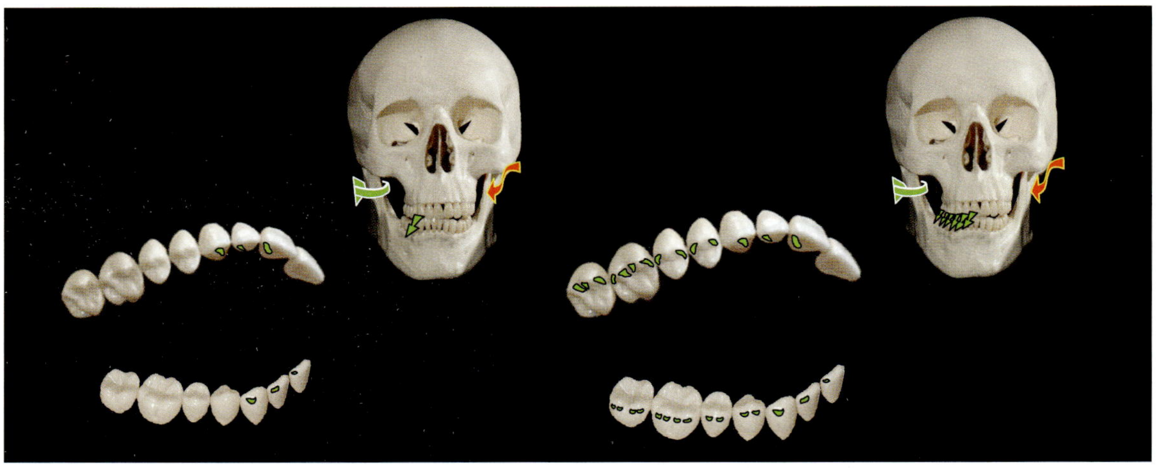

Fig 3-2-31 Left: canine guidance contacts, which may or may not include centrals and laterals. Right: group function FOA against inner guiding inclines.

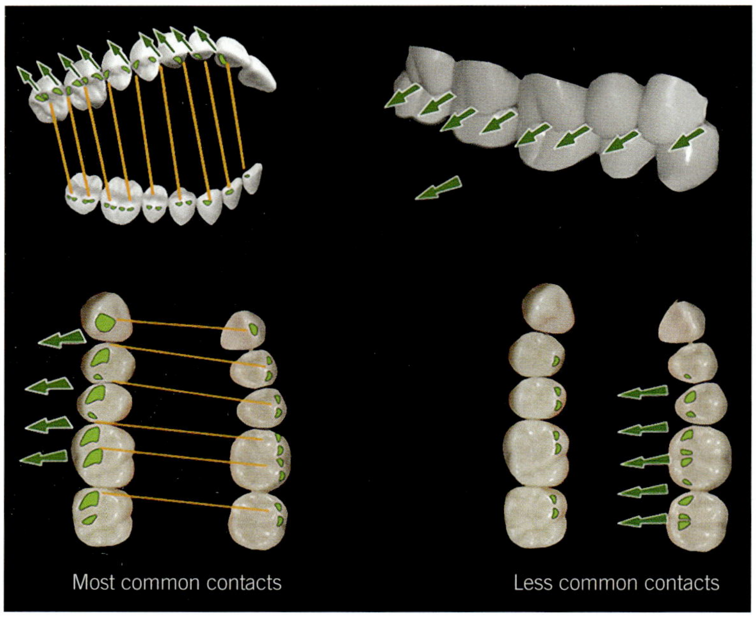

Fig 3-2-32 Potential working-side contacts. FOA of supporting cusps against inner guiding inclines of guiding cusps. Most common working-side contacts: FOA of lower buccal cusps against inner inclines of upper buccal cusps. Less common "cross-tooth contacts": FOA of upper palatal cusps against inner inclines of lower lingual cusps. Arrows indicate direction of movement of mandibular cusps relative to the maxillary teeth.

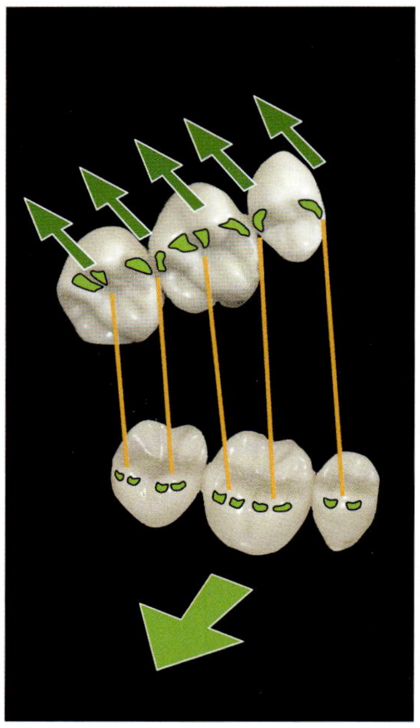

Fig 3-2-33 Potential working-side contacts: FOA of supporting cusps against the inner inclines of the guiding cusps.

Slide in centric

When the mandible is retruded to the point of initial contact in centric relation and then squeezed closed, the resulting "slide in centric," occurs between the mesial inclines of the maxillary tooth or teeth in contact against the distal inclines of the opposing mandibular tooth or teeth (Figs 3-2-17, 3-2-18, and 3-2-36). When the maximal intercuspal position coincides with centric relation, there is no slide in centric.

Factors of occlusion

Occlusal scheme

When restoring the dentition, a suitable occlusal scheme has to be established. The "occlusal scheme" consists of the intercuspal relation and the protrusive, lateral, and laterotrusive range of contacts from MI to edge-to-edge relations. The dynamic contacts are also called the "occlusal pattern" or "occlusal scheme." In restoring the occlusion, many case-specific factors that interrelate must be diagnosed, analyzed, and taken into consideration for each individual case. These include the occlusal determinants and additional esthetic, phonetic, biome-

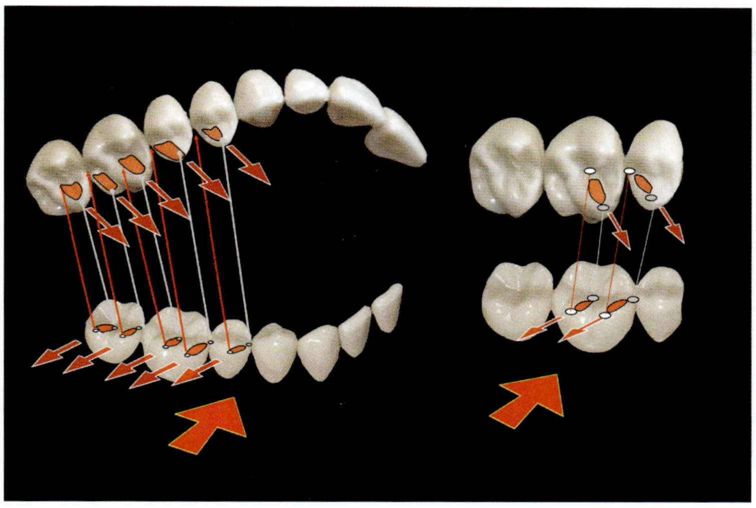

Fig 3-2-34 Potential non-working side contacts. Inner inclines of opposing supporting cusps. Small arrows indicate direction of movement of the opposing supporting cusp inner inclines as they pass one another. Non-working potential contacts are maxillary inner supporting inclines against opposing mandibular inner supporting inclines.

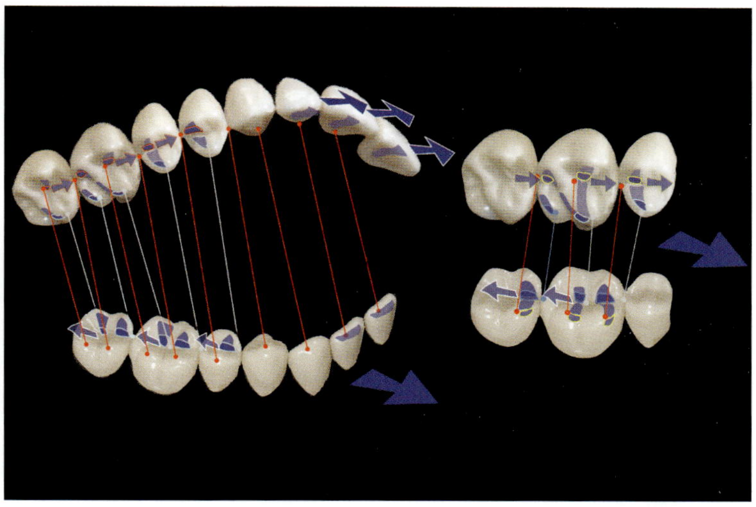

Fig 3-2-35 Potential protrusive contacts. Palatal inclines of maxillary incisors against mandibular incisal ridges. Posterior potential contacts of distal maxillary inclines against mesial mandibular inclines. Distal upper against mesial lower inclines.

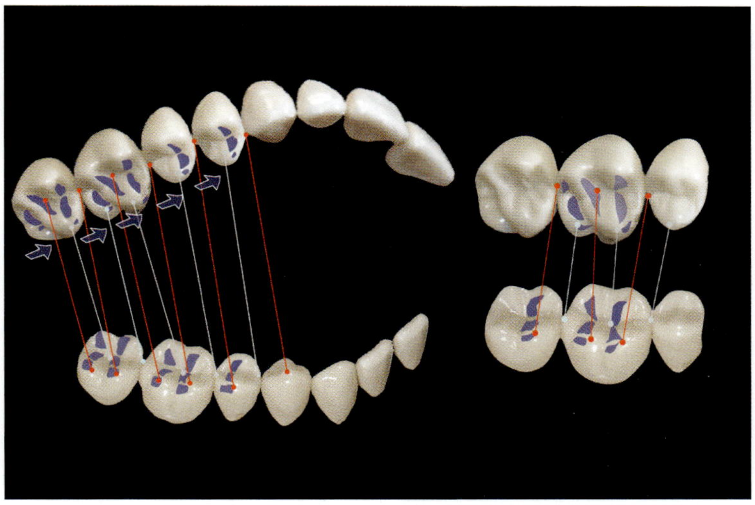

Fig 3-2-36 Potential contacts in slide between centric relation and MI. Mesial maxillary inclines contact opposing distal mandibular inclines.

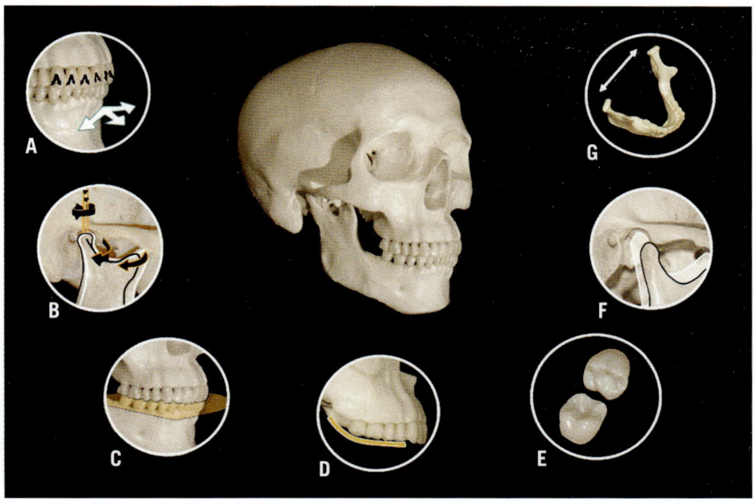

Fig 3-2-37 Factors of occlusion (from top left anti-clockwise): **A** anterior guidance, **B** side shift, **C** occlusal plane, **D** anteroposterior curvature (compensating curve), **E** cusp height and angulation, **F** condylar guidance, **G** intercondylar distance.

chanical, prosthetic, and individual case-specific determinants. Occlusal factors that influence the dynamic tooth contact pattern are called the "factors of occlusion" or "occlusal determinants" (Fig 3-2-37). There are also vertical and horizontal determinants.

Vertical determinants

The vertical determinants were historically first described as the "Hanau's Quint"[2,4] and included the protrusive condylar guidance, the protrusive incisal guidance, the occlusal plane, the anteroposterior occlusal curvature, and the posterior cusp height and angulation (Fig 3-2-38). These were first described in relation to planning balanced occlusions in full dentures. The fixed or unalterable factors that cannot be changed are the condylar determinants. In tooth- or implant-borne restorations, the other factors may or may not be alterable depending on whether the prosthetic restorations are to be tooth borne, implant borne, fixed, or removable. The vertical factors in the sagittal plane determine if there is contact on the incisal guidance alone with posterior disocclusion or simultaneous anterior and posterior contact, known as balanced occlusion (Figs 3-2-39 and 3-2-40). The steepness or flatness of the protrusive guidance and the timing of the disocclusion as immediate or delayed have clinical implications and are determined by these factors. During lateral excursions, vertical and horizontal factors interrelate to determine whether there will be anterior canine guidance or group function with non-working disocclusion. The steepness or flatness of the working side tooth cuspal guidance is significant. The unalterable factors here are the non-working condylar guidance inclination or pathway and the nature of the lateral side shift.

Disocclusion by working canine guidance and non-working condylar guidance

In a class I occlusion with canine guidance, the lateral tooth-guided movement from MIP to the lateral edge-to-edge position is guided by the inclines of the maxillary canine teeth. The non-working condyle is guided by the inclination of the non-working eminence. Tooth contact on the non-working side is separated by the combined guidance of the canine and non-working guidance. The disoccluding effect nearer the guiding element is more pronounced. Thus, the effect of separating the non-working side teeth is greater closer to the non-working condylar guidance. Similarly the separation of the posterior working side teeth is

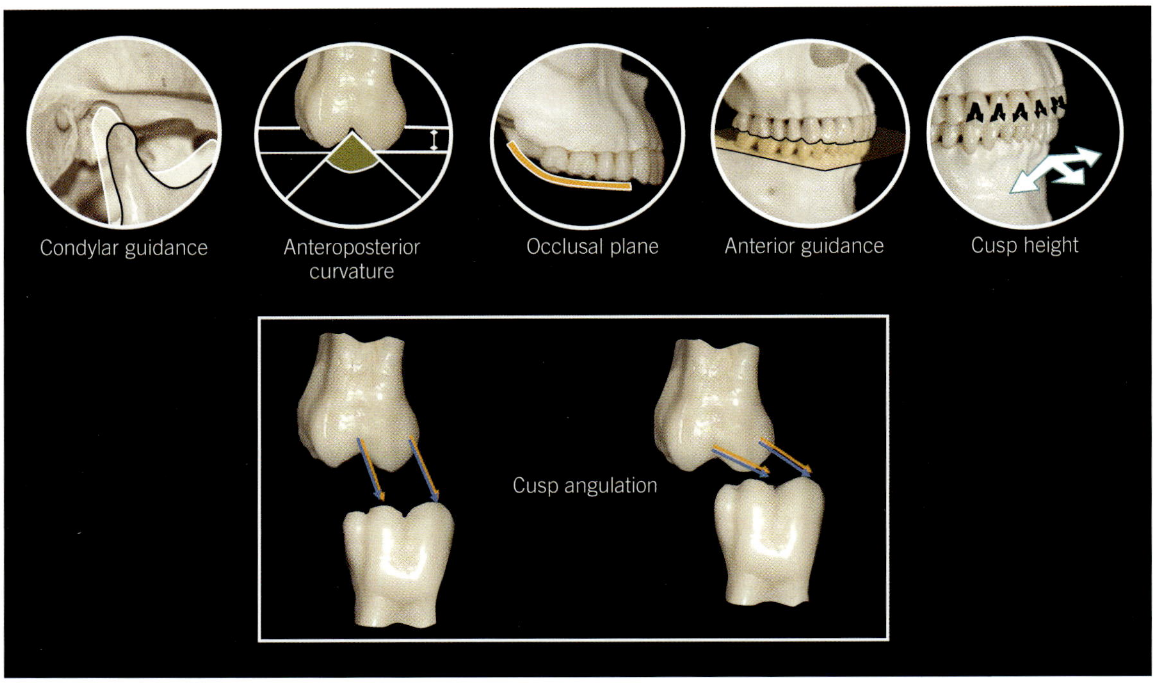

Fig 3-2-38 Vertical protrusive factors of occlusion (top left to right): condylar guidance, anteroposterior curvature, occlusal plane, anterior guidance cusp height, and cusp angulation. The interrelation of all factors determines the degree of vertical or horizontal posterior tooth separation or disclusion.

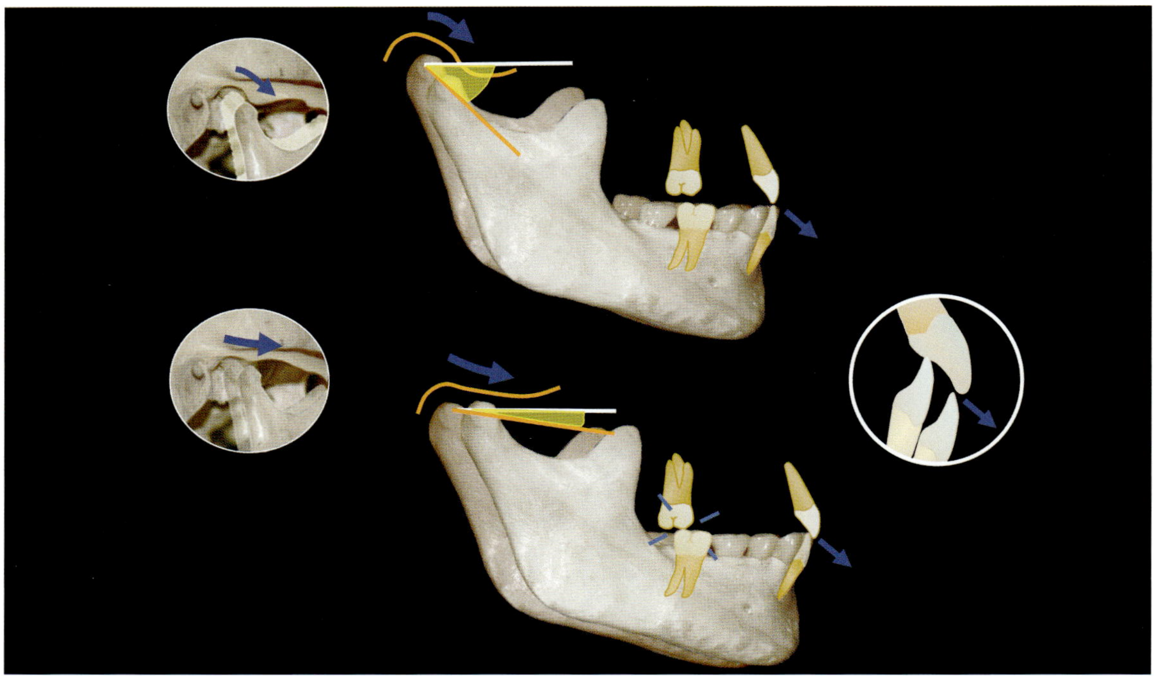

Fig 3-2-39 With the same incisal guidance, steep condylar guidance (top) discludes posterior molars and flat condylar guidance (bottom) does not separate posterior molars.

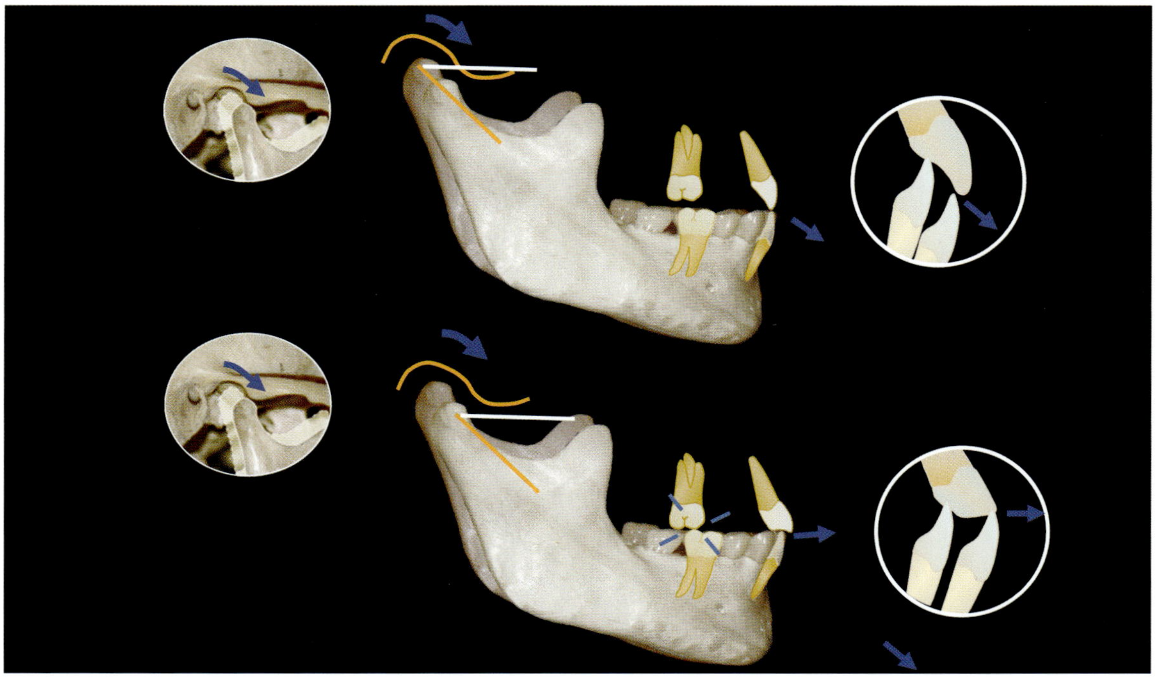

Fig 3-2-40 With the same condylar guidance, steep incisal guidance (top) discludes posterior molars and flat incisal guidance (bottom) does not separate posteriors.

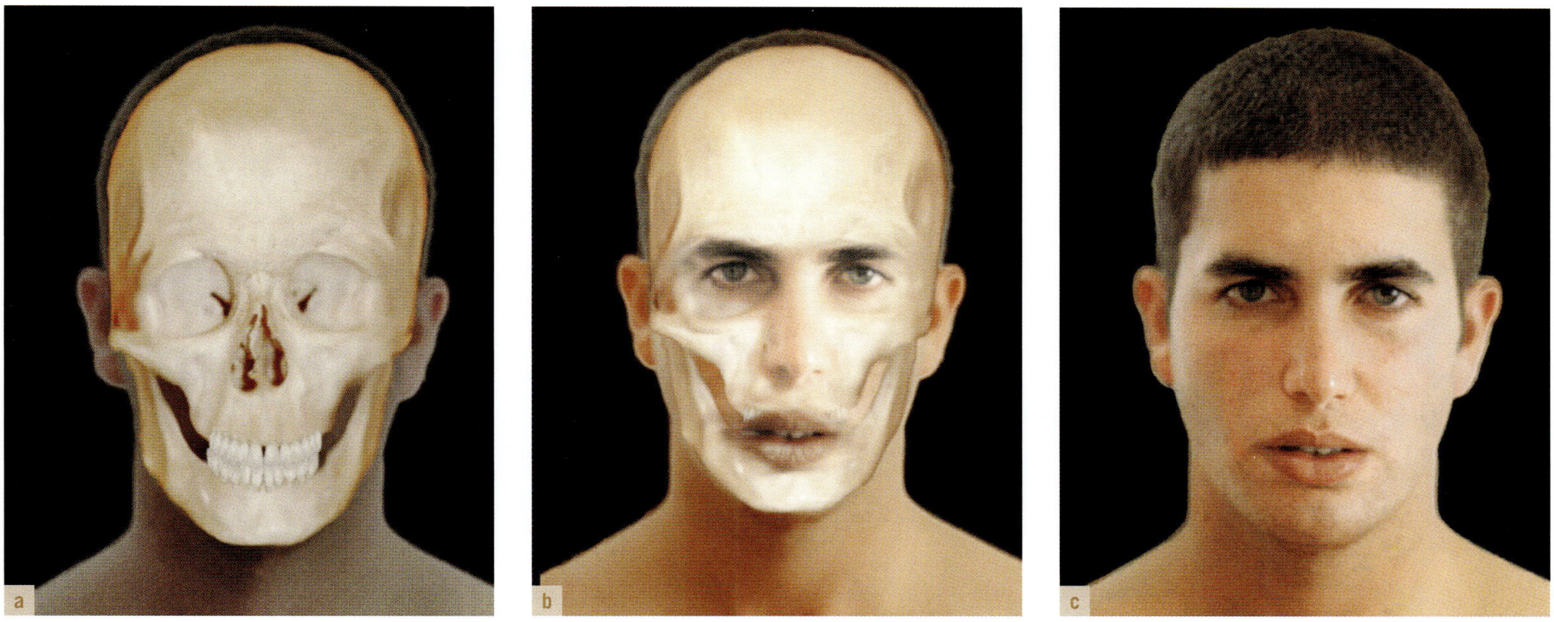

Fig 3-3-5 Frontal view at rest. Facial form is determined by the underlying skeletal morphology.

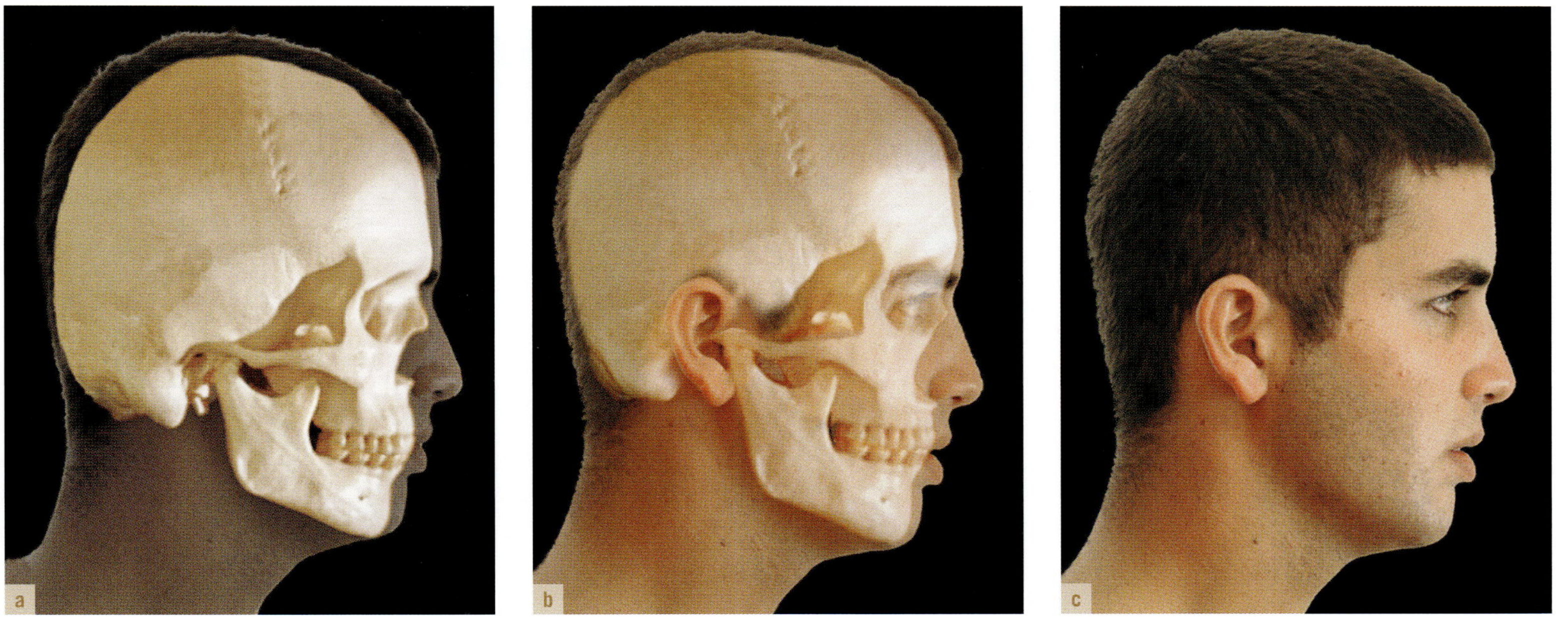

Fig 3-3-6 Sagittal view at rest. Class I orthognathic. Facial form and anteroposterior skeletal mandibular maxillary relations determine the facial appearance, particularly in profile.

degree of anteroposterior or lateral skeletal variation is excessive, the facial appearance may come to be perceived as unesthetic. Normal variations in anteroposterior skeletal relations are seen in Figs 3-3-7 and 3-3-8. Variations from common to more extreme anteroposterior relations are seen in Fig 3-3-9.

Evolutionary psychology of facial beauty

Why the appearance of the more extreme variants becomes perceived as unpleasing and engenders feelings of antipathy and discomfort is not clear, but may be linked to atavistic and ancient tribal perceptions engendering social acceptability and threats posed by non-normative social group members.[4,5] The average face is generally perceived to be the most esthetic.[6] Degrees of facial asymmetry are linked to attractiveness judgments.[4,7]

Averageness, symmetry, and sexual dimorphism are considered as strongly influencing biologically based standards of beauty that determine evolutionary preference in mate selection.[5,6] Averageness is favorably perceived as proximity to a spatially average face for a population. Symmetry manifests as bilateral facial symmetry and sexual dimorphism as feminine traits in female faces and masculine traits in male faces. Facial beauty is considered to be anchored in biology and survival of the species because it relays signals about reproduction and internal health. Fixed neuroanatomical arrangements in the human brain must be in place to extract the biological relevance of beauty.[7] A preference for beautiful faces is seen in infants. Other theories propose that concepts of attractiveness may be by-products of the way brains process information. A preference for average (and symmetric) faces could also be a by-product of their subjective familiarity and a preference for familiar stimuli.[6,7] It is argued that both kinds of selection pressures may have shaped our perceptions of facial beauty.[6]

As skeletal and dental relations deviate from the class I orthognathic model, the dental and occlusal relations become affected. Intercuspal relations change with variation in posterior support. The vertical and horizontal overlap of the anterior teeth may vary considerably with corresponding alterations in the excursive guidance. Vertical variants can effect occlusal relations with differences in the interarch distance and face height.[8-10]

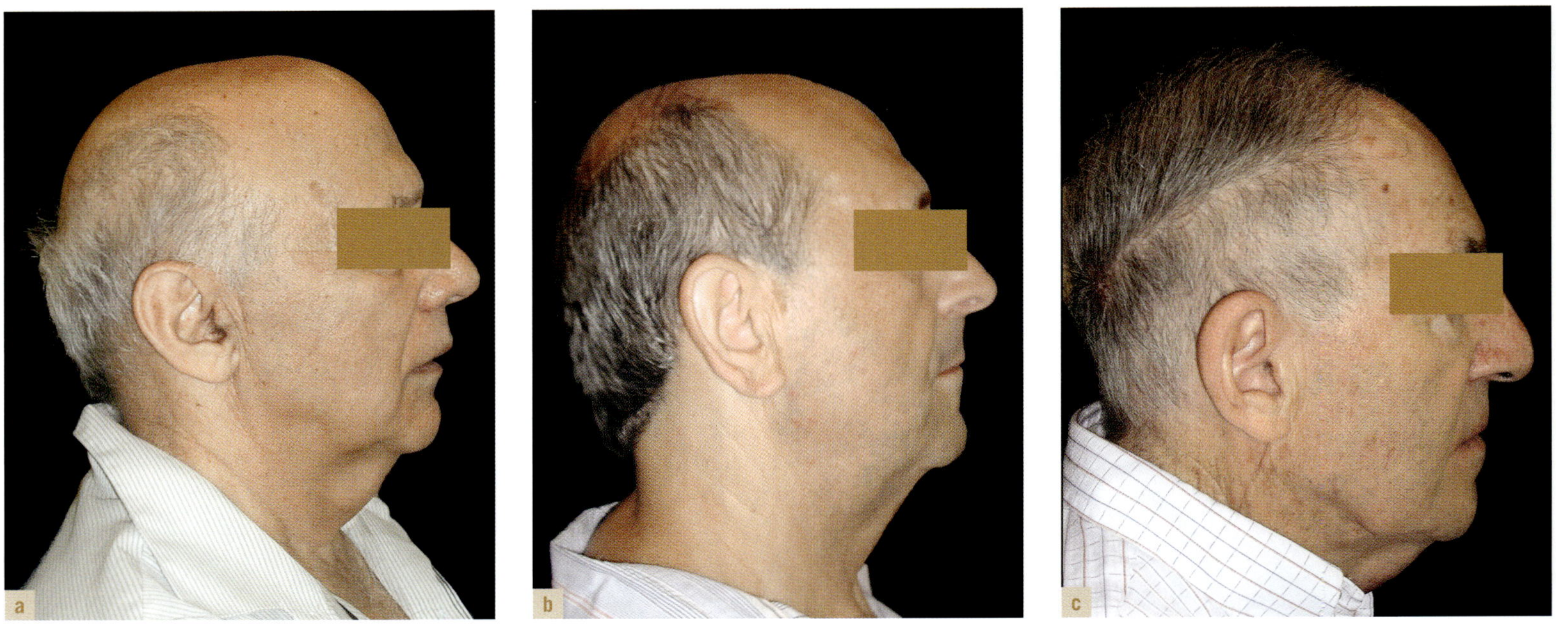

Fig 3-3-7 Normal variations in profile due to a class II retrognathic, b class I orthognathic, and c class III prognathic skeletal relations.

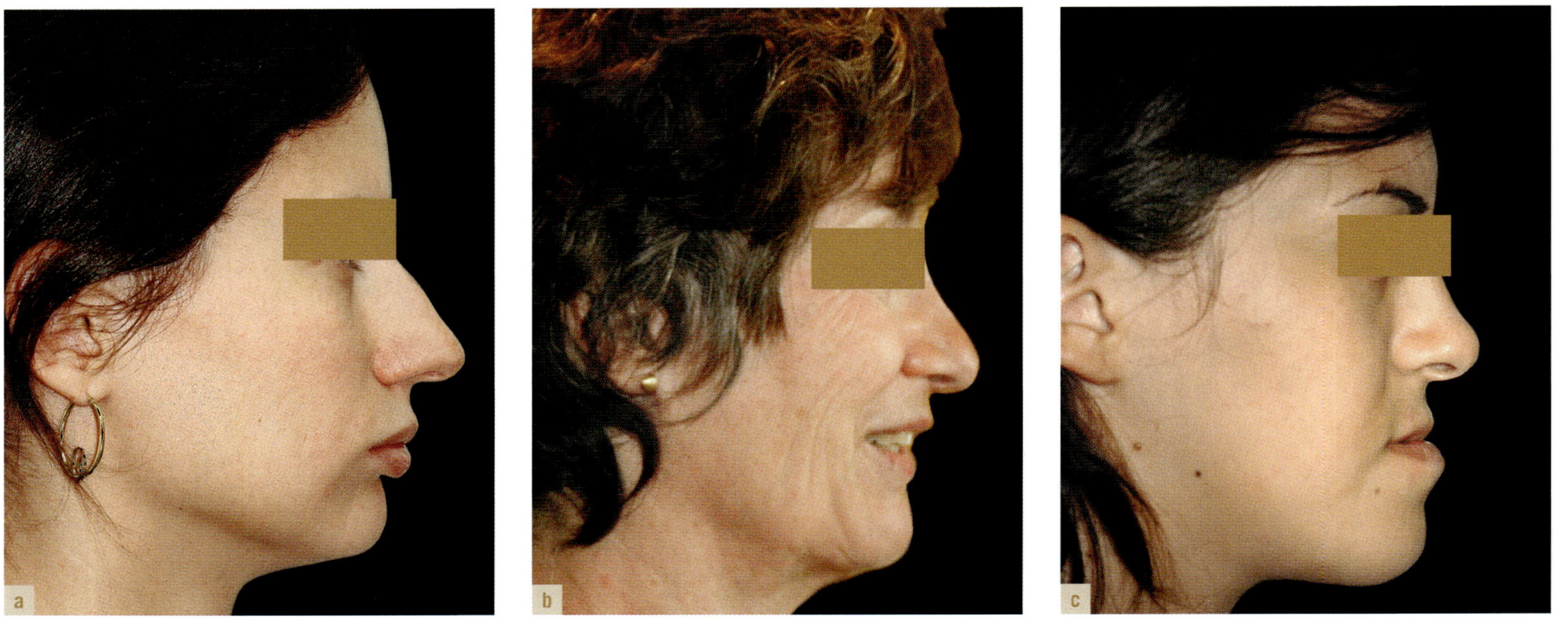

Fig 3-3-8 Normal variations in profile due to a class II retrognathic, b class I orthognathic, and c class III prognathic skeletal relations.

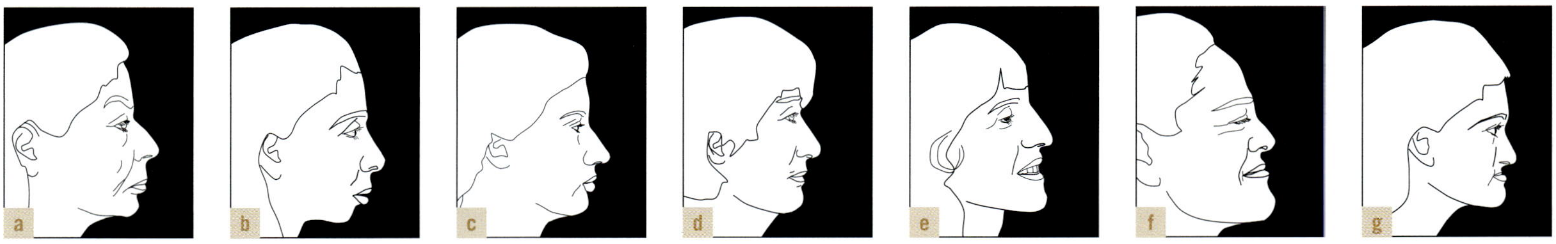

Fig 3-3-9a to c Class II retrognathic, d class I orthognathic, and e to g class III prognathic skeleton relations. As skeletal relations vary anteroposteriorly facial appearance becomes progressively more divergent from the class I norm.

For example, in class II division 1 cases, the retrognathic relation of the mandible creates an often severe horizontal overlap of the anterior incisors and canines. This can cause pronounced tooth display at rest, and more so on smiling. When severe, this can be perceived as retrognathic with the lower lip folded or "trapped" behind the maxillary incisors, as seen in Fig 3-3-10.

Facial proportions and face height

Vertical face height varies considerably according to individual genetic makeup. The face consists of the unalterable components of the upper two-thirds – from the lips upwards, and the lower third –from the lips down to the chin. The lower third varies with posture from occlusion in maximum intercuspation (MI) to various degrees of opening. Esthetic evaluations are commonly made with the lips at rest, the mandible in a

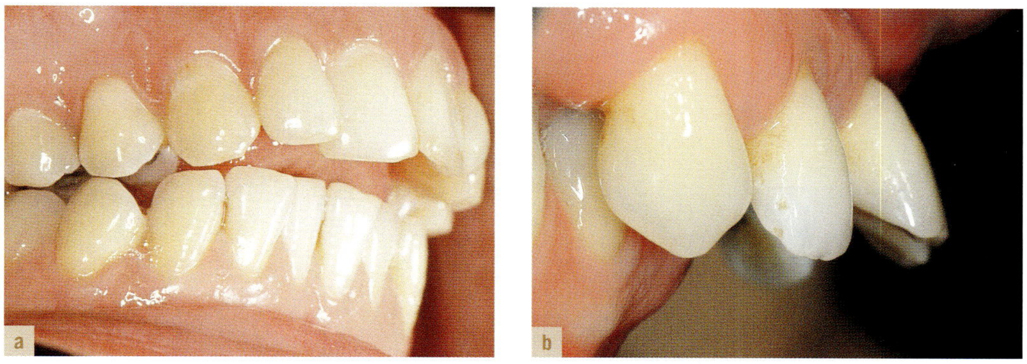

Fig 3-4-55 Severe class II division 1 Increased horizontal overlap.

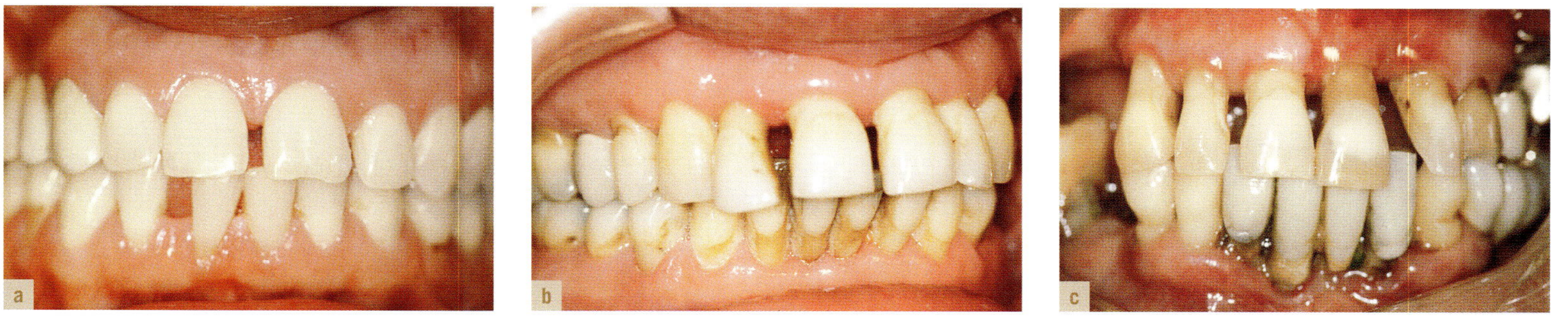

Fig 3-4-56 Anterior flaring, a mild, b moderate and c severe.,

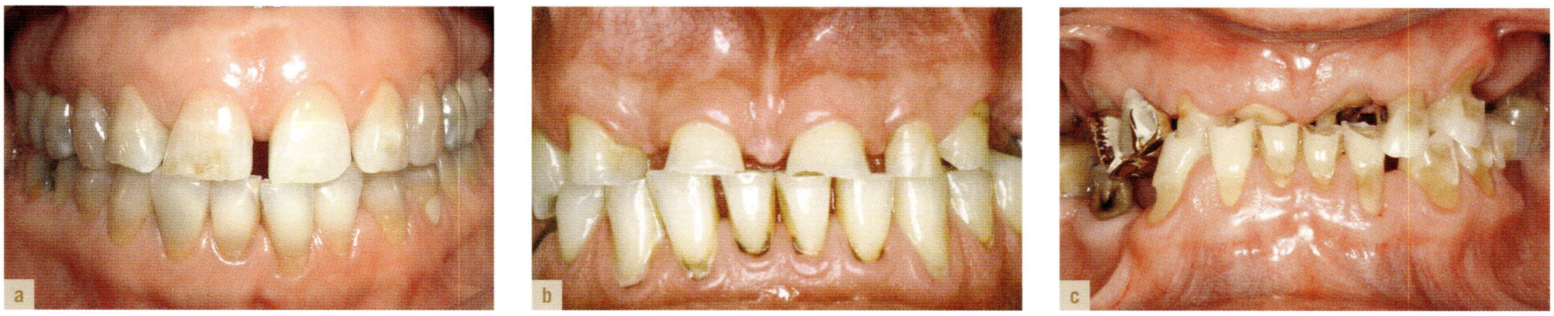

Fig 3-4-57 Anterior wear, a mild, b moderate, and c severe.

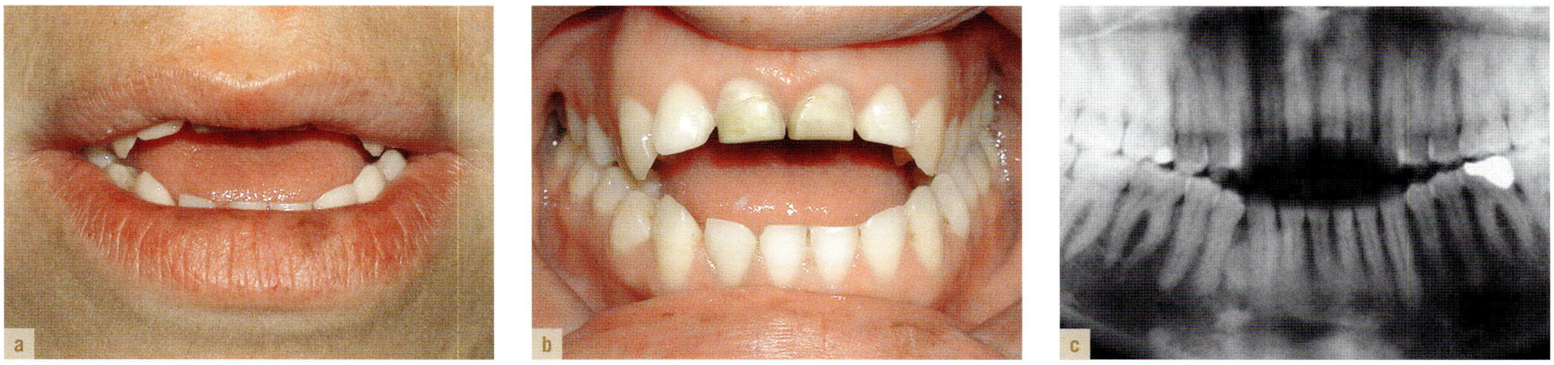

Fig 3-4-58 Anterior erosion, gastroesophageal reflux, anterior open relation, anterior open bite, esthetic impairment.

Box 3-4-8 Anterior relation discrepancies

- Anterior open bite
- Reversed anterior plane (reverse curve)
- Reverse anterior horizontal overlap, crossbite
- Complete vertical overlap, complete overbite
- Severe class II horizontal overlap overjet
- Anterior flaring, anterior tooth migration
- Anterior wear

Esthetic variants

Esthetic variants or impairments may be classified by particular elements that differ from the class I "alpha smile" (Fig 3-4-59). This is a descriptive classification with objective values. The objective measure of a variant may be described as the extent of the deviation from the norm. Mild, moderate, and severe are clinically useful gradations.

Esthetic or cosmetic variations may be minimal or may be considerable and clearly noticeable. Variations listed in Box 3-3-1 in Chapter 3.3 describe single particular variants. In many cases several variants are

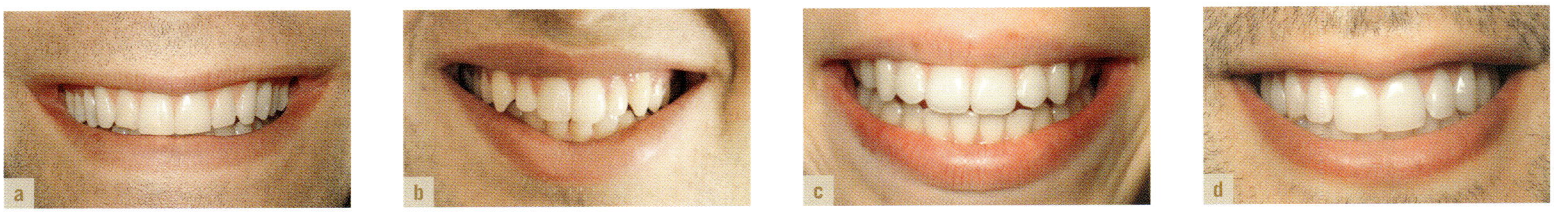

Fig 3-4-59 Alpha smiles. Idealized smiles with classic reference determinants of shape, arrangement, and harmony of the teeth in the smiling orofacial window.

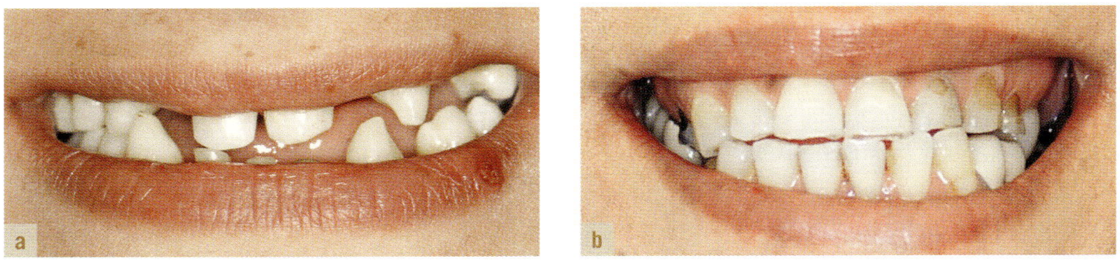

Fig 3-4-60 Asymmetry of the orofacial window, a with spacing and asymmetry of form, and b with asymmetric gingival planes, asymmetric posterior tooth display, and asymmetry of form.

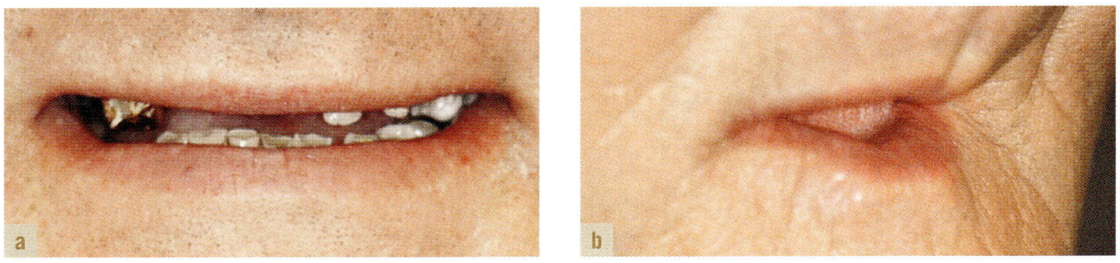

Fig 3-4-61 Lack of lip support. Inadequate tooth display.

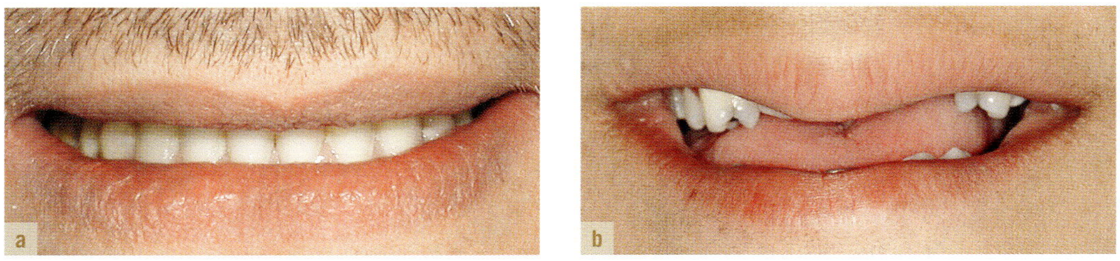

Fig 3-4-62a Diminished anterior maxillary tooth dimension and display with moderate reduction in crown height. b Diminished anterior tooth display.

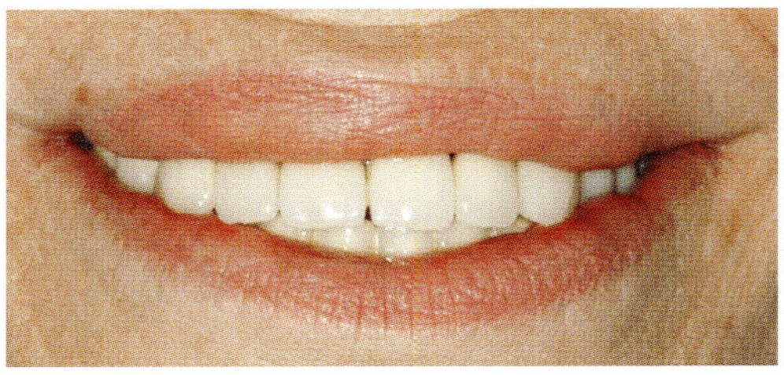

Fig 3-4-63 Excessive tooth display.

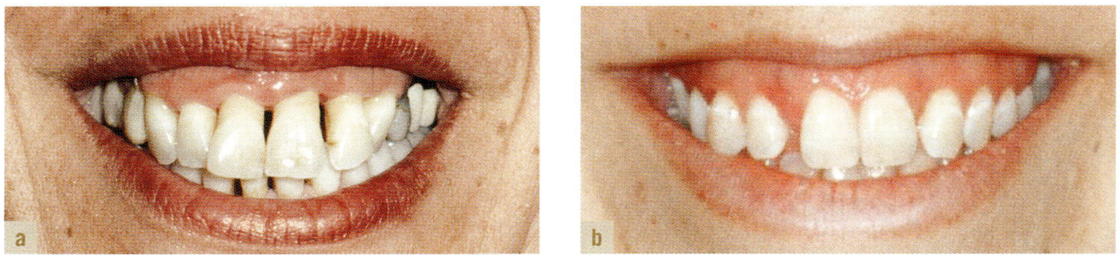

Fig 3-4-64 Excessive gingival display.

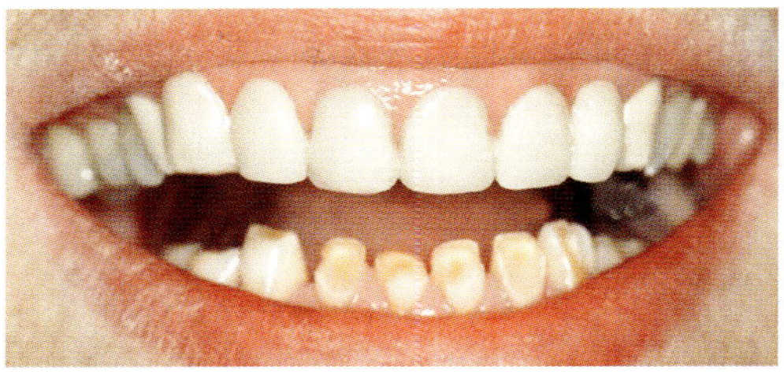

Fig 3-4-65 Disharmony of occlusal planes with lip lines and gingival lines.

apparent in the same dentition. Examples of variations and their diagnostic descriptions are shown in Figs 3-4-60 to 3-4-70.

Diagnostic classification of morphologic variants

Diagnosis of disease

Diagnosis is defined as the process of recognizing a disease or condition by its outward signs and symptoms and analyzing the physiological/biochemical cause(s). The *Shorter Oxford English Dictionary* defines disease as "a disorder of structure or function that produces specific symptoms."[65] The *Merriam-Webster Dictionary* defines disease as "a condition that impairs normal functioning and is typically manifested by distinguishing signs and symptoms."[66]

GPT8 defines diagnosis as "the determination of the nature of a disease."[40] Dentitions present with a large variety of morphologic variation, as described above. These may be due to or present together with dental disease, and/or occlusal parafunction and are strongly related to the individual patient's perception and adaptation.

When does a dental and occlusal variant become considered to be a disease or a disorder?

Morphologic variations in the occlusion and skeletodental complex shown in this chapter are not diseases according to the above definitions. However, they may be related to functional, esthetic, and adaptive difficulties that may require therapy. The question then arises as to which morphologic variant or occlusal-related dental conditions require therapy and how are these diagnosed?

4 Posterior Support

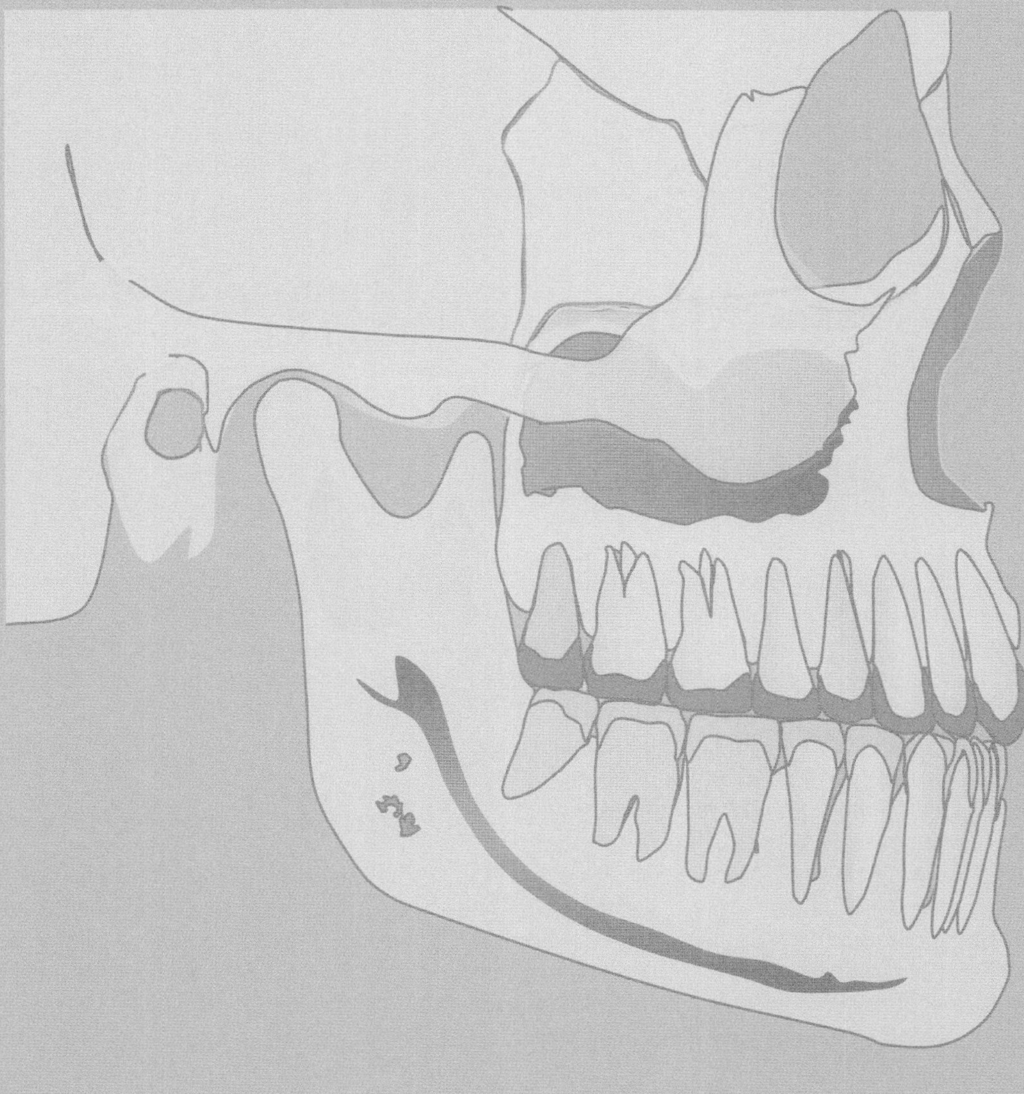

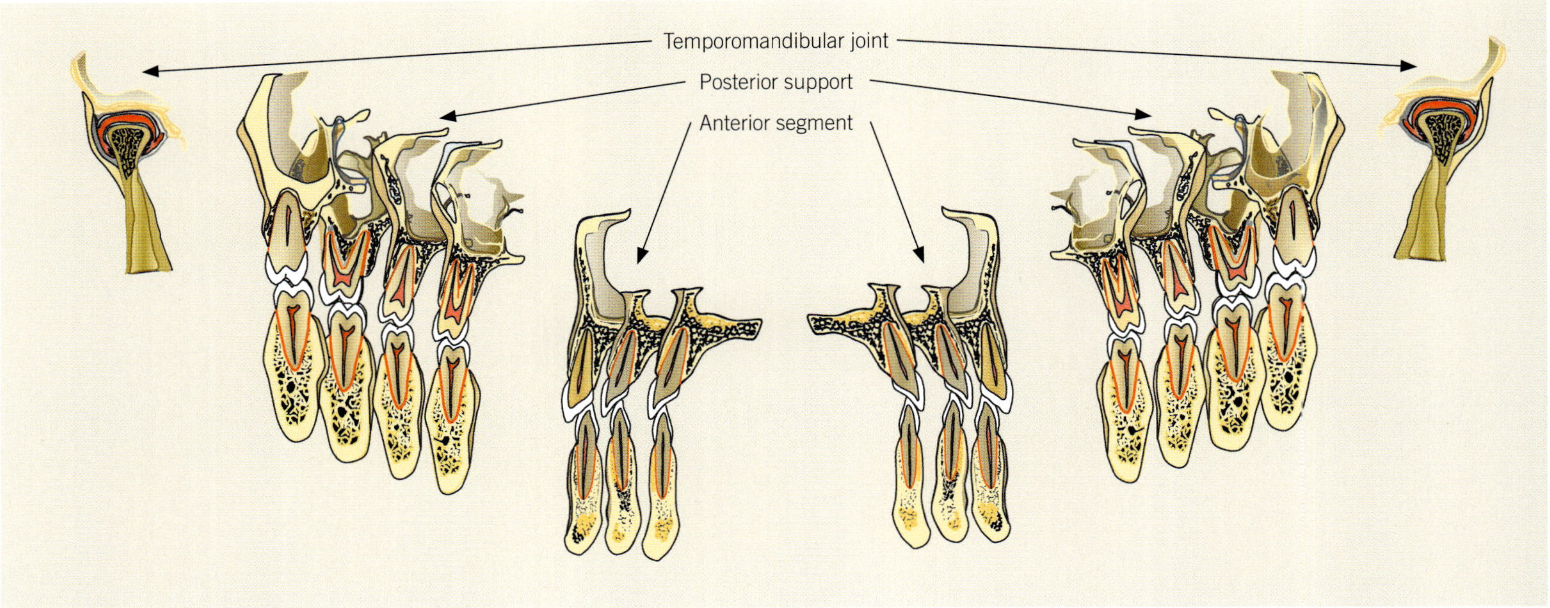

Fig 4-1 The functional load-bearing elements of the masticatory system: the posterior support ; the temporomandibular joints; and the anterior segment.

Contents

Definition of posterior support

Mastication, swallowing, and occlusal parafunction generate considerable forces that are transferred to the bony structures of the skull. The maxilla and facial skeleton are hollow structures, with hollow maxillary sinuses and nasal cavities situated directly above the maxillary teeth. The principal functional load-bearing elements of the masticatory system are the posterior teeth and their alveolar bone, the temporomandibular joints (TMJs) and the anterior teeth (Figs 4-1 and 4-2). The bulk of the occlusal support is provided by the posterior teeth and is termed the "posterior support." The intercuspal relation is the end point of mandibular closure, where occlusal forces pass via the roots of the teeth to be dissipated to the supporting structures of the facial skeleton. The TMJs have a minor load-bearing role that is increased when the posterior teeth are lost. The support provided by the anterior dental segment is significantly less than that by the posterior segment, and will depend on the skeletal relation and the horizontal and vertical overlap of the anterior teeth.

Functions of the posterior support

There are three principal functions of the posterior support:

1. To support the forces of swallowing, mastication, and occlusal parafunction.
2. To maintain the occlusal vertical dimension (OVD).
3. To provide sufficient occluding masticatory surfaces for masticatory comfort and efficiency (Fig 4-3).

Each dentition may vary in its ability to provide masticatory support and function depending on the individual components of the posterior support.

Components of the posterior support

There are three components of the posterior support:

- The number of occluding contacts.
- The number of supporting teeth and tooth or implant abutments.
- The amount of supporting bone (Fig 4-4).

The number of occluding contacts in a full complement of opposing standing teeth may be the same as the number of occluding contacts in opposing fixed partial dentures (FPDs) with reduced numbers of supporting abutments. The amount of alveolar bone support may also vary in the standing teeth and abutments, reducing the functional capacity of the posterior segment.

Reduced posterior support

The posterior support may become reduced with progressive loss of opposing dental units but may still be able to support function and maintain the OVD. Opposing pairs of remaining premolars may be able to provide sufficient support and function.

A distinction must be made between reduced posterior support and lost posterior support. In the case of reduced posterior support, there is a reduced capacity to support the functional and parafunctional forces of occlusion and to maintain the OVD. The comfort of the patient and the ability to chew effectively may also be significantly compromised. The clinician and patient must decide whether function, comfort, and longevity are not adversely affected as in the case of remaining premolar occlusion (Fig 4-5). Alternatively, it may be decided to restore or reinforce diminished posterior support either with fixed or removable prostheses, to supply additional implant abutments, or to replace lost alveolar bone by bone augmentation.

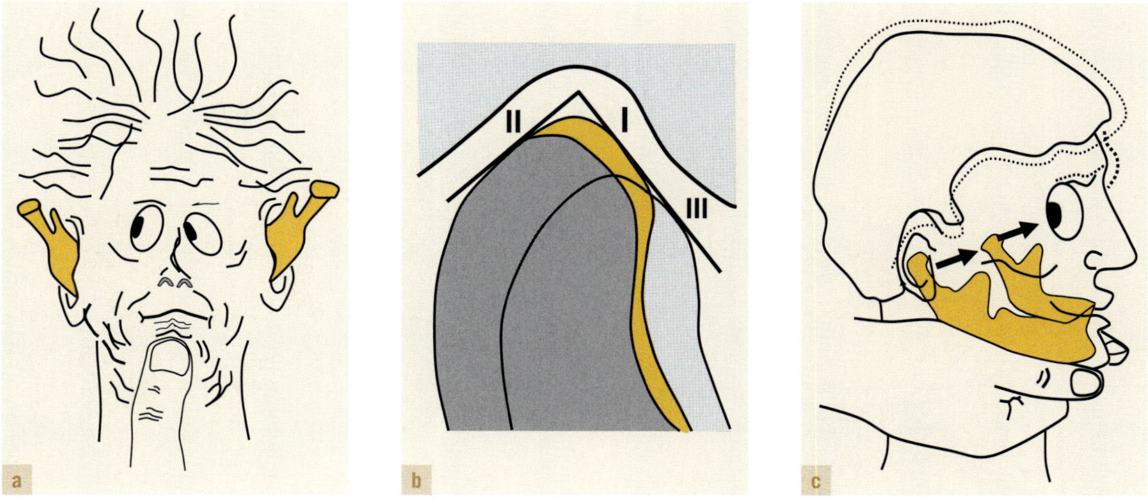

Fig 4-44 Conceptual condylar relations with mandibular manipulation in centric relation.
a Rearmost, uppermost, midmost purported to cause excessive distal force from chin point guidance.
b "I" optimal anterior superior relation, "II" distally displaced, "III" anterior displaced. (Redrawn from Celenza and Nasedkin.[98])
c Bimanual guidance is purported to raise the condyles anteriorly, seating the discs against the eminence.

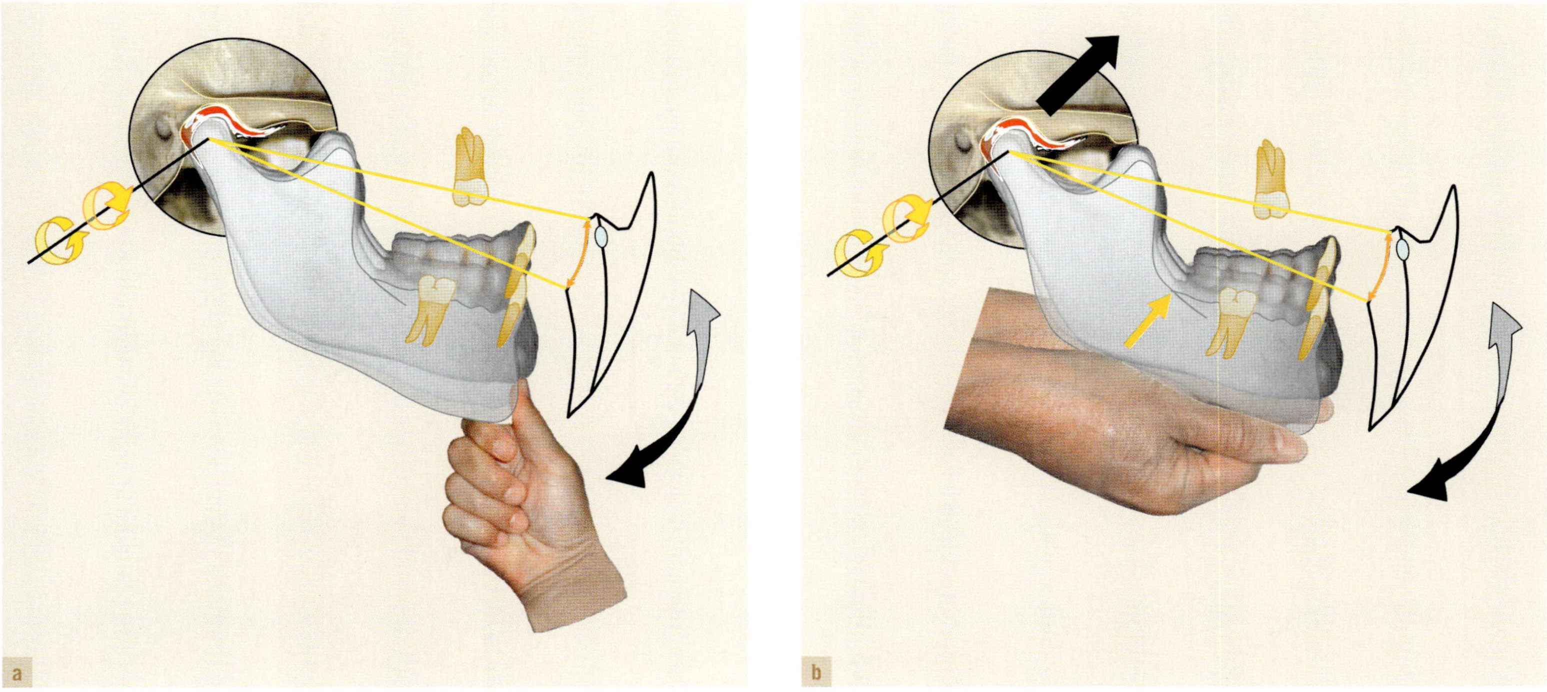

Fig 4-45 Centric relation manipulation techniques. a Chin point guidance rotates the mandible in a terminal hinge relation with muscles relaxed. b Bimanual guidance rotates the mandible around the terminal hinge while pressing the condyles anteriorly and superiorly against the eminentiae.

- Conceptual
- Anatomical (post mortem)
- Clinical recording systems
- Radiographic imaging

Conceptual

The conceptual and semantic description of the optimal condyle fossa relation has received much attention, and the many varying definitions and concepts seen in the GPT8, reviews, and dedicated texts attest to its once controversial nature.[2,98] The optimal condyle fossa relation has been described semantically as the "rearmost, uppermost, midmost position" of the condyle in the fossa. This was changed to the "uppermost midmost" and finally to the "uppermost, anteriormost position." The seating of the anterior aspect of the condyles on the mid-section of the discs against the eminence was also added to the definition in various semantic formats.[2,98] The various conceptual definitions were related to corresponding clinical manipulative techniques (Fig 4-44). Chin point guidance was claimed to create excessive distal pressure. Bimanual manipulation is claimed to seat the condyle anterosuperiorly in a functional relation to the disc. A graphic conceptual representation of condylar relation is shown in Fig 4-44b.[98] 'I' was described as the optimal relation, with 'II' as distally related and 'III' as anteriorly related.[98]

All definitions of centric relation hold that the mandible is rotated around its terminal hinge axis in an arc of 20 to 25 mm. They also describe centric relation as the most distal unforced mandibular relation from which eccentric movements can be made (Fig 4-45). The horizontal expression of the relation is the apex of the gothic arch tracing (Fig 4-46).

Anatomical post mortem relations

Sagittal sections of the condyle relation show that the relation of the condyle to the eminence reflects the most recent glossary definition, with the condyle functionally related to the distal slope of the eminence.[2,99-103]

Relations shown in MI depict the condyle position of centric relation with the assumption that for an MI to CR discrepancy of 1 to 1.5 mm, the condyle will be more distally related by 0.5 mm.

Anatomy of terminal hinge rotation

Post mortem examination of the condyle disc assembly in centric relation is difficult, since the mandible cannot be manipulated into centric

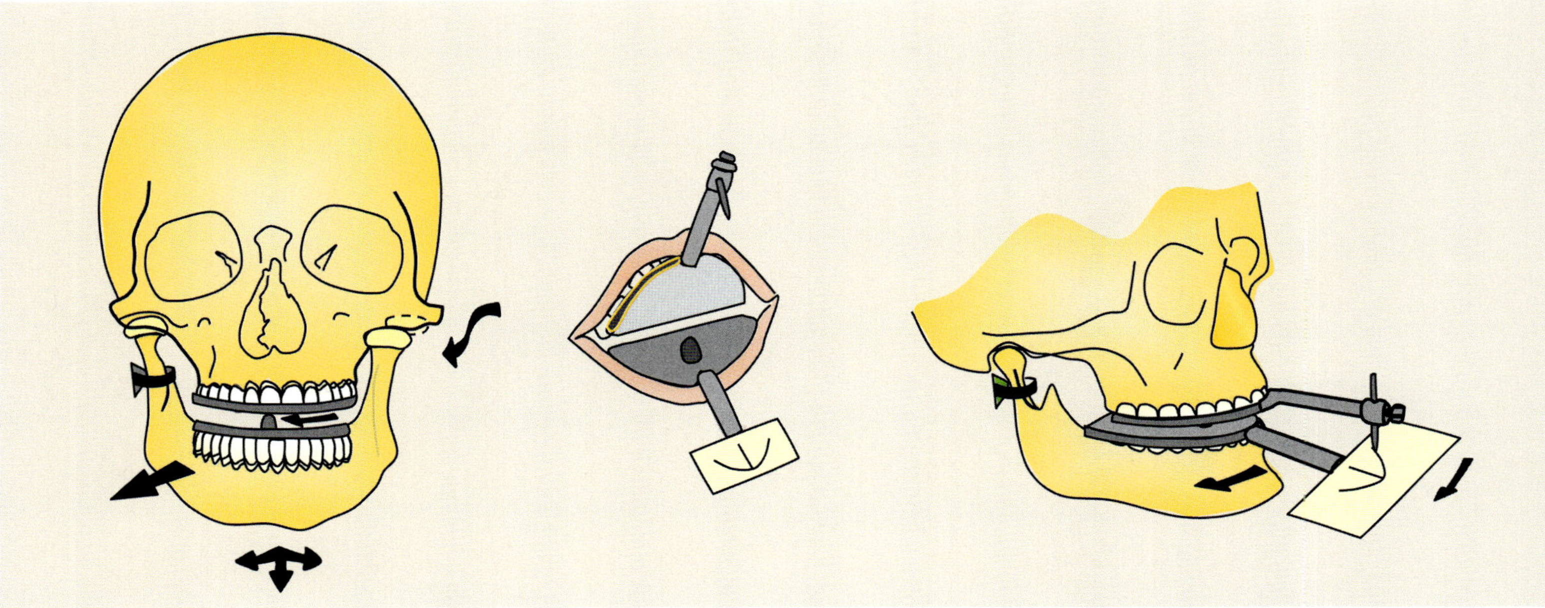

Fig 4-46 Gothic arch tracing. The apex of the gothic arch represents the horizontal expression of centric relation as the terminal position from which lateral movements may be made at a given vertical dimension.

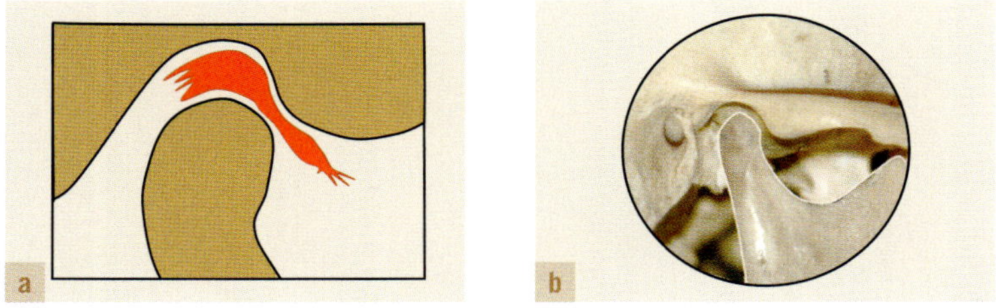

Fig 4-47a Condyle eminence relation from cadaver skull in MI.[103] b Dry skull relation of condyle to eminence in MI.

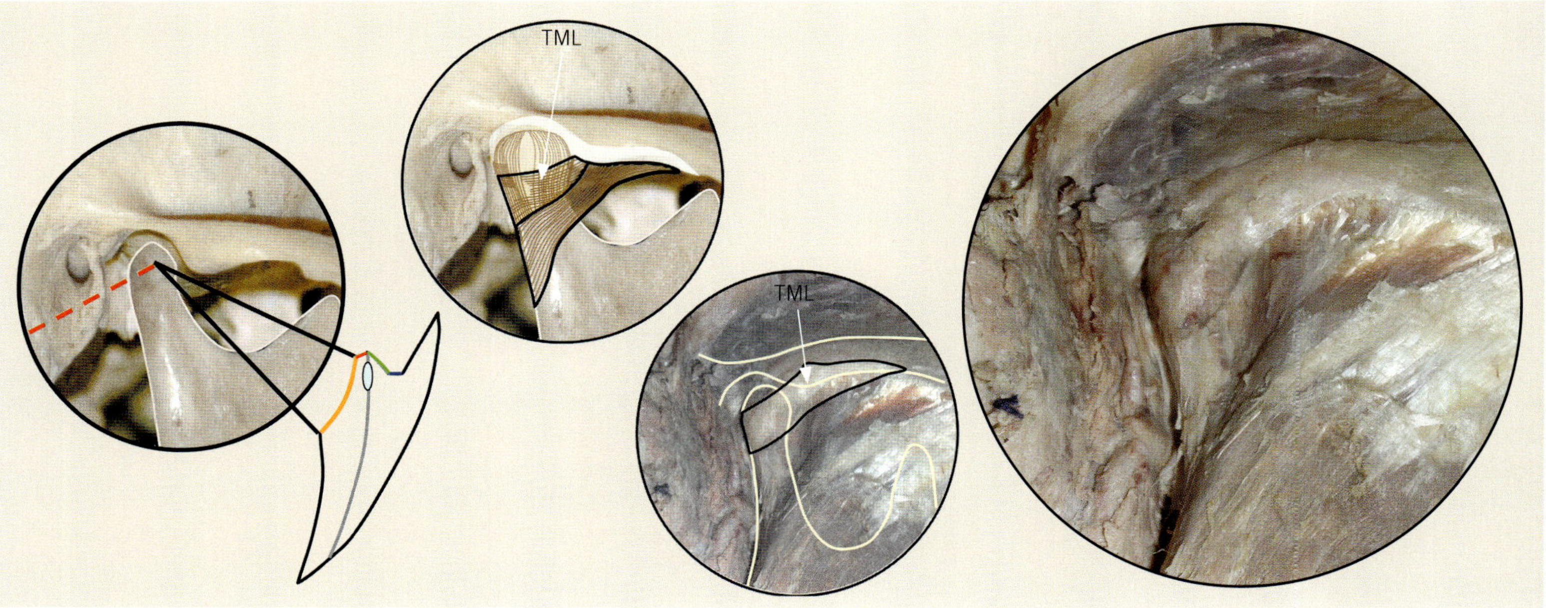

Fig 4-48 Rotation in centric relation. Temporomandibular ligaments (TML) limit distal movement and provide the mechanism for rotation around the terminal hinge axis.

relation (Figs 4-48 and 4-49). One study obtained a sagittal section with the teeth wired together in the intercuspal relation. This gave a sagittal histological image, which is illustrated diagrammatically in Fig 4-47a.[103] The histological section in Fig 4-49b is not in centric relation. These images show that there is no distal stop with soft areolar connective tissue distally. Gross anatomy dissections and histological sections show that the lateral temporomandibular ligament provides the distal restraining mechanism that facilitates rotation of the condyle against the eminence around a horizontal axis (Figs 4-48 and 4-49). On examination of these and other anatomical images of the disc, it becomes apparent that the movement of the condyle 0.3 mm distally up the eminence is within the normal range of joint function and not likely to be of any clinical significance. This is the range of difference reported to result from differences in condylar relation due to varying manipulation techniques (Figs 4-49 to 4-53).[100-105]

Clinical recording systems

Clinical registration of centric relation is carried out using several methods. These include interocclusal registrations (occlusal records,[2] wax

5 Occlusal Vertical Dimension

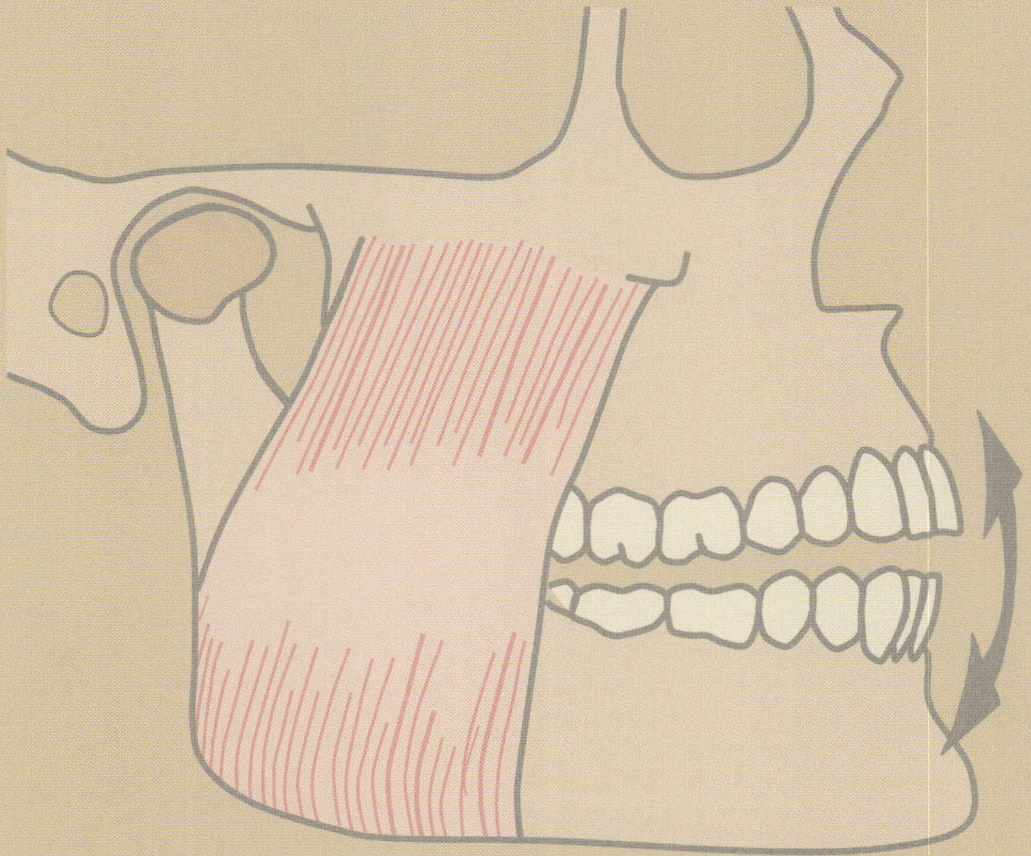

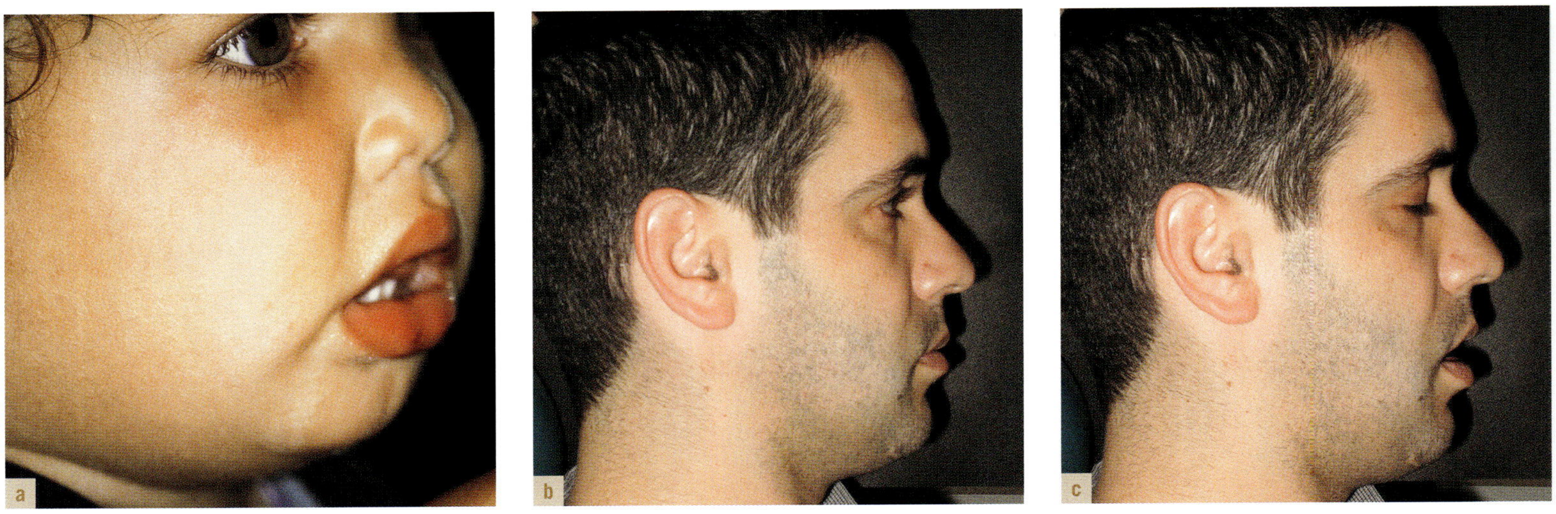

Fig 5-1a to c Mandibular resting posture varies with body posture, sleep, alertness, lip contact, and many other variables.

Contents

Growth and development

The restoration and maintenance of the occlusal vertical dimension (OVD) is an important part of clinical dentistry. Clinical questions relating to this important aspect of oral rehabilitation are addressed in this chapter.

OVD is established as a result of ordered growth and development of the teeth, skull, and facial structures through the primary, mixed, and permanent dentition stages of genetically determined maturation. The posterior teeth maintain the OVD, together with the anterior teeth, with the exception of class II division 1, severe complete vertical overlap in class II division 2, and anterior open bite situations.

During growth, the mandible develops, assuming resting postural relations from which oral respiration, speech, and all other normal daily and nocturnal functions occur. Postural relations progressively adapt to the changes of occluding vertical relations during growth through primary, mixed, and permanent dentitions to adulthood (Figs 5-1 and 5-2).[1]

Compensatory eruption

In some cases with loss of tooth structure from wear or breakdown or opposing tooth loss, tooth eruption or segmental eruption may occur. This process has been ascribed a compensatory role to maintain OVD, however the mechanism is not well understood.[2,3]

In a dry skull study of 337 aboriginal skulls, comparing moderate and severe wear cases, compensatory tooth eruption and generalized alveolar bone growth compensated for 50% of the loss in face height due to the loss of occlusal surface height from wear.[2]

Skeletal face height is maintained by the vertical stops of the occluding teeth. The appearance of the face is primarily perceived in postural resting relations (Fig 5-1). Loss of OVD by tooth loss, wear or breakdown

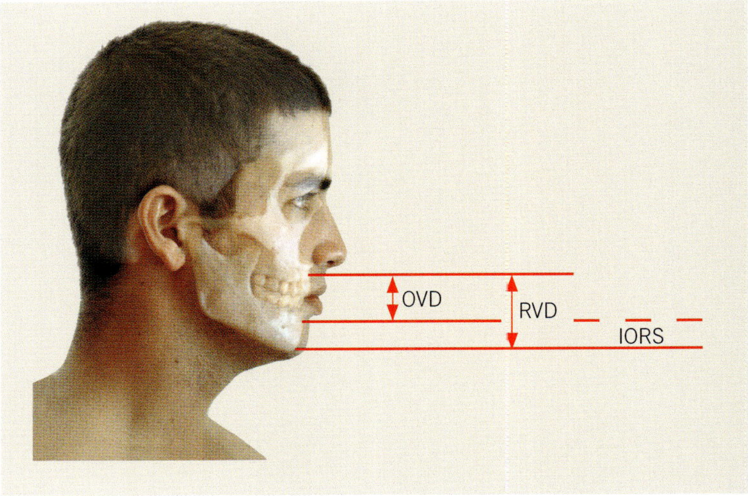

Fig 5-2 Occlusal vertical dimension (OVD). Rest vertical dimension (RVD). Interocclusal rest space (IORS), formerly termed the "freeway space." This is the distance between the occlusal surfaces of the teeth when the mandible is in its postural resting relation. This is commonly measured as the amount of vertical separation of the incisors from maximum intercuspation (MI).

will reduce occluding skeletal face height and may sometimes alter the facial appearance on closure and in postural relations. Facial height may not always reflect skeletal loss of OVD.

Mandibular posture, postural rest, rest position

For many years, clinicians grew up with the concept that there was one single immutable and unalterable rest position, independent of feedback from intercuspation and primarily dependent on the physiologic resting lengths of the muscles. Resting face height was considered to be established at an early age and was thought to be immutable and constant.[4-10]

Constancy of face height concept

This "constancy of face height concept"[6] held sway for many years. It was thought that encroachment on the "freeway space" would cause the muscles to attempt to reestablish OVD resulting in trauma to the alveolus intrusion and mandibular dysfunction.[4-10] This was considered

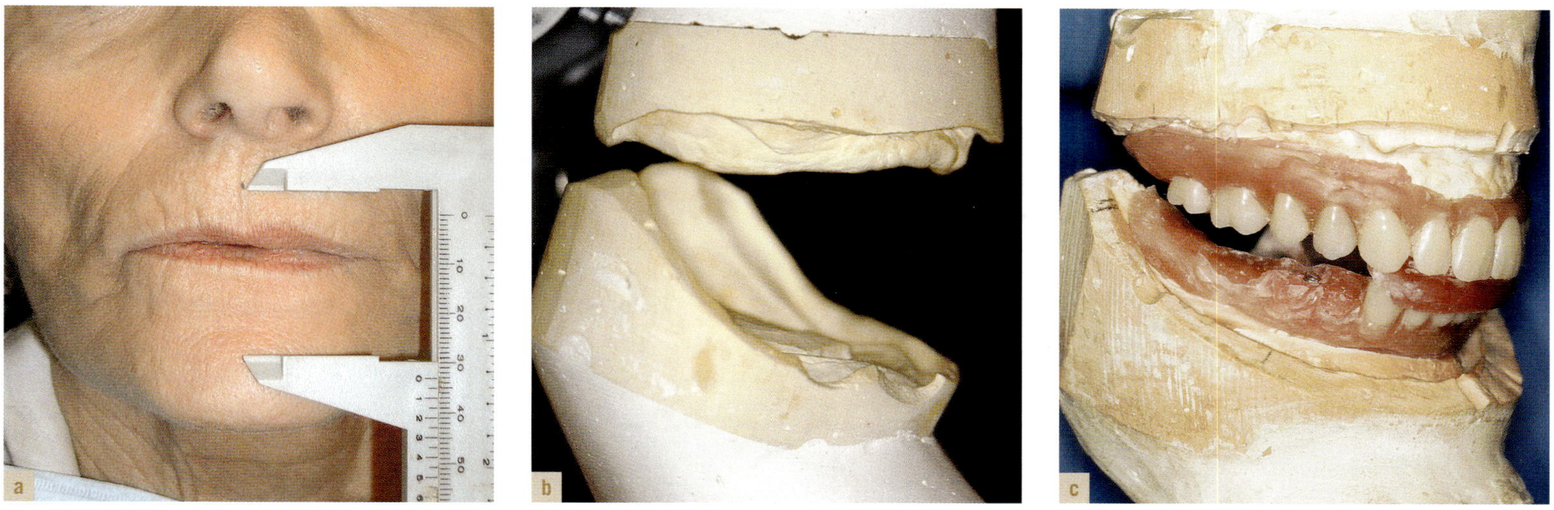

Fig 5-3a to c Resting postural relation and the "clinical rest position" (CRP) have been traditionally used as the starting reference relation for establishing a new OVD in complete edentulism. RVD is initially established from facial reference points. With the aid of trial bases and occlusal rims, OVD is established with the distance between the same facial reference points reduced by 2 to 3 mm on closure.

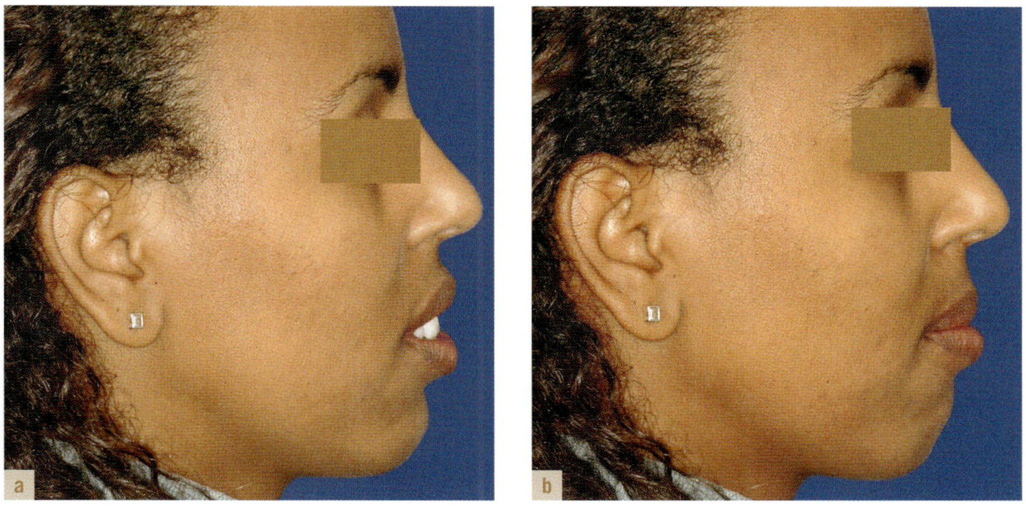

Fig 5-4a and b The lower chin skin reference point is significantly affected by contraction of the mentalis muscle, lip posture, and facial expression.

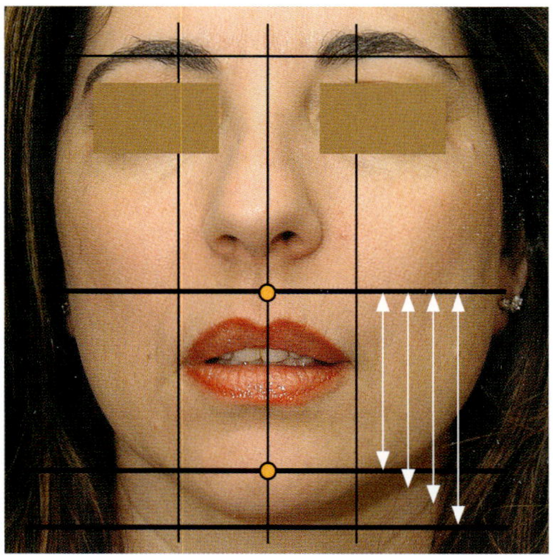

Fig 5–5 Postural rest position is difficult to define since there are multiple possible postural resting mandibular relations that may be assumed.

to be true for both partially edentate and fully edentulous dentitions. It was considered important to restore lost OVD without encroaching on the "freeway space" and exceeding the "rest position." Exceeding the original face height was thought to cause temporomandibular disorders (TMDs).[4-18]

Rest position, interocclusal rest space – measurement of the rest position

Resting postural relation and the "clinical rest position" have been traditionally used as the starting reference relation for establishing a new OVD for complete dentures in total edentulism. Resting vertical dimension is initially established from facial reference points. With the aid of trial bases and occlusal rims, OVD is established with the distance between the same facial reference points reduced by 2 to 3 mm on closure (Fig 5-3).

The lower chin skin reference point is generally positioned over the mentalis muscle. Slight contractions of the mentalis and variations in lip posture and facial expression can significantly change the position of this skin reference point (Fig 5-4).

The postural rest position continues to be used as a vertical reference relation for restoring the OVD in prosthodontics. However, controversy remains regarding the ability to define, establish clinically, and measure a repeatable postural relation that fits this role. Mandibular posture occurs at multiple possible instantaneous positions constantly moving in response to changes in posture, respiration, swallowing, stress, lip competence, and speech (Figs 5-1, 5-4, and 5-5). The distance between the teeth with the mandible at rest, formerly the "freeway space," is now termed the "interocclusal rest space" (IORS) (Fig 5-2).[19] This is the distance between the upper and lower teeth in the incisor region with the mandible in the rest position.

Glossary definitions of rest position

Definitions have varied over the years with differing editions of the *Glossary of Prosthodontic Terms*.[19,20]

Restoration of the fully edentulous dentition with complete dentures has traditionally been carried out using the vertical dimension of rest as the primary vertical reference relation. The rest OVD is established with the patient seated upright and instructed to rest the mandible by a variety of techniques.[11,13-16]

Methods of establishing the clinical rest position

This postural relation or position was termed the clinical rest position (CRP) as it was established clinically.[13] Methods employed in establishing CRP include:[11,13-16]

- Phonetic method: The patient is seated in an upright position and is instructed to phonate letters and words such as M, S, or Mississippi and then relax the jaw. The rest vertical dimension (RVD) is immediately recorded by measuring the distance between two premarked points on the skin in the midline, one over the chin of the mandible, and the second in the subnasal philtrum or on the nose (Fig 5-3). The phonetic method elevates the mandible to the level of the closest speaking distance, after which it is relaxed.[14]
- Command: The patient is seated upright and instructed to look ahead, close or tap (on command) the teeth together, and then relax the jaw. The RVD is measured immediately as the distance between the two arbitrary maxillary and mandibular reference markings.[21,22]
- Swallowing: The patient is seated in an upright position and instructed to swallow, lick the lips, and relax the mandible.[11,13-16,19,21]

These three methods have a common feature in that they get the mandible elevated close to the maxilla by phonation, swallowing, or tooth closure and then it is immediately relaxed by relaxing the elevators. The degree of relaxation following this mandibular elevation is uncontrolled but presumably influenced by the recent elevation event. In a study comparing these three methods in 20 fully dentate healthy young students, a remarkable degree of similarity was found. The mean IORS was 1.7 mm ± 1.28.[22] Table 5-1 shows the range of CRP values from various studies using different methods.

RVD and OVD

The current glossary definition of RVD is:

- Rest vertical dimension: "The distance between two selected points (one of which is in the middle of the face or nose and the other of which is on the lower face or chin) measured when the mandible is in the physiologic rest position" (Fig 5-3).[19]
- Occlusal vertical dimension: "The distance measured between two points when the occluding members are in contact" (Fig 5-2).[19]

These are clinical definitions designed to compare rest and closure in the same sitting, originally in denture fabrication.

Closest speaking space

The closest speaking space is the distance between the anterior teeth needed to enunciate certain letters and words. The anterior teeth must be separated sufficiently to allow air to pass through this space and create the desired sound. The degree of opening is influenced by the vertical overlap of the anterior teeth. Teeth with a deep vertical overlap (class II division 2) will need to open more than incisors with class III or class I relations. If measurements are made from these speaking procedures they will differ between the various vertical overlaps between patients. The closest speaking space is additionally used as a clinical tool to assess vertical relations. The closest speaking distance and the IORS are different phenomena, although their dimensions in some cases may be similar.[14]

Difficulty in defining a single postural "rest position"

Look up "rest position" in the *Glossary of Prosthodontic Terms* and you are referred to see the definition "Physiologic rest position." Physiologic rest position (PRP) has been defined over the years with small variations between editions.[19,20]

All these definitions include the supposition that the muscles are in a state of "of minimal contractual activity," of "tonic equilibrium," and "in equilibrium in tonic contraction." This had not been substantiated by any neurophysiologic study, and in light of the purported precise nature of rest position as a single critical point, clinicians were left in a quandary with many unanswered issues. There has never been reference in these glossary definitions to the term "clinical rest position" and the clinical methods used in its location.[11,13,22-25]

Clinical rest position was a postural reference position described in clinical texts and used to establish a new vertical dimension for complete dentures in edentulous patients. This was established by phonetic command or swallowing, without measuring the degree of muscle contraction.[22] The Glossary's concepts of "tonic equilibrium," "equilibrium in tonic contraction," or "minimal contractual activity" were not referenced. With the development of electromyography (EMG), many studies were carried out in an attempt to resolve this issue (reviewed in the following sections).

Mechanism of postural rest and baseline EMG

Muscular determined (servo control), passive tissue elasticity (viscoelastic effect,) or both

Mandibular posture is maintained by a combination of the passive viscoelastic tension of the soft tissues and by low levels of activity in the elevator muscles. Without this activity – as in sleep – the jaw drops open (Fig 5-1).[26] During walking or running, stretch reflexes in the jaw-closing muscles limit the movement of the mandible, with both passive forces and active reflex responses maintaining jaw posture within narrow limits during brisk head movements.[26,27]

Body postural reactions are coordinated tonic and triggered actions that are controlled by a central program, and it is speculated that mandibular position is controlled in a similar manner.[26,28,29]

The neuromuscular system regulating muscle tone has been described as a servo control mechanism employing neuromuscular feedback.[30] A servo mechanism, or servo, is an automatic device that uses error-sensing feedback to correct the performance of a mechanism. Tonic baseline EMG levels have been attributed to tonic stretch unitary firing of type I fibers deep in masseter and anterior temporal, with background motor neuron excitation and tonic firing in the fusimotor system.[26,30] In sleep and during general anesthesia, contraction of the jaw elevators is reduced or abolished, as the connective tissues primarily support the mandible. The level of tonic EMG activity can vary from minimal levels during general anesthesia, sleep, hypnosis, autogenic relaxation, biofeedback, or relaxation. EMG levels rise with increased levels of alertness and stressed vigilance.[30-38] EMG masseter and anterior temporal resting levels were reduced with body posture, eye closure, and ambient light intensity levels.[30,37,38] Normative resting minimal EMG levels have been compared with raised EMG levels with myofascial pain dysfunction and craniomandibular disorder groups, with varying results.[39-45] Values of EMG have been reported and serve as reference values (see Chapter 2.3).[42,46] The levels of minimal baseline resting EMG are subject to the degree of relaxation

65. Monaco A, Sgolastra F, Ciarrocchi I, Cattaneo R. Effects of transcutaneous electrical nervous stimulation on electromyographic and kinesiographic activity of patients with temporomandibular disorders: A placebo-controlled study. J Electromyo Kinesio 2012;22:463–468.
66. Manns A, Miralles R, Palazzi C. EMC bite force and elongation of the masseter muscle under isometric voluntary contractions and variations of vertical dimension. J Prosthet Dent 1979,42:674–682.
67. MacKenna BR, Türker KS. Jaw separation and maximum incising force. J Prosthet Dent 1983;49:726–730.
68. Lindauer SI, Gay T, Rendell J. Electromyographic-force characteristics in the assessment of oral function. J Dent Res 1991;70:1417–1421.
69. Rivera-Morales WC, Mohl ND. Relationships of occlusal vertical dimension to the health of the masticatory system. J Prosthet Dent 1991;65:547–553.
70. De Boever JA, Carlsson GE, Klinberg IJ. Need for occlusal therapy and prosthodontic treatment in the management of temporomandibular disorders. Part II. Tooth loss and prosthodontic treatment. J Oral Rehabil 2000 27:647–659.
71. Ekberg EC, Vallon D, Nilner M. The efficacy of appliance therapy in patients with temporomandibular disorders of mainly myogenous origin. A randomized, controlled, short-term trial. J Orofac Pain 2003;17:133–139.
72. Kovaleski WC, De Boever J. Influence of occlusal splints on jaw musculature in patients with temporomandibular joint dysfunction. J Prosthet Dent 1975;33:321–327.
73. Manns A, Miralles R, Santander H, Valdivia J. Influence of the vertical dimension in the treatment of myofascial pain dysfunction syndrome. J Prosthet Dent 1983;50:700–709.
74. Dahl BL, Krogstad O. Long-term observations of an increased occlusal face height obtained by a combined orthodontic/ prosthetic approach. J Oral Rehabil 1985;12:173–176.
75. De Boever JA, Adriaens PA, Seynhaeve TM. Raising the vertical dimension of occlusion with fixed bridges (abstract). J Dent Res 1989;68:902.
76. Kohno S, Bando E. Functional adaptation of masticatory muscles as a result of large increase in the vertical occlusion. Dtsch Zahnarztl Z 1983;38:759–764.
77. Christensen I. Effect of occlusion-raising procedures on the chewing system. Dent Practit Dent Rec 1970;20:233–238.
78. Carlsson GE, Ingervall B, Kocak G. Effect of increasing vertical dimension on the masticatory system in subjects with natural teeth. J Prosthet Dent 1979;41:284–289.
79. Hellsing G. Functional adaptation to changes in vertical dimension. J Prosthet Dent 1984;52:867–870.
80. Magnusson T. Change in recurrent headache and mandibular dysfunction after treatment with new complete dentures. J Oral Rehabil 1982; 9:95–105.
81. Wilding RIC, Owen CP. The prevalence of temporomandibular joint dysfunction in edentulous non-denture wearing individuals. J Oral Rehabil 1987;14:175–182.
82. Ramfjord SP, Blankenship JR. Increased occlusal vertical dimension in adult monkeys. J Prosthet Dent 1981;45:74–83.
83. Yaffe A, Tal M, Ehrlich J. Effect of occlusal bite raising splint on electromyogram motor unit histochemistry and myoneuronal dimensions in rats. J Oral Rehabil 1991 Jul;18:343–351.
84. Akagawa Y, Nikaido T, Tsuru H. Histologic changes in rat masticatory muscles subsequent to experimental increase the occlusal vertical dimension. J Prosthet Dent 1983;50:725–732.
85. Goldspink G. The adaptation of muscle to a new functional length. In: Anderson DJ, Matthews B (eds). Mastication. Bristol, UK: John Wright & Sons, 1976:90–99.
86. Yabushita T, Zeredo JL, Fujita K, Toda K, Soma K. Functional adaptability of jaw muscle spindles after bite raising. J Dent Res 2006;85:849–853.
87. Bell WH, Scheideman G. Correction of vertical maxillary deficiency: stability and soft tissue changes. J Oral Surg 1981;39:666–670.
88. Ellis E 3rd, Carlson DS, Frydenlund S. Stability of midface augmentation: an experimental study of musculoskeletal interaction and fixation methods. J Oral Maxillofac Surg 1989;47:1062–1068.
89. Hunt NP, Cunningham SJ. The use of kinesiography to assess mandibular rest positions following corrective orthognathic surgery. J Craniomaxillofac Surg 1998;26:179–184.
90. Tallgren A. The continuing reduction of the residual alveolar ridges in complete denture wearers: a mixed- longitudinal study covering 25 years. J Prosthet Dent 1972;27:120–132.
91. Lambadakis J, Karkazis HC. Changes in the mandibular rest position after removal of remaining teeth and insertion of complete dentures. J Prosthet Dent 1992;68:74–77.
92. Kois IC, Phillips KM. Occlusal vertical dimension: alteration concerns. Compend Contin Educ Dent 1997;18:1169–1177.
93. Mack MR. Vertical dimension: A dynamic concept based on facial form and oropharyngeal function. J Prosthet Dent;1991;66:478–485.
94. Ricketts RM. The biologic significance of the divine proportion and Fibonacci Series. Am J Orthod 1982;81:351–370.
95. Rufenacht CR. Fundamentals of esthetics. Chicago: Quintessence Publishing, 1990.
96. Gross MD, Nissan J, Ormianer Z, Dvori S, Shifman A. The effect of increasing occlusal vertical dimension on face height. Intl J Prosthodont 2002;15:353–357.

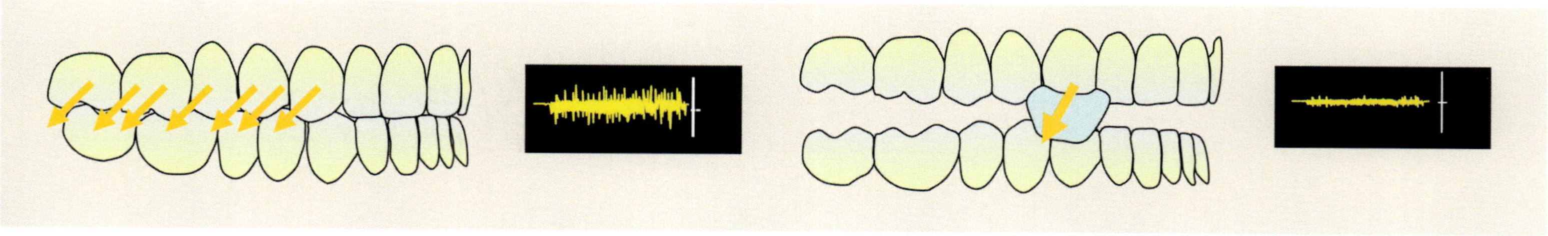

Fig 6-2-9 Two studies on natural teeth with overlays varying canine and group function guidance. Both reported less EMG temporalis and masseter activity on laterotrusive maximum voluntary clench and gliding movements with the overlays.[12,21]

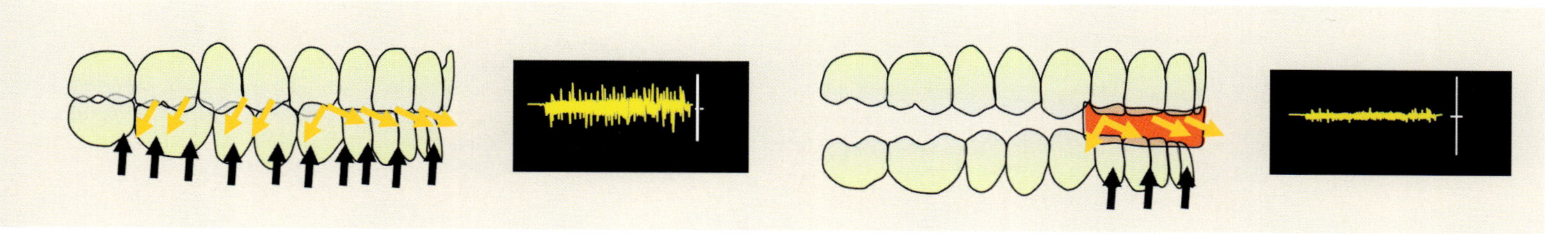

Fig 6-2-10 An "anterior bite stop" had a significant effect in decreasing EMG activity for both clenching muscle activity for the anterior and posterior temporalis and masseter during clenching and grinding.[20]

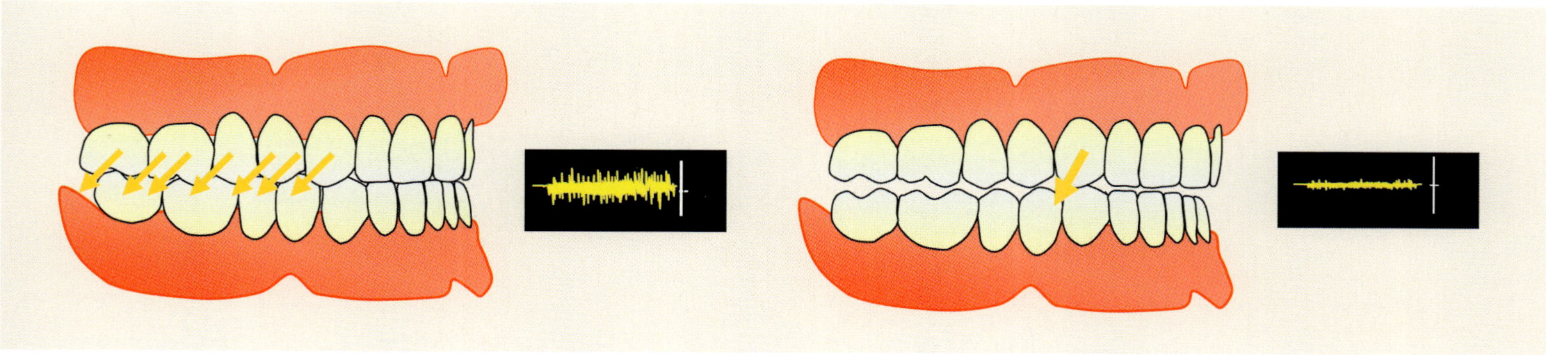

Fig 6-2-11 In a study of full dentures, Miralles et al[22] reported less EMG activity with canine guidance than with a fully balanced occlusion.

spectively. The steeper the guidance, the less the EMG activity. Vertical dimension changes were shown to have no effect between anterior and posterior blocks, and between unilateral anterior and intermediate and posterior blocks. An anterior jig with a flat guiding surface reduced clenching and grinding EMG levels (Fig 6-2-10).[20]

One study reported no difference in masseter EMG activity between canine guidance and group function for edge-to-edge lateral clenching with maxillary splints in normal subjects. Altering the occlusal balance significantly reduced muscle activity.[16] Another study found the same masseter and anterior temporalis EMG activity for canine guidance and first molar guidance patterns during lateral movement and during lateral clenching on maxillary splints (Fig 6-2-8).[18]

Natural teeth

In a study comparing group function and canine overlays, "canine protected occlusions" did not significantly alter muscle EMG activity during mastication but significantly reduced muscle EMG activity during voluntary lateral clenching.[12] In another study comparing simulated canine guidance with group function, less EMG activity was recorded in all muscles with canine overlay versus natural group contact (Fig 6-2-9).[21]

Dentures

In a study of nine full denture subjects (one man, eight women; mean age 59 years) anterior temporal and masseter EMG activity were recorded in maximum voluntary clench in MI and in edge-to-edge laterotrusion. Canine guidance was compared with full balance. Lower EMG activity was recorded with canine guidance as compared with a fully balanced occlusion (Fig 6-2-11).[22]

Conclusions

The evidence for a neuromuscular protective mechanism is not strong. The contention is that the anterior guidance and anterior tooth contact possess a neuromuscular protective mechanism that reduces loading of the anterior teeth. This argument is given as one of the justifications to provide protrusive and lateral disocclusion in fixed restorations. The mechanism for this process has not been demonstrated. Increased numbers of pressoreceptors in the canines have been shown. Suggestions of periodontal ligament (PDL) receptors and muscle proprioception have been made. Most of the EMG studies show reduced activity for anterior versus group laterotrusive clenching. Laterotrusive clenching on maxillary splints is not a convincing analogy of parafunction in natural teeth. Two studies showed reduced EMG activity in natural teeth between canine guidance and group function.[12,21] The objective of a "protective" anterior guidance would be to reduce excusive parafunctional loading, since this is the activity causing most damage to the teeth and the supportive structures. However, voluntary edge-to-edge protrusive clenching is different from daytime and nighttime clenching and grinding. Nighttime grinding is the most potentially damaging parafunction activity and there is no evidence to correlate voluntary laterotrusive clenching in edge-to-edge relations with nighttime grinding.

Table 6-2-1 EMG studies

Authors	Occlusal testing model	Subjects	Occlusal scheme and method	Results	Study authors' conclusions
Williamson & Lundquist[15]	Maxillary acrylic splint. Posterior disclusion vs contacts in eccentric movement	5 women, 4 men 7/9 4/5 history of TMD	Lateral gliding movement with simultaneous closing force	For all subjects, as the posterior teeth disocclude during lateral or protrusive movements, EMG activity suddenly drops. This did not occur when the posterior teeth contacted in eccentric movements	Posterior disclusion in eccentric movements involuntarily reduces muscle EMG activity
Shupe et al[17]	Maxillary occlusal splint. Flat canine guidance, steep canine guidance, posterior group function, contact of premolars and first molars on acrylic splint in excursions	9 healthy adults (23–41) Healthy class I dentitions, no dysfunction	Maximum voluntary clench 10 s increments. Max voluntary lateral grinding 10 s. Gum chewing 90 s	Grinding and chewing on maxillary acrylic splint shows least EMG activity with steep canine guidance, more with flat canine guidance and most EMG activity with group function	
Belser & Hannam[12]	1.Maxillary canine cast overlay vs group guidance on natural teeth 2. Self-cured acrylic overlay on first molar producing working side interference and non-working hyperbalance vs group guidance scheme of subject's natural dentition	12 healthy adults (34–45) Complete natural dentition with worn canines and some balancing molar contacts	EMG anterior and posterior temporal and masseter. Lateral clench. Lateral movement. Unilateral gum chewing	1. In lateral clench, less EMG in all muscles with canine overlay vs natural group contact (but different vertical dimension 2. In lateral clench, same EMG with single molar overlays as natural group function. Chewing no difference 3. Clench with non-working side interference also does not reduce EMG but changes bilateral EMG patterns	Canine protected occlusions do not significantly alter muscle EMG activity during mastication but significantly reduces, muscle EMG activity during voluntary lateral clenching.
Manns et al[11]	Maxillary acrylic occlusal splint. Three separate blocks in the maxillary arch. Posterior group contact from canine to second molar vs canine guidance. Maxillary splint split into 3 – 1 anterior, 2 posterior	6 healthy adults (17–35) Complete natural occlusion. No dysfunction	EMG anterior and posterior temporal and masseter. Maximum voluntary clench in centric relation and also during dynamic lateral excursions.	Canine guidance produces consistent and significant reduction in muscle EMG activity under all conditions relative to group function Non-working temporal more reduced than non-working masseter Working masseter EMG more reduced than temporal	1. Fewer contacts. The fewer the contacts, the lower the threshold of periodontal receptor activation, which then inhibits muscle EMG activity (Extrapolation dubious, the inhibitory mechanism is speculated and extrapolated from the nocioceptive reflex.) 2. Claims that canines are more sensitive to pressure than posterior teeth 3. Decreased stability inhibits force: with canine guidance, decreased mandibular stability inhibits muscle EMG activity
Graham & Rugh[18]	Maxillary acrylic splint. Canine guidance versus single molar guidance with identical vertical dimension increase	10 healthy adults (23–32)		No difference between canine guidance and single molar guidance	"The observed reduction in EMG activity with both guidance patterns is most likely caused by central neural commands that relax the jaw-closing muscles to allow the necessary jaw opening to achieve lateral movement."
Miralles et al[22]	Complete dentures Fully balanced occlusion and canine guidance	9 subjects (41-71)	EMG anterior and posterior temporal masseter. Maximum voluntary clench in maximum intercuspation and in laterotrusion	Lower EMG activity in canine guidance compared to group function	
Visser et al[23]	Stabilization splints 2mm thickness, 3mm thick and on protrusive repositioning splint	10 healthy subjects 10% and 50% maximal clench		Less EMG activity in protrusion	
Manns et al[24]	Maxillary unilateral acrylic overlay split into 3 sections. First section lateral incisor and canine, second contacting both premolars, and third with both molars in contact	8 healthy adults (21–26) Ipsilateral (working side) masseter and anterior temporal surface electrodes	1. Group function lower lateral to molar 2. Canine edge-to-edge lateral 3. Steeper and higher lateral canine edge-to-edge	Elevator EMG activity with the anterior blocks was significantly lower than the intermediate and posterior blocks. No difference between intermediate block alone, intermediate plus posterior block, and all three blocks together	
Borromeo[16]	Maxillary acrylic splint	10 normal subjects (20–35)	Maximum laterotrusive clench	No difference between canine guidance and group function. Same reduction in masseteric EMG, relative to centric relation	Change in muscle length and increase in vertical dimension reduce EMG activity
Becker et al[20]	Anterior acrylic jig	30 subjects	EMG of anterior and posterior temporalis, masseter, and anterior digastric during clenching and grinding tasks	Decreasing EMG activity for both clenching and grinding for all tested elevator muscles	
Okano et al[21]	Metal and acrylic overlays on natural teeth Metallic overlays simulated canine guidance, group function, and balanced occlusion (one balancing contact)	20 healthy adults		Less EMG in all muscles with canine overlay vs natural group contact	EMG activity in the anterior temporalis significantly increased in the simulated group function occlusion and the simulated bilateral balanced occlusion compared with the simulated canine-protected occlusion
Scott et al[25]	Protrusive maximum clench compared to maximum clench in MI relation	10 subjects Natural teeth	Measured and compared anterior and posterior temporal activity	In maximum clench in MI, high EMG values with no difference between anterior and posterior. In protrusive clench, little or no activity in both locations	

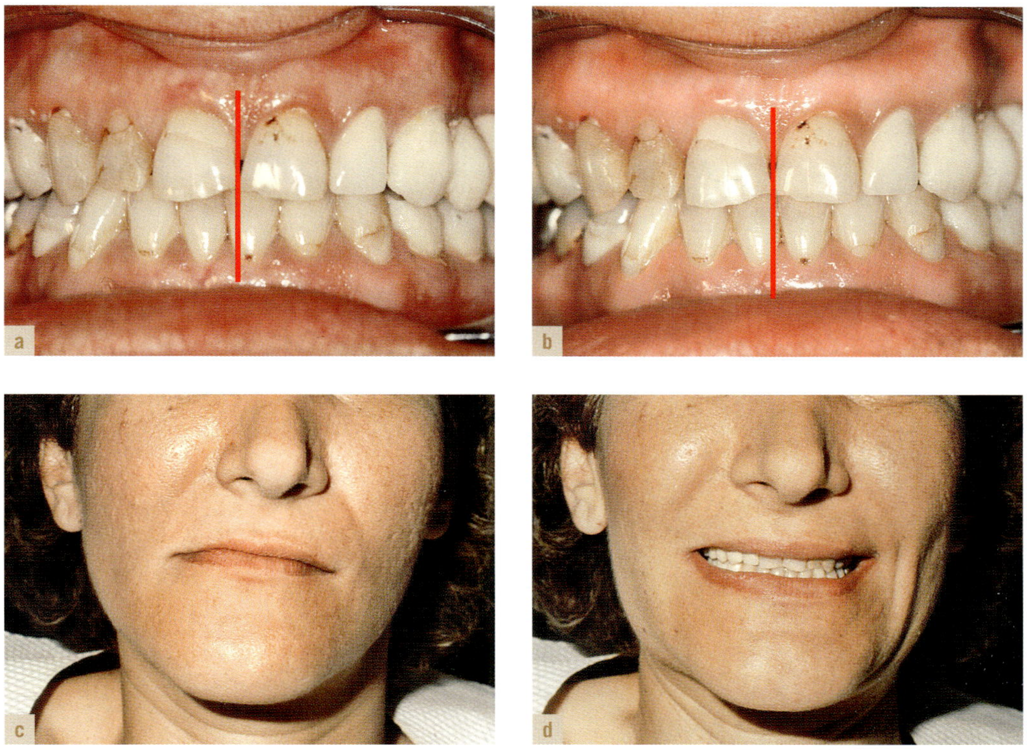

Fig 6-2-23a to d This patient was unable to close in a centered MI position. She could only close in a lateral relation. Efforts to close in MI causeD severe muscle pain and discomfort. The muscles were in co-contraction (or splinted) and very tender to pressure. Symptoms arose after placing the upper left temporary fixed partial denture. A deflective contact was seen in the partial denture. Symptoms resolved over several weeks after removal of the deflective contact and provision of a night guard. The etiological effect of deflective contact, stress, pain modulation, and musculoskeletal predisposition are difficult to separate. It is rare to find such a severe reaction apparently to a small occlusal discrepancy.

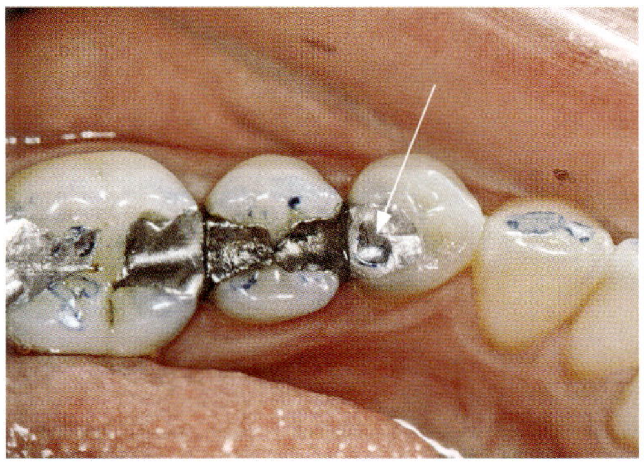

Fig 6-2-24 A newly introduced interference or "high" contact. A patient received a new amalgam restoration on the lower right first premolar and complained of discomfort from the tooth, and muscle pain for 3 days. Symptoms disappeared spontaneously after 5 days. The shiny facet indicates that the patient "sought out" and ground on the new "interfering" restoration. In this context, the SEPOC "interfered" with comfort.

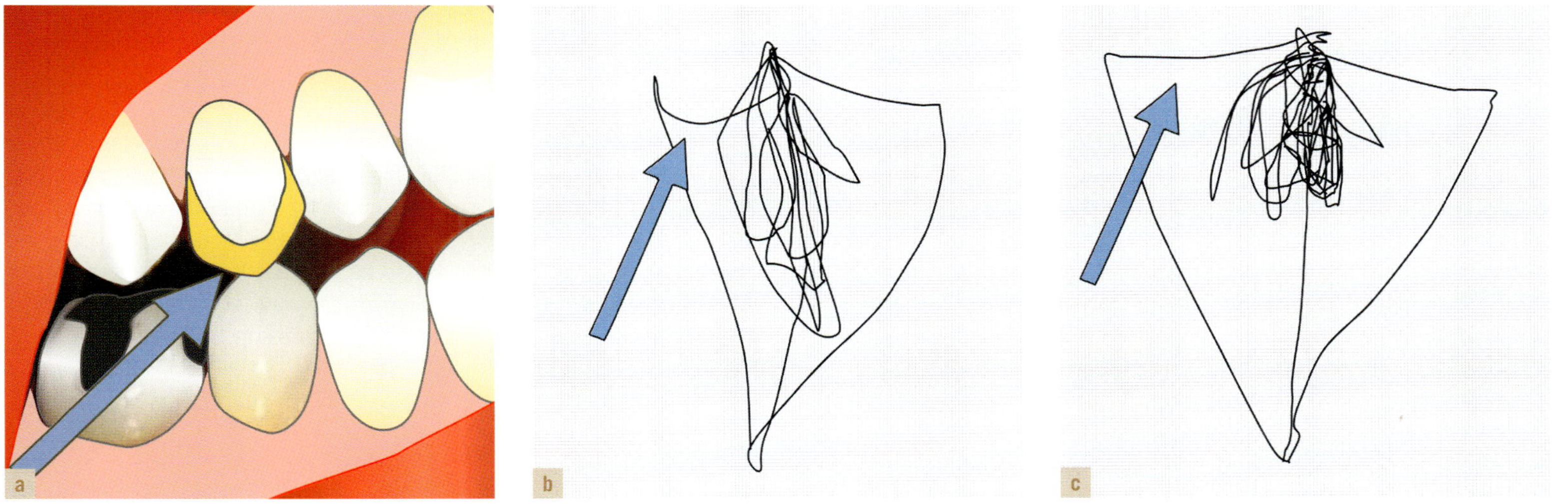

Fig 6-2-25a New restoration on the second premolar creates a new working guidance/interference. b Change in right closing angles of chewing cycles. c Original guidance restored after reduction of premolar contact. Original chewing cycles restored. (Image courtesy of Professor Arthur Levin.)

been evaluated in human subjects by observing clinical signs and symptoms, and neuromuscular responses by EMG or jaw tracking.

Occlusal trauma (animal studies)

Animal studies have been carried out through the years by placing high crowns or high restorations with arch wires and elastics that jiggled the tooth back and forth. Conclusions of these studies were that (in the absence of periodontal inflammation) these interferences induced a lesion of trauma with initial bone loss, subsequent repair, a widened periodontal ligament, tooth mobility, and no loss of cervical connective tissue periodontal attachment (Table 6-2-4).[105-107] Occlusal trauma became defined as injury to the attachment apparatus due to excessive occlusal forces.[30] When occlusal trauma and periodontitis were combined, a co-destruction theory was proposed,[108-110] with periodontitis and occlusal trauma together causing greater loss than periodontitis alone in Beagle dogs. Squirrel monkey studies did not fully substantiate

Table 6-2-3 Risk factors for temporomandibular disorders

Risk factors for TMDs	Occlusal risk factors	Occlusal deficiencies not qualified as risk factors
Gender/hormonal factors[72]	Anterior open bite[143] *f* Js	Deflective contacts[37-39,62],
Depression/somatization[72]	Unilateral crossbite[143] *f* Js	Occlusal interferences[37-39,62,70-72,88,124]
Multiple pain conditions/widespread pain[72] Ms Js	Overjet > 6–7 mm *f* Js [143,146,148]	Excessive vertical dimension[62]
Bruxism/oral parafunction Self-reported bruxism[71,72,130] Js	More than 5–6 missing posterior teeth[143] *f* Js	Overclosure
Trauma[130]	RCP–ICP slide >2 mm *f* Js[143]	Lack of posterior support No association[124,132] *f*
Vulnerable genotypes[131]	Dental wear[71]	Overbite/overjet No association[62,143,144]
	Loss of posterior support[132] *m* Js & Ms	
	Mandibular instability in ICP *f*[88] *m*[132]	

Key: f: female; m: male; Js: joint-related signs and symptoms; Ms: muscle-related signs and symptoms

Table 6-2-4 Animal occlusal trauma studies

Study	Animals	Experimental model	Time	Findings
Gottlieb and Orban[105]	Dogs n = 33	High crowns	12 hours to 13 months	Alveolar resorption after 24 hours
Box[106]	Sheep	High crown Periodontitis uncontrolled	104 days	Increased mobility Deepened pockets
Wentz et al[107]	Monkeys Maxillary second molar	Jiggling forces by high crown lingual arch wires. Periodontitis uncontrolled	2 to 6 months	Alveolar resorption and inflammation short term Adaptation widened PDL 3 to 6 months
Glickman & Smulow[108]	Rhesus monkey			Proposed co-destruction theory
Svanberg and Lindhe[109]	Beagle dogs n =14	Jiggling forces plus ligature induced periodontitis against controls	7, 24, 39, 280 days	Adaptation in non-periodontitis group. Inflammation and bone loss in periodontitis group
Lindhe & Svanberg[110]	Beagle dogs	Jiggling forces plus ligature-induced periodontitis against controls	10 months	Short term: no interaction Long term: 6 months increased bone loss periodontal lesion plus lesion of occlusal trauma
Meitner[111]	Squirrel monkeys n = 4	Tipping by elastics plus ligature periodontitis	20 weeks	No attachment loss when tipping and periodontitis were simultaneous Increased attachment loss due to addition of elastics
Polsen & Zander[112]	Squirrel monkeys n = 10	10 weeks of ligature periodontitis plus 10 weeks of elastics jiggling	10 weeks	Trauma (elastics) superimposed on existing infrabony pockets increased bone loss but did not affect the connective tissue attachment
Polson et al[113]	Squirrel monkeys	Jiggling (elastics) with and without ligature periodontitis	10 weeks and 20 weeks	Existing marginal inflammation inhibited the potential for bone regeneration from jiggling trauma
Ericsson & Lindhe[114]	Beagle dogs n = 8	Ligature periodontitis with and without jiggling trauma	12 months	Enhanced rate of destruction of the periodontium Periodontitis plus jiggling occlusal trauma

this theory (Table 6-2-4).[111-113] Beagle dog studies supported the theory of a zone of co-destruction occurring in the crestal attachment area when occlusal trauma and periodontitis were concurrent, together with increasing mobility.[110,114,115] The path of inflammation is altered with occlusal trauma, increasing mobility and periodontitis in the zone of co-destruction. This facilitates the spread and alters the pathway of plaque-associated inflammation into the deeper periodontal structure. A dog study showed increased bone loss and loss of cervical connective tissue attachment when jiggling trauma was combined with ligature periodontitis as compared with periodontitis alone for a prolonged time period.[114] There was increased periodontal ligament width, a reduced percentage of tissue volume of collagen, and an increased volume of vascular structure and leukocytes. Extrapolation of these findings to human occlusal trauma has been guarded. Some controversy remains regarding co-destruction. It is accepted that the superimposition of the lesion of occlusal trauma onto the lesion of inflammatory periodontitis will result in more bone loss than from periodontitis alone, but not necessarily with increased attachment loss.[110,112,115-117] Studies of excessive contacts in implants are varied. One dog study showed increased marginal bone loss with occlusal overload plus ligature peri-implantitis compared with peri-implantitis alone[118] (see Chapter 7).

In the year 2000, the American Academy of Periodontology published parameters of care on the diagnosis and treatment of periodontal diseases.[117] The following parameters were proposed: "Failure to treat occlusal traumatism appropriately in patients with chronic periodontitis may result in progressive loss of bone and an adverse change in prognosis." "The lesion of trauma from occlusion may occur in conjunction with, or independent of, inflammatory periodontal diseases." "Although trauma from occlusion and inflammatory periodontal disease may occur concurrently, each condition may be treated separately. The treatment goals and end points for each condition may be independent of each other. Occlusal therapy is generally addressed following, or in conjunction with, procedures to resolve the inflammatory lesions."[117]

Supporting tissue response to experimental occlusal interferences (EOIs) in humans

Clinically placed single restorations with premature or deflective contacts in MI can have an adverse effect on the supporting alveolar tissues.[39] The premature tooth may become sensitive primarily from periodontal and, more rarely, endodontic inflammation. The lesion of occlusal trauma may develop in the periodontium with compression, resorption, and eventual widening of the periodontal ligament space, widened lamina dura, condensing osteitis, and tooth mobility.

In single teeth, this effect may be transient, from several days to several weeks. Movement of the traumatized teeth away from the adverse occlusal force is described as pathologic tooth migration. If teeth are jiggled back and forth by alternating occlusal parafunctional forces they may remain mobile with increased mobility. No loss of connective

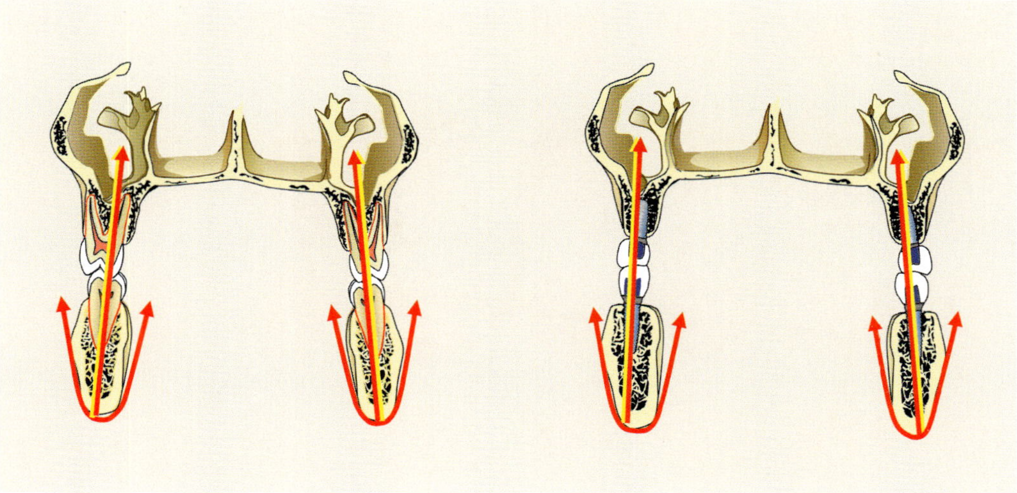

Fig 7-9 Loading of implants and teeth in maximum intercuspation. Direction and dissipation of force has conventionally been considered to be axial to the loaded implants. This is influenced by the relative intensity and synchronicity of the closing muscles and several other factors.

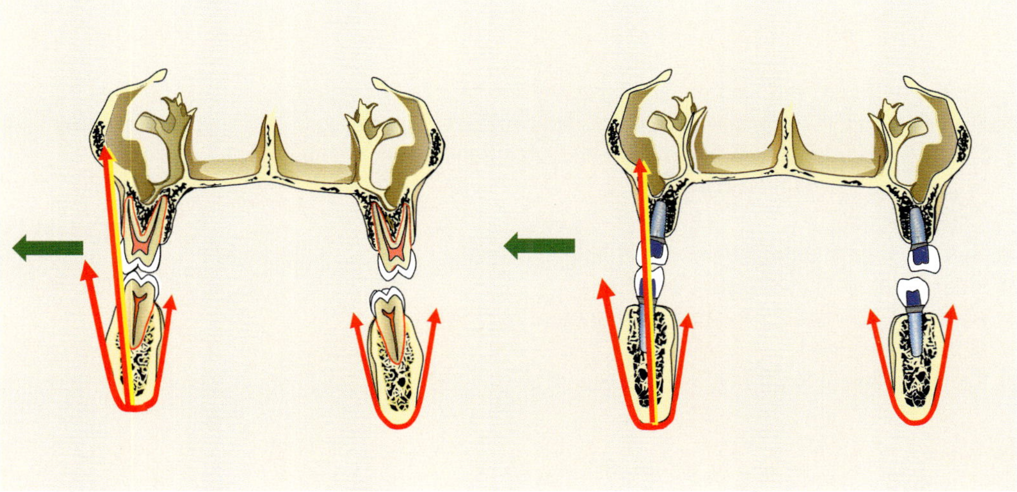

Fig 7-10 On lateral tooth-guided contact forces are directed to the buccal supporting structures for both teeth and implants.

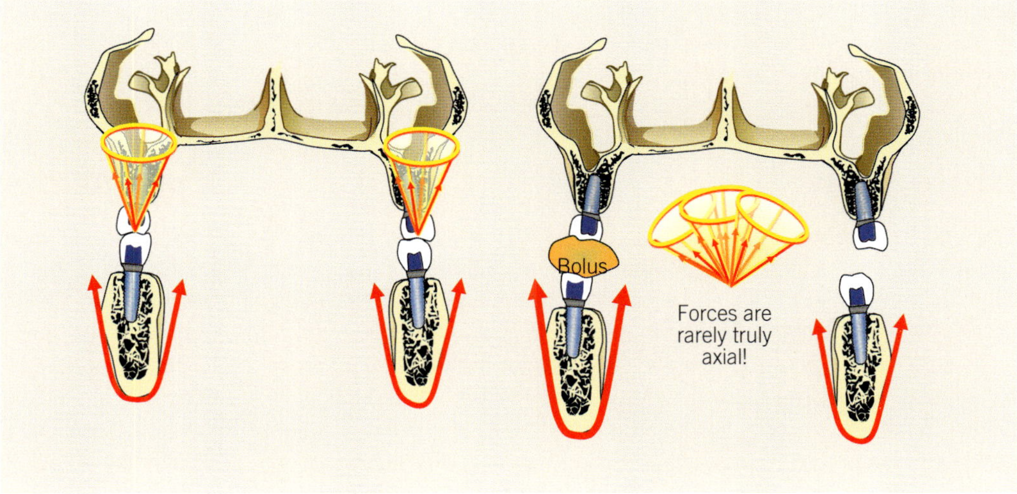

Fig 7-11 Axial force direction is rarely truly axial and is dependent on supporting interarch relations, alveolar and skeletal morphology, intensity of elevator muscular contraction, the relative degree of contraction and coordination between elevator muscles, and cuspal morphology. Forces may be multidirectional, as represented by all possible directions within cones (illustrated). Mastication of a bolus, incision and crushing, and excursive parafunction all increase the intensity and lateral direction of the occlusal forces.[29]

Implant neck geometry

Neck geometry and collar surface finish have been implicated as factors in marginal bone loss.[36,37] Neck geometry has varied over the years with straight, tapered, threaded and medialized with so-called platform switching and invagination.[38,39] The rationale of threaded necks was designed to improve the stress distribution at the neck in the cortical bone region and hence reduce load-induced cervical marginal bone loss. Following initial bone loss these become more prone to plaque accumulation.

Early marginal bone loss in the integration and healing phase

Some marginal bone loss around oral implants during the first year of function is a common observation.[40] This is seen radiologically as a horizontal reduction or a "saucerization" down to and often beyond the first threads with vertical loss of round 1 to 1.5 mm. A subsequent steady state with minimal bone loss of 0.2 mm per year is described.[30]

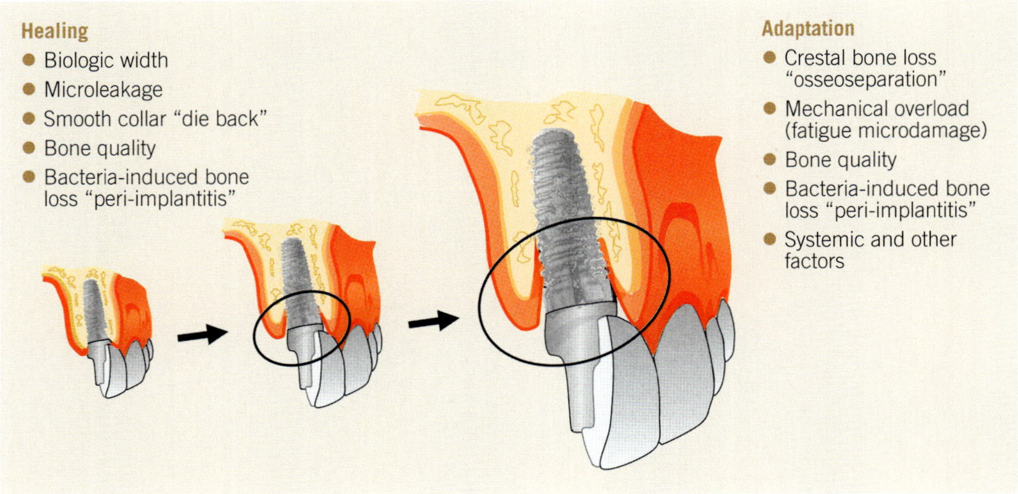

Fig 7-12 Initial marginal bone loss commonly occurs in the healing phase during first year of functional loading. Subsequent crestal bone loss in the subsequent adaptation phase can occur from a variety of factors.[40]

Several different possible causes have been postulated as possible contributory factors of early marginal bone loss in the healing phase (Fig 7-12). Their interaction with the foreign body reaction has been considered contributory to this early bone loss.[18]

These include:

- Surgical preparation of the implant bed
- Establishment of a biological width
- Apicocoronal level of the abutment/implant microgap
- Occlusal overload
- Configuration and surface finish of the implant neck

Additional bone density factors, bone volume, and buccolingual bone thickness have been implicated.[20,25,40] Following the healing phase the integrity of the bone–implant interface is maintained by a continuous process of adaptation. Crestal bone loss in the adaptation phase can occur from several factors,which may include mechanical overload and bacterial induced bone loss (Fig 7-12).

Biologic width

The interface between the implant, bone,and the gingiva has been shown to develop a biologic width that has been likened to the biologic width of teeth. An epithelial and connective tissue dimension has been demonstrated of varying lengths in several animal and human models.[41-43] The biologic need to establish a seal of the integument from the crestal BIC establishes this biologic seal.[41] With a reduction of gingival dimension, crestal bone was seen to resorb apically, which was described as a process that reestablished the biologic width. Initial bone resorption in clinical conditions has been ascribed to the biologic need to create biologic width.[41] This has also been shown to occur in models with no abutment–implant microgap interface. The question of whether the tissue can grow coronally or if the bone has to resorb apically is not clear.[41-44]

Smooth collar "dieback"

The necks of screw-type implants were traditionally left smooth and machined to reduce plaque retention and peri-implant inflammation. However, when the collar was placed below the crestal level of the bone, bone did not integrate to the flat machined surface and invariably resorbed down to either the first thread in machined screw-type implants or down to the machined rough surface border in implants with rougher surface axial walls. This process was formerly called "dieback".[44] The surface finish of the collar consequently has varied and has been machined and microtextured over varying time frames. Some implants were made with very short machined necks, others with machined necks and the first three threads, and yet others with microtextured surfaces up to the implant rim, according to the pervading concept.

Abutment implant interface microleakage

An additional variable purportedly affecting marginal bone loss is microgap microleakage. Several studies have shown that the internal chamber of implants is infected with viable bacteria and that fluid and bacterial interchange (microleakage) via the implant–abutment interface (microgap) is unavoidable.[45-47] This was shown to cause an inflammatory reaction at the implant–abutment interface in dogs.[47] The distance of the microgap to the bone crest was shown to affect the amount of bone loss in monkeys.[48] This microleakage was considered by some to have an effect on the bone loss down to the first thread in the first year of loading.

Platform switching

The concept of platform switching or medialization of the interface uses an abutment that is narrower than the implant platform and cervical diameter. The claim is that the increased distance of the microgap from the bone crest and medialization of the biologic width avoids the need for the bone to recede, creating a biologic width and reduces possible effects of microleakage.[38,39] Clinical outcome studies of the effects of these variables are varied and generally not supportive of any particular scheme over any other.

Frost's mechanostat model

The bone response to normal and excessive loading is significant in maintaining osseointegration.[21,23,49-53] A model of bone response to varying load intensity was proposed by Wolff; later the mechanostat model was developed by Frost (Fig 7-13).[21,51,52] This model is based on the response of a long bone and quantifies levels of load in physiologic, mild overload, and pathologic overload ranges. In the physiologic range, remodeling occurs. Remodeling is the process of continuous bone turnover, maintaining the morphology of the bone in a steady state. Modeling refers to a change in shape of the bone in response to mild overload. Positive modeling may occur as an increase in dimension or hypertrophy. Negative modeling may manifest as a decrease in dimension or resorption. This model is often extrapolated to the bone–implant interface.[21,49] Physiologic load of 800 to 1,500 μstrain is considered to maintain remodeling of the interface in a steady state.[23] Higher values

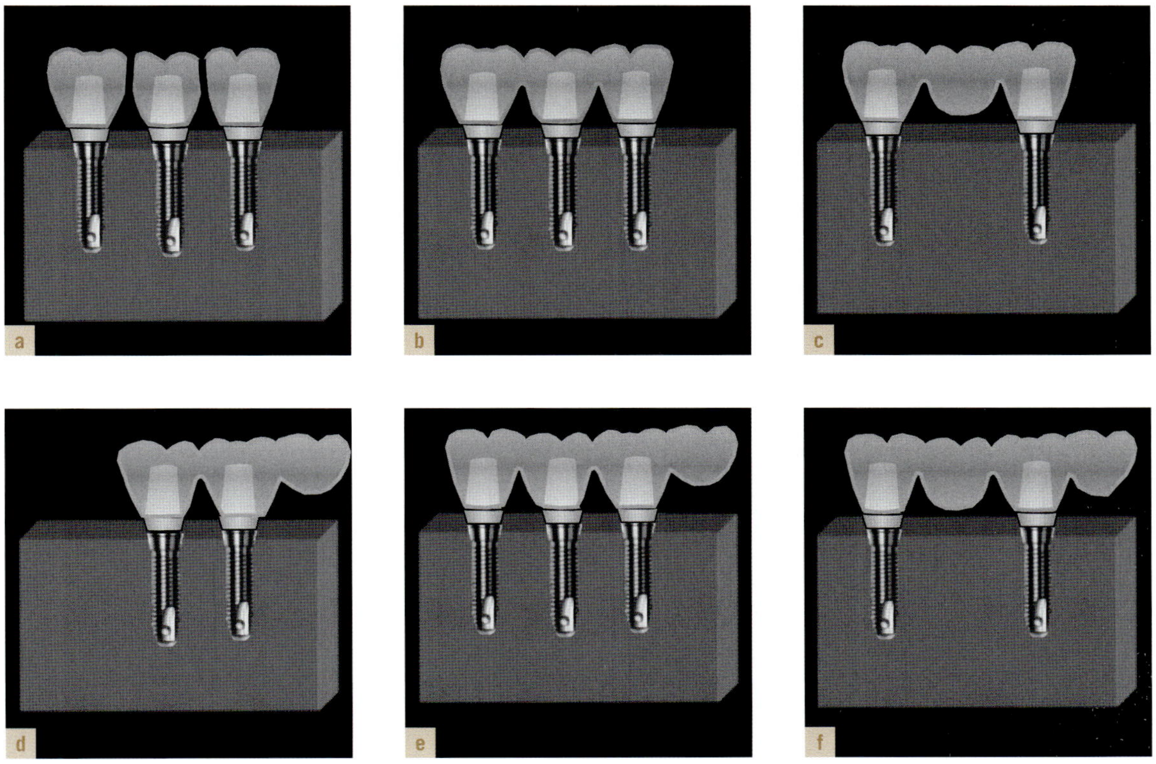

Fig 7-74 Varying superstructure designs. a Unconnected single restorations. b Three adjacent connected restorations. c Two spaced with interposed pontic. d Two adjacent wih cantilever. e Three adjacent connected with cantilever. f Two spaced with interposed pontic and cantilever.

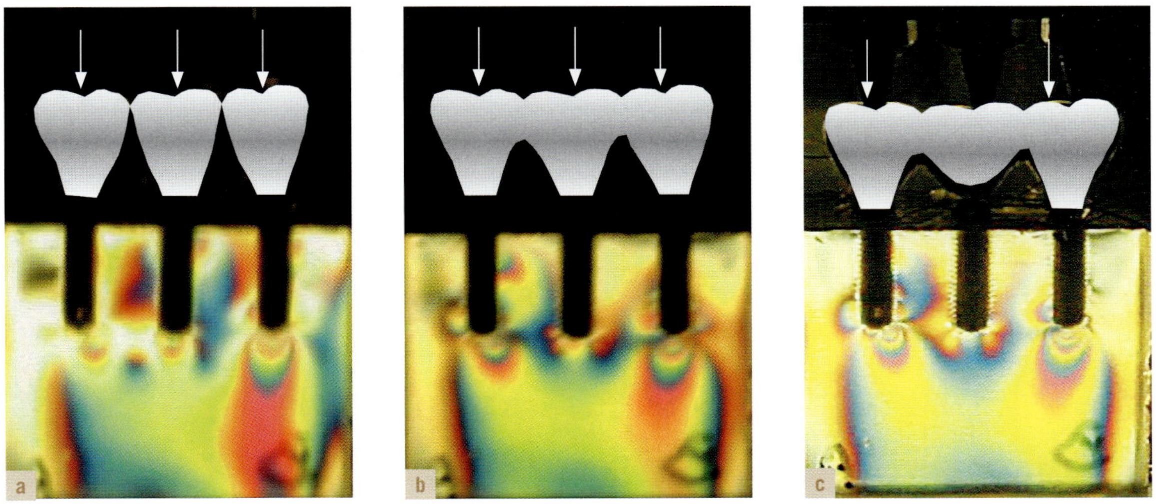

Fig 7-75 Photoelastic block models on axial loading showed less stress at implant apices for non-connected restoration a versus connected b Connected also showed greater stress than spaced with interposed pontic, c while non-connected showed the least stress of all three configurations.

strain gauges adhered to the implant necks. Different superstructure designs were loaded in a custom-loading frame axially and at 30 degrees. Abutment distribution, pontic and cantilever designs, C/I ratio, axial and non-axial loading, connected and unconnected restorations were tested.

Loading of 20 kg was simultaneous in the center of each implant restoration and pontic (Figs 7-73 to 7-79).[130,131]

30 degrees off-axis versus axial

Strain values from 30 degrees off-axis loading were significantly greater for all implants and for all restorations, compared with vertical loading ($P < 0.001$). The total strain for non-axial loading was eight times greater than for axial loading.

Spaced versus adjacent implants

Loaded models showed a tendency for spaced implants to produce similar if not better strain distributions than adjacent connected implants (Figs 7-75, 7-78, and 7-79).

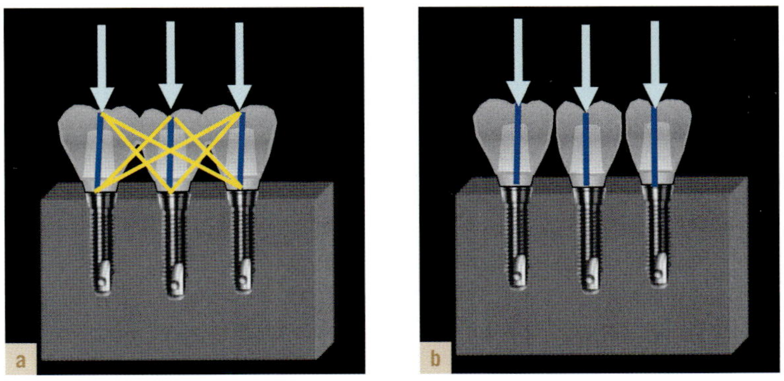

Fig 7-76a and b Increased moment arms (yellow) in connected restorations would cause greater strain levels at implant necks and supporting structures.

Crown-to-implant ratio

A 10-year clinical study showed that implant restorations with high C/I ratios, even in the range of 1:2 and 1:3, may be successful.[91] Splinting may reduce the deleterious potential of unfavorable C/I ratios.[49] Crown height space (CHS) may be more significant than C/I ratio. A CHS greater

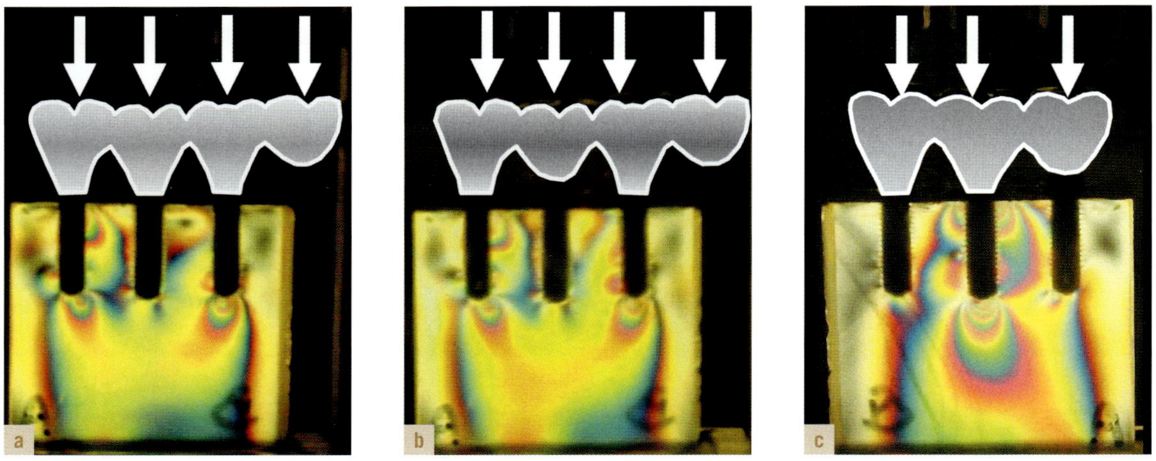

Fig 7-77 Photoelastic model shows the greatest stress is seen around the implant adjacent to the cantilever for two adjacent implants.

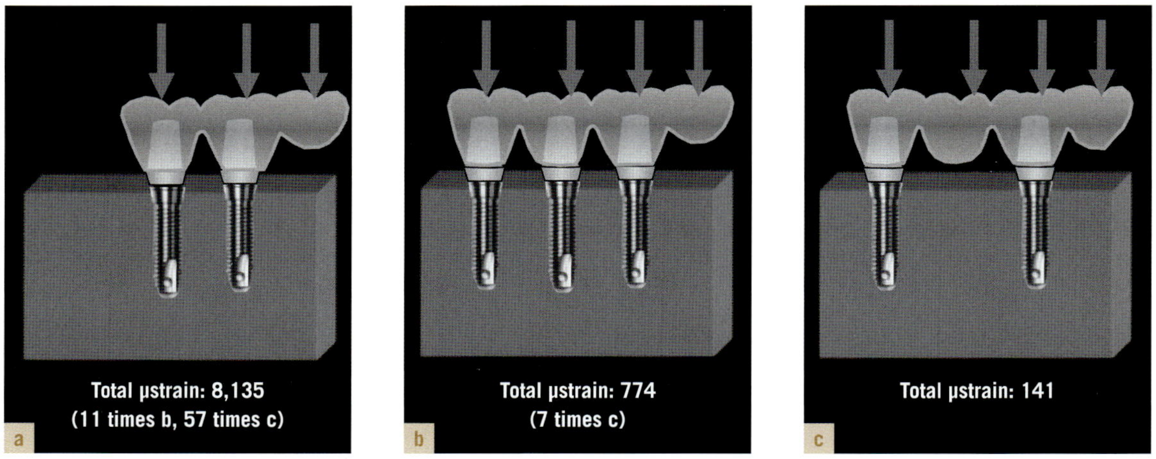

Fig 7-78 Total cervical strain values in µstrains for vertical loading of cantilevered restorations. a 8,135 µstrain for two adjacent, b 774 µstrain for 3 adjacent, and c 141 µstrain for spaced with interposed pontic. Total strain for spaced with mid pontic and cantilever (c) was 57 times less than for two implants adjacent to the cantilever.

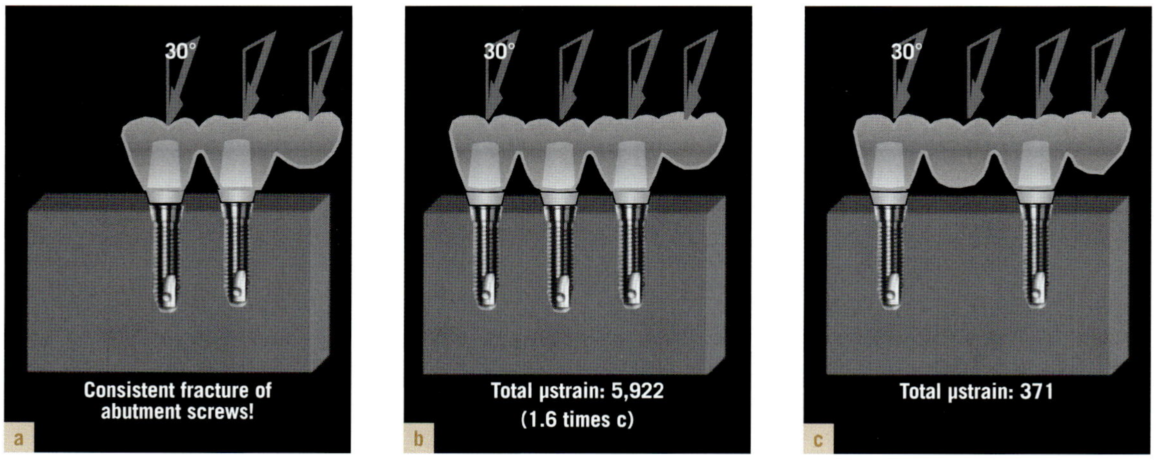

Fig 7-79 Total cervical strain values for 30 degree off-axis loading of cantilevered restorations. a Configurations with two adjacent implants suffered catastrophic failure with fracture of abutment screws at each loading b 5,922 µstrain for three adjacent implants, and c 371 µstrain for spaced implants (16 times less strain).

than 15 mm has been described as biomechanically unfavorable.[92] The results of the study (Fig 7-73) showed that crowns with low C/I ratio transferred lower stress than crowns with a higher C/I ratio up to 1:1.5. Force application at 30 degrees in cases with C/I ratio of 1:1.75 and 1:2 resulted in fracture of the abutment screw followed by dislodgement of the crowns. Crown height ranged from 10 to 20 mm. Failures were noted at crown height >15 mm when force application was at 30 degrees. Splinting increased cervical stresses and could not prevent prosthetic failure.

For both connected and unconnected restorations with C/I ratios greater than 1:1.5, the abutment screws fractured consistently.

Connected/unconnected crowns

Lower stresses were recorded for the unconnected crowns than for the connected crowns ($P < 0.001$). This may be explained by the fact that loading connected implants created moment arms on adjacent implants, as illustrated in Fig 7-76.

Cantilevers

For vertical loading of the FPD with a cantilever for different supporting implant numbers and distribution, the most unfavorable combination was on the two implants adjacent to the cantilever. The total strain at the implant necks for the two adjacent implants with a cantilever was 8,135 µstrain, as compared to 774 µstrain for three adjacent implants and 141 µstrain on two spaced implants (Fig 7-78). The load on the two adjacent implants was 11 times more than on three adjacent implants. While load on the two spaced implants was seven times less than on the three adjacent and 57 times less than on the two adjacent implants. For 30-degree loading, configurations with two adjacent implants had consistent fracture of the abutment screws. Total strain on three adjacent implants was 5,922 µstrain and 371 µstrain for the spaced implants, showing 16 times less strain (Fig 7-79).

8 Dental Articulators

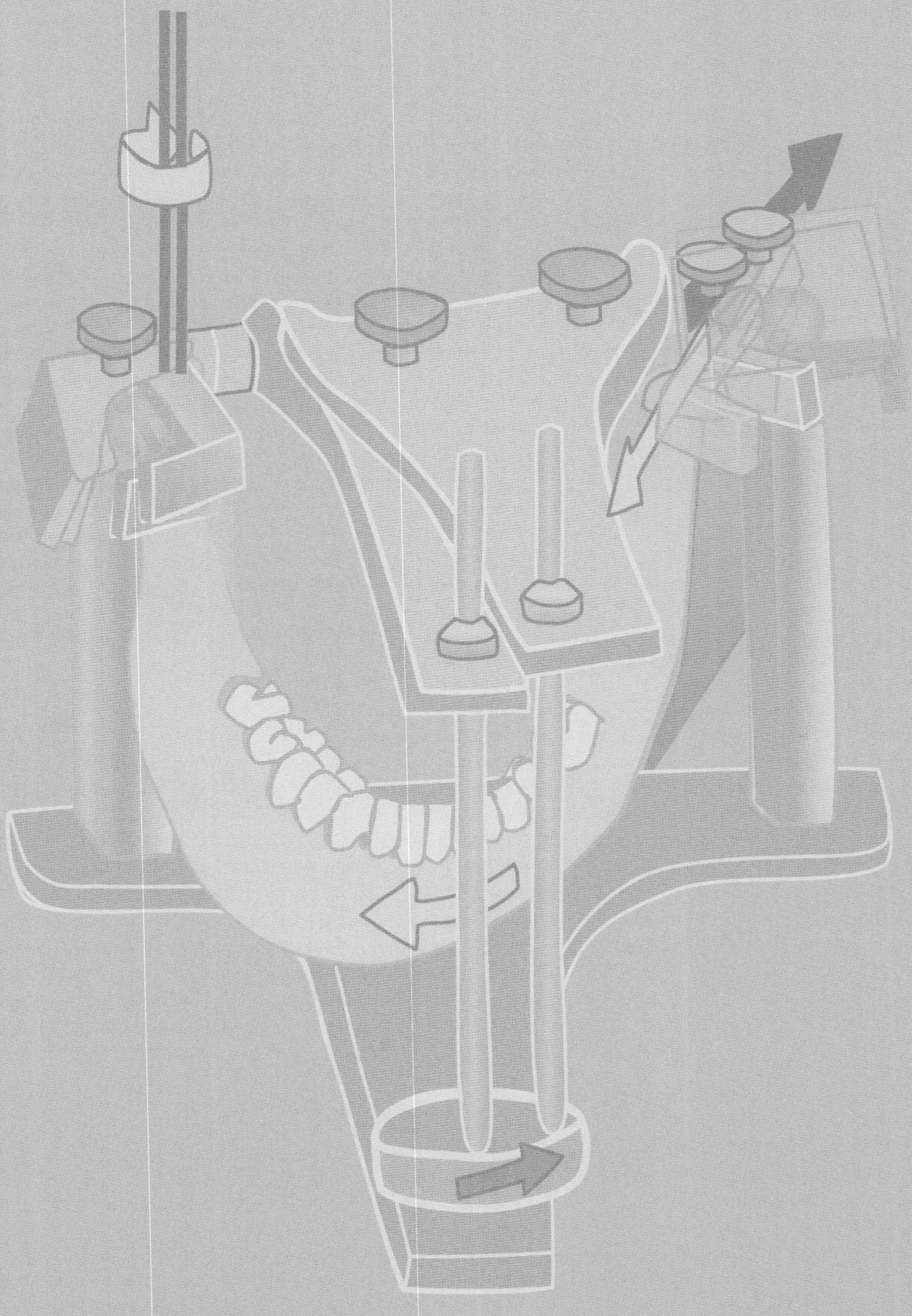

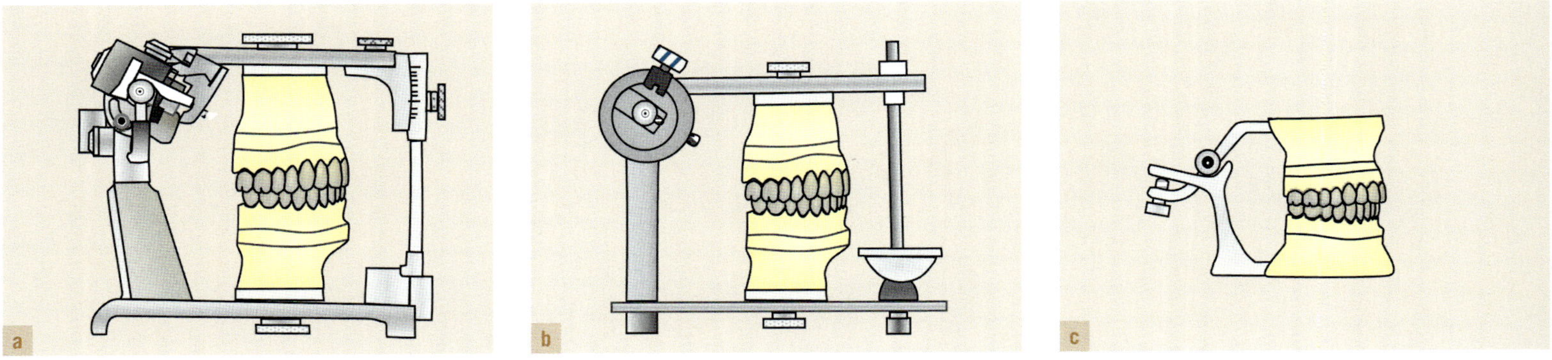

Fig 8-1 Articulators may be classified into three basic types: a fully adjustable, b semi-adjustable, and c plane line.

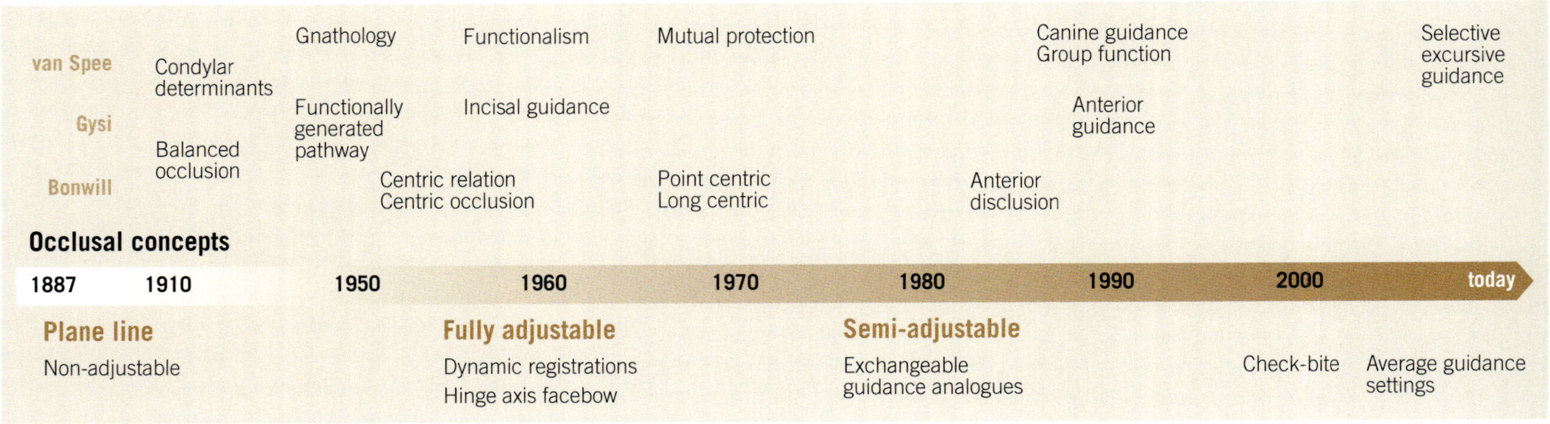

Fig 8-2 Evolution of occlusal concepts and articulators developed in conjunction. Conceptual paradigms regarding the clinical efficacy of articulators have been changing, with a trend away from complex articulator systems.

Contents

Articulator types

Dental articulators were developed as tools for use in the restoration of lost and missing components of the dentition. Three basic articulator types emerged: plane line, non-adjustable, semi-adjustable and fully adjustable (Fig 8-1). The development and use of each type of articulator grew and receded with an associated therapeutic concept. Plane line instruments have fixed condylar guide mechanisms on a plane line and are generally small and do not have a facebow transfer facility. Semi-adjustable instruments have a facebow transfer facility and mostly have flat condylar guide mechanisms with sagittal condylar guidance inclination and Bennett angle adjustments. These can be adjusted according to protrusive and lateral interocclusal registrations. Fully adjustable instruments were developed with condylar guide mechanisms set according to mechanical pantographic, stereographic, and later electronic dynamic registration systems.[1-3] Virtual digital systems are in the developmental stages for application with other digital technologies.

Definitions

Many different articulators are available today. They may be classified in various ways according to their analogical properties, or according to their ability to vary some of the determinants of mandibular movements. A useful division is of fully adjustable, semi-adjustable, and plane line articulators.[1-7]

Evolution of dental articulators and occlusal concepts

Over the years, articulators have been used in prosthodontics as analogues of mandibular closure and movement for the restoration of lost and depleted dentition. As occlusal concepts developed, instruments changed from initial plane line non-adjustable to semi-adjustable and fully adjustable. Generally, occlusal concepts came to be associated with particular articulator types (Fig 8-2).

The manufacturing of these three basic varieties of articulator has continued to date, although with modifications. From 1887 to 1920, occlusal concepts centered around denture occlusion. Balanced occlusion emerged as the optimal occlusion model for complete dentures. This required an articulator that moved in excursions, with some semblance of condylar guidance.

The need to reproduce the condylar guidance led to the development of semi-adjustable instruments that were set using protrusive and lateral interocclusal registrations.

The era of fully adjustable articulators with dynamic registrations and condylar settings passed through a mechanical stage to an electronic stage and has seen a gradual recession in popularity. These were associated with concepts of so-called "gnathologists," who believed that the accurate articulator settings of condylar determinants and the mandibular side shift had to be incorporated into the guiding inclinations of restorations. It was believed that freedom to reach the borders of movement was important and that the incorporation of these determinants would prevent dysfunction and avoid so-called occlusal-related problems.[8-18] Intermediate systems with replaceable curved condylar guide mechanisms set from dynamic registrations are still in use.

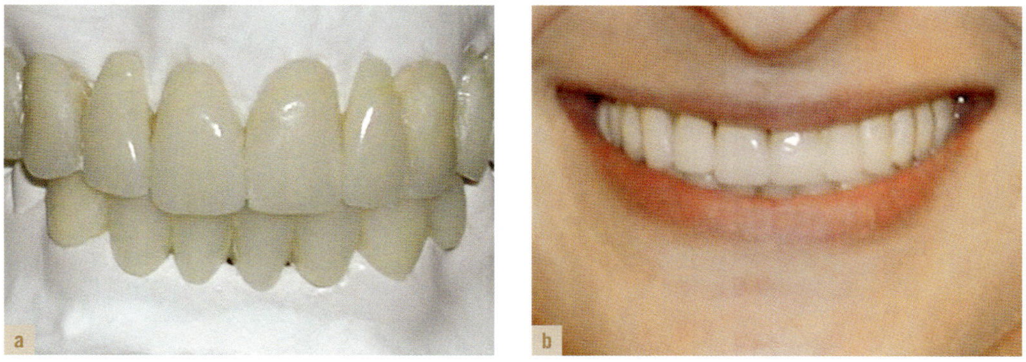

Fig 10-35a Corrective wax-up for provisional restorations with anterior vertical overlap with esthetic anterior and posterior occlusal planes. b Provisional restorations fitted, showing esthetic appearance.

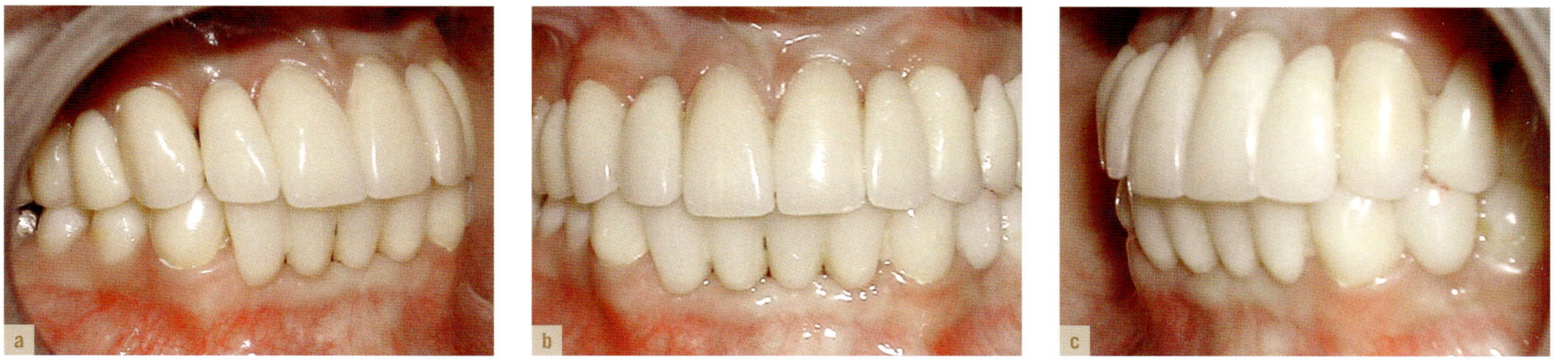

Fig 10-36a to c Provisional restorations in the mouth.

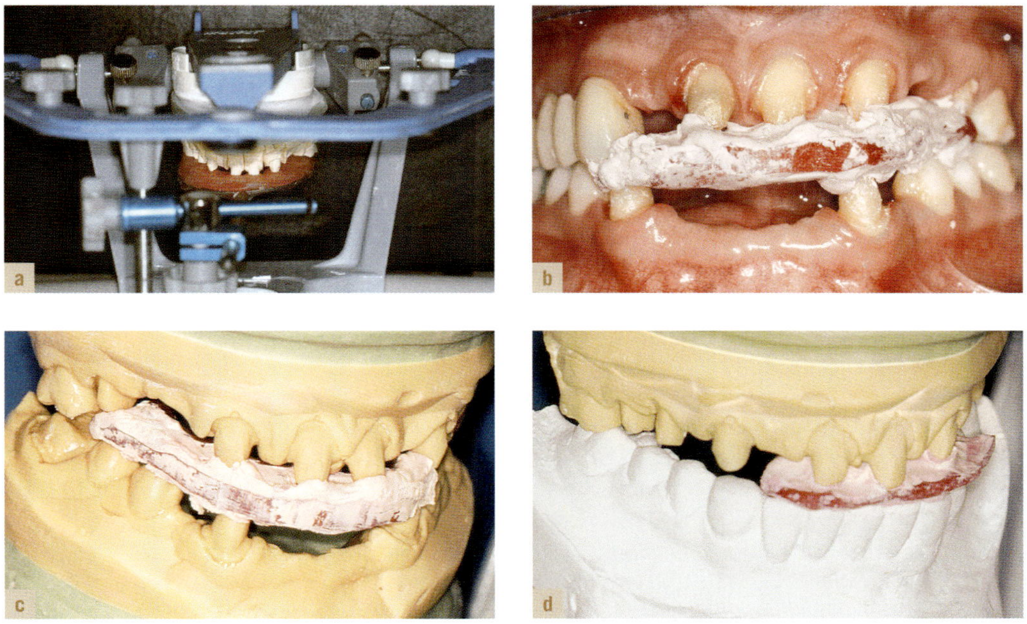

Fig 10-37a Facebow mounting of the maxillary working cast. b Centric relation record at the correct vertical dimension. c Working casts mounted in centric relation. d Upper working cast cross-mounted in CR against the lower provisional cast.

The treatment protocol is based on periodontal, esthetic, and prosthetic considerations. In this case, normal preparation and crown margins were used.[60,61]

Provisional restorations

A corrective wax-up for the provisional restorations was made with an anterior vertical overlap. Protrusive and lateral guidance were waxed in relation to anterior esthetically dictated crown length and vertical overlap and to condylar articulator guidance set by protrusive check records (Fig 10-35a). Provisional restorations were fabricated and fitted (Figs 10-35 and 10-36). Esthetics and occlusion were adjusted and the patient allowed to function with the provisional restorations for several months. With the patient happy with her esthetics and function, the determinants were transferred from the provisional restorations to the final restorations (Figs 10-37 to 10-43).

Provisional restorations to final restoration

Full-arch impressions and final working casts with appropriate die indexing and margin identification were made. The maxillary cast was mounted to a semi-adjustable articulator using an ear-piece facebow with a nasion third reference point. Centric relation records were taken at the original OVD and the working mandibular cast mounted against the maxillary working cast (Fig 10-37). A process of cross-mounting was

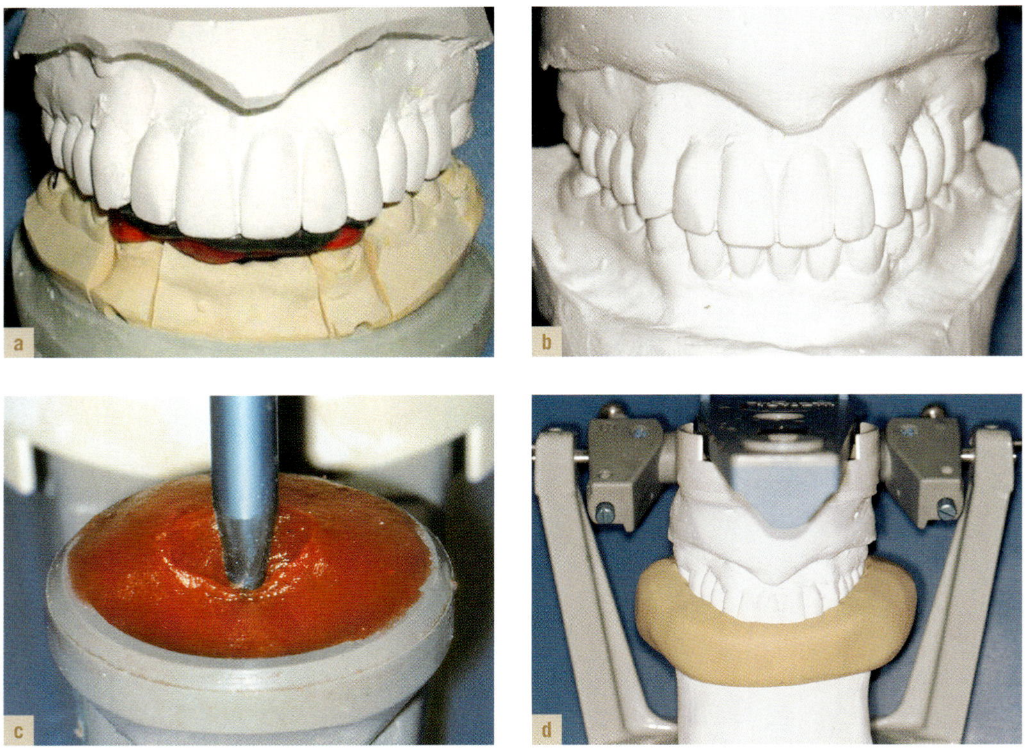

Fig 10-38a Lower working cast cross-mounted against upper provisional cast. b Upper and lower provisional casts are now mounted in centric relation. c Custom incisal guidance table molded in acrylic from excursive movements of the provisional casts. d Occlusal silicone index is made from opposing provisional casts.

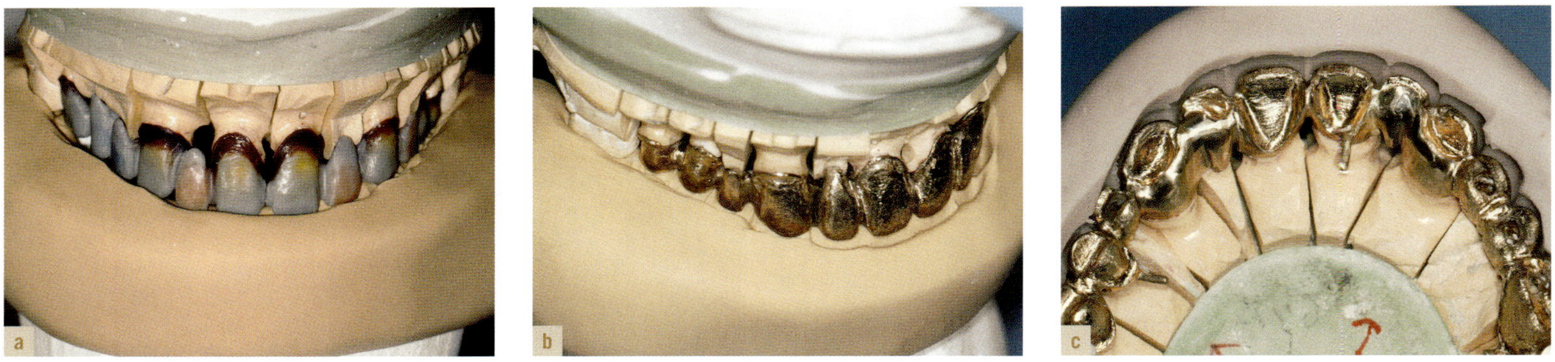

Fig 10-39a Maxillary cast cross-mounted with lower provisional and occlusal silicone index of upper provisional. Wax-up of maxillary restoration relative to the provisional maxillary occlusal index b Metal castings in relation to the occlusal index. c Metal castings in relation to the facial index.

then carried out, which allowed for the correct relation of the working casts to the opposing casts of the provisional restorations. Intraoral interocclusal records were made in centric relation at the correct vertical dimension of the maxillary prepared teeth against the lower provisionals *in situ*. The cast of the mandibular provisionals was mounted against the maxillary working cast (Fig 10-37d). Interocclusal CR records were also made of the mandibular prepared arch without the provisional against the upper arch with the provisionals in position. The lower working cast was then mounted against the maxillary provisional cast (Fig 10-38a). With the whole cross-mounting process carried out accurately, the provisional casts were accurately related in centric relation/MI (Fig 10-38b). The casts were interchanged with accurate relation of both working casts to opposing casts of the provisional restorations. A custom incisal guidance index was molded in acrylic as the incisal guide pin was moved with the upper articulator member guided in all lateral, lateroprotrusive, and protrusive excursions by the provisional casts (Fig 10-38c). Buccal and occlusal silicone indexes were fabricated from the mounted casts of the provisional restorations. The buccal index was made by pressing silicone putty up against the buccal surfaces of the mounted maxillary and mandibular provisional casts. The occlusal index was made by placing a roll of putty on the occlusal surfaces of the lower provisional cast and closing the upper provisional cast down against the lower provisional cast (Fig 10-38d). The occlusal index contained the occlusal imprint of both provisional casts and can be related at will to opposing working casts. One provisional cast was replaced with the corresponding working cast that was in correct relation to the mounted buccal or occlusal silicone index (Figs 10-39 and 10-40). Restorations could then be waxed up by additive or cut-back techniques related to the appropriate silicone indices and their castings tested to verify desired dimensions and space for porcelain (Fig 10-39). Final porcelain veneers were then created, also in relation to the desired facial and occlusal relations of the provisional casts as created by the buccal and occlusal indexes and by occlusion with the cross-mounted provisional casts (Fig 10-40). Esthetic corrections and occlusal fine tuning was carried out intraorally in the bisque stage. The final restoration can be seen in Figs 10-41 to 10-43.

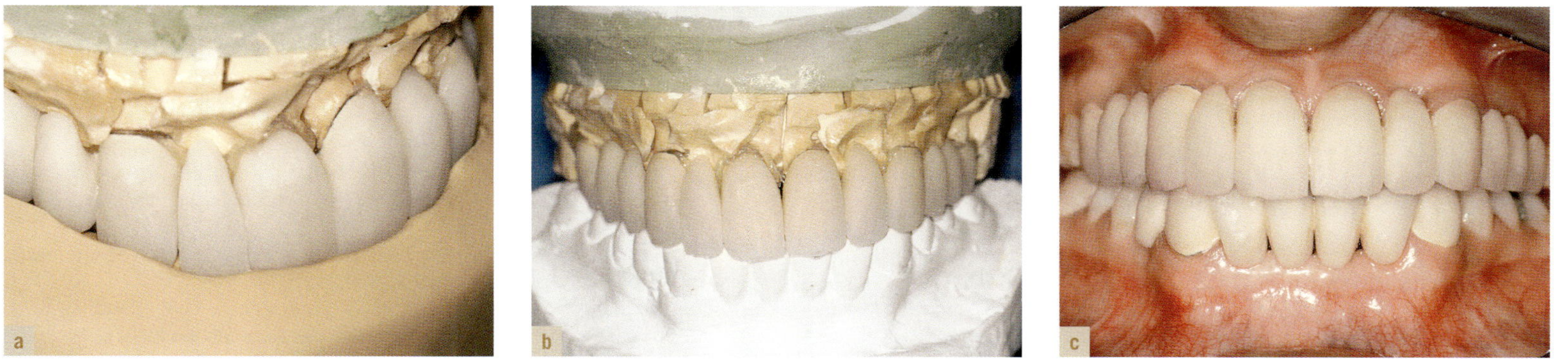

Fig 10-40a and b Porcelain fabricated in relation to occlusal silicone index, and to opposing cross-mounted cast of provisional restoration c Bisque try-in of porcelain for esthetic adjustment and occlusal fine tuning.

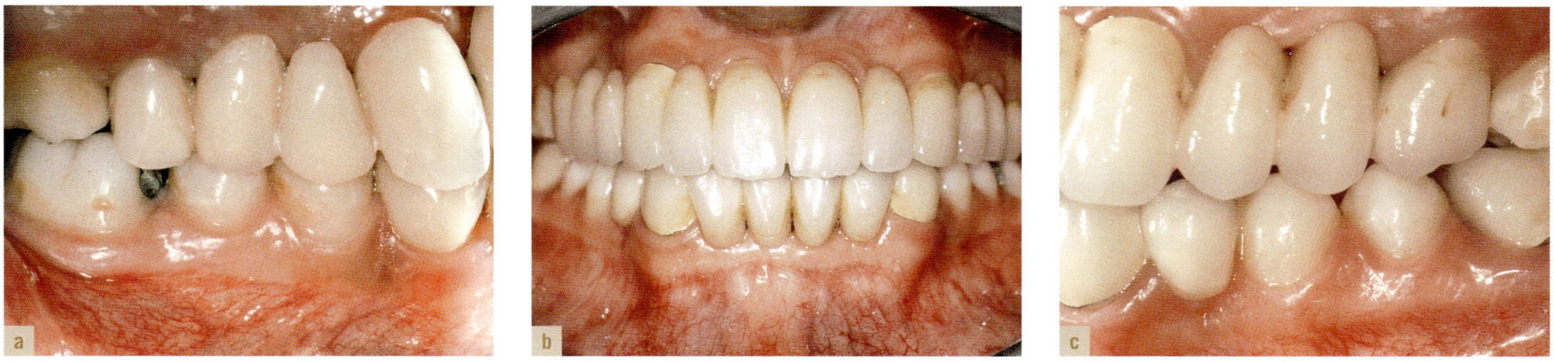

Fig 10-41a to c Final porcelain restorations in maximum intercuspation.

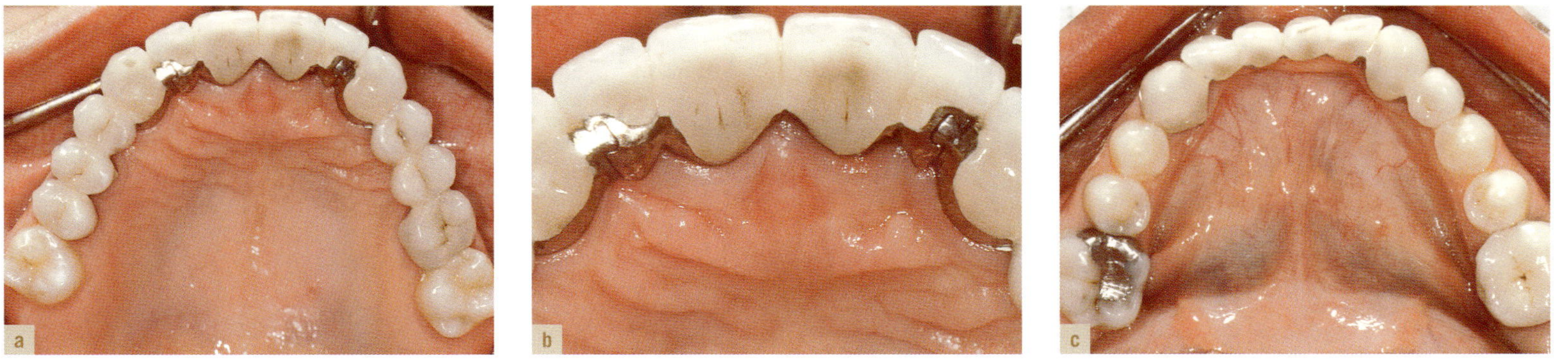

Fig 10-42a to c Occlusal views of final restorations. Interlock attachments on distal of maxillary second incisor pontics.

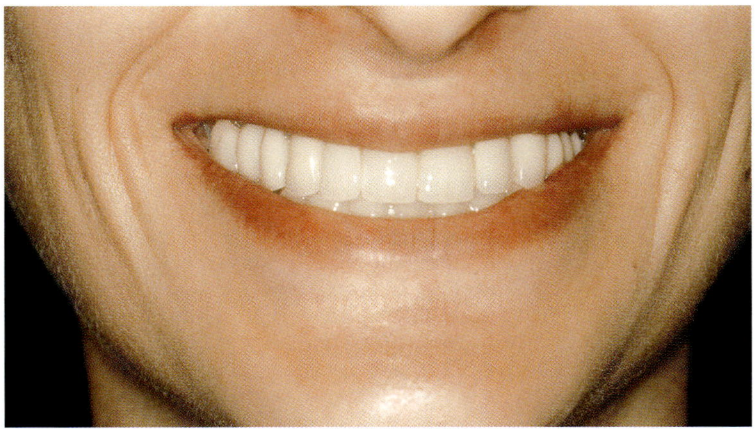

Fig 10-43 Final esthetic result. (Images courtesy of Dr O Ghelfan.)

References

1. Dunn WJ, Murchison DF, Broome JC. Esthetics: patient's perceptions of dental attractiveness. J Prosthet Dent 1996;5:166–171.
2. Fraedani MD, Barducci G. Esthetic Rehabilitation in Fixed Prosthodontics. Chicago: Quintessence Publishing, 2008.
3. Chiche GJ. Esthetics of Anterior Fixed Prosthodontics. Chicago: Quintessence Publishing, 1994.
4. Goldstien R. Esthetics in Dentistry Volume I: Principles, Communications, Treatment Methods. Hamilton: BC Decker, 1998.
5. Schmidt KL, Cohn JF. Human facial expressions as adaptations: Evolutionary questions in facial expression research. Am J Phys Anthropol 2001;116:[Suppl 33]:3–24.
6. Rich B, Goldstein GR. New paradigms in prosthodontic treatment planning: A literature review. J Prosthet Dent 2002;88:208–214.
7. The glossary of prosthodontic terms. J Prosthet Dent 2005;94:10–92.
8. American College of Prosthodontists. Parameters of care for the specialty of prosthodontics. J Prosthodont 2005;14(Suppl 1):1–103.
9. Stohler CS. Clinical decision-making in occlusion: a paradigm shift. In: McNeill C (ed). Science and Practice of Occlusion. Chicago: Quintessence Publishing, 1997:294–305.
10. Ash MM. Paradigmatic shifts in occlusion and temporomandibular disorders. J Oral Rehabil 2001;28:1–13.
11. Pokorny P, Weins JP, Litvak H. Occlusion for fixed prosthodontics – a historical perspective of the gnathological influence. J Prosthet Dent 2008;99:299–313.
12. Klineberg I, Kingston D, Murray, G. The bases for using a particular occlusal design in tooth and implant-borne reconstructions and complete dentures. Clin Oral Implants Res 2007;18(Suppl 3):151–167.
13. Beyron H. Characteristics of functionally optimal occlusion and principles of occlusal rehabilitation. J Am Dent Assoc 1954;48:648–656.
14. Beyron H. Occlusion: point of significance in planning restorative procedures. J Prosthet Dent 1973;30:641–652.
15. Beyron H. Optimal occlusion. Dent Clin North Am 1969 Jul;13:537–554.
16. Klineberg I, Stohler CS. Study group report and discussion. Int J Prosthodont 2003;16(Suppl):89–90.
17. Milner M. Musculoskeletal disorders and the occlusal interface. Int J Prosthodont 2005;18:297–299.
18. Carlsson GE. Some dogmas related to prosthodontics, temporomandibular disorders and occlusion. Acta Odontol Scand 2010;68:313–322.
19. Mohl ND. Diagnostic rationale: an overview. In: Mohl N, Zarb GA, Carlsson GE, Rugh JD (eds). A Textbook of Occlusion. Chicago, IL: Quintessence; 1988:179–184.
20. Eckert SE, Choi YG, Koka S. Methods for comparing the results of different studies. Int J Oral Maxillofac Implants 2003;18:697–705.
21. Jacob RF, Carr AB. Hierarchy of research design used to categorize the "strength of evidence" in answering clinical dental questions. J Prosthet Dent 2000;83:137–152.
22. Lang NP, Pjetursson BE, Tan K, Bragger U, Egger M, Zwahlen M. A systematic review of the survival and complication rates of fixed partial dentures (FPDs) after an observation period of at least 5 years. II. Combined tooth implant-supported FPDs. Clin Oral Implants Res 2004;15:643–653.
23. Libby G, Arcuri MR, LaVelle WE, Hebl L. Longevity of fixed partial dentures. J Prosthet Dent 1997;78:127–131.
24. Scurria MS, Bader JD, Shugars DA. Meta-analysis of fixed partial denture survival: prostheses and abutments. J Prosthet Dent 1998;79:459–464.
25. Lindquist E, Karlsson S. Success rate and failures for fixed partial dentures after 20 years of service: Part I. Int J Prosthodont 1998;11:133–138.
26. Pjetursson BE, Lang NP. Prosthetic treatment planning on the basis of scientific evidence. J Oral Rehabil 2008;35(Suppl 1):72–79.
27. Torbjörner A, Fransson B. A literature review on the prosthetic treatment of structurally compromised teeth. Int J Prosthodont 2004;17:369–376.
28. de Backer HG, Decock V, van der Berghe L. Long-term survival of complete crowns, fixed dental prostheses, and cantilever fixed dental prostheses with post and cores on root canal-treated teeth. Int J Prosthodont 2007;20:229–234.
29. Walton TR. An up to 15-year longitudinal study of 515 metal-ceramic FPDs: Part 1. Oucome. Int J Prosthodont 2002;15:439–445.
30. Shillingburg HT Jr, Hobo S, Whitsett LD, Jacobi R, Brackett SE. Fundamentals of Fixed Prosthodontics, ed 3. Chicago: Quintessence Publishing, 1997:85–118.
31. Oruc S, Eraslan O, H. Alper Tukay A, Atay A, Stress analysis of effects of non rigid connectors on fixed partial dentures with pier abutments. J Prosthet Dent 2008 Mar;99:185–192.
32. McGuire MK. A long-term survey of 100 treated periodontal patients under maintenance care. J Periodontol 1991;62:51–58.
33. McGuire MK, Nunn ME. Prognosis versus actual outcome II: the effectiveness of commonly taught clinical parameters in developing an accurate prognosis. J Periodontol 1996;67:658–665.
34. McGuire MK, Nunn ME. Prognosis versus actual outcome III: the effectiveness of clinical parameters in accurately predicting tooth survival. J Periodontol 1996;67:666–674.
35. Faggion CM Jr, Petersilka G, Lange DE, Gerss J, Flemmig TF. Prognostic model for tooth survival in patients treated for periodontitis. J Clin Periodontol 2007;34:226–231.
36. Ante IH. The fundamental principles, design and construction of crown and bridge prosthesis. Dent Item Int 1928;50:215–232.
37. Lulic M, Bragger U, Lang NL, Zwahlen M, Salvi M, GE. Ante's (1926) law revisited: a systematic review on survival rates and complications of fixed dental prostheses (FDPs) on severely reduced periodontal tissue support. Clin Oral Implants Res 2007;18(Suppl 3):63–72.
38. Leles CR, Morandini W, Silva ET, Nunes MF, Freire MC. Assessing perceived potential outcomes of prosthodontic treatment in partial and fully edentulous patients. J Oral Rehabil 2008;35:682–689.
39. Libby G, Arcuri MR, LaVelle WE, Hebl L. Longevity of fixed partial dentures. J Prosthet Dent 1997;78:127–131.
40. Scurria MS, Bader JD, Shugars DA. Meta-analysis of fixed partial denture survival: prostheses and abutments. J Prosthet Dent 1998;79:459–464.
41. Lindquist E, Karlsson S. Success rate and failures for fixed partial dentures after 20 years of service: Part I. Int J Prosthodont 1998;11:133–138.
42. Palmqvist S, Soderfeldt B. Multivariate analyses of factors influencing the longevity of fixed partial dentures, retainers, and abutments. J Prosthet Dent 1994;71:245–250.
43. Greene C. Concepts of TMD etiology: effects on diagnosis and treatment. In: Laskin DM, Greene C, Hylander WL (eds). TMDs: An Evidence-based Approach to Diagnosis and Treatment. Chicago: Quintessence Publishing, 2006.
44. Dawson PE. Position paper regarding diagnosis, management, and treatment of temporomandibular disorders. J Prosthet Dent 1999;81:174–178.
45. De Boever JA, Carlsson GE, Klineberg IJ. Need for occlusal therapy and prosthodontic treatment in the management of temporomandibular disorders. Part I. Occlusal interferences and occlusal adjustment. J Oral Rehabil 2000;27:367–379.
46. Svensson P, Jadidi T, Arima L, Baad-Hansen, Sessle B. Relationships between craniofacial pain and bruxism. J Oral Rehabil 2008;35:524–547.
47. Marklund S, Wanman A. A century of controversy regarding the benefit or detriment of occlusal contacts on the mediotrusive side. J Oral Rehabil 2000;27:553–562.
48. Clark GT, Tskiyama Y, Baba K, Watanabe T Sixty-eight years of experimental occlusal interference studies: What have we learned. J Prosthet Dent 1999;82:704–713.
49. Bush F. Occlusal etiology of myofascial pain dysfunction syndrome. In Laskin D: The President's Conference on the Examination, Diagnosis and Management of Temporomandibular Disorders. Michigan: University of Michigan,1982:98–103.
50. Jorgensen KD. The relationship between retention and convergence angle in cemented veneer crowns. Acta Odontol Scand 1955;13 35–40.
51. Wiskott HW, Nicholls JI, Belser UC. The relationship between abutment taper and resistance of cemented crowns to dynamic loading. Int J Prosthodont 1996;9:117–130.
52. Gilboe DB, Teteruck WR. Fundamentals of extracoronal tooth preparation. Part I. Retention and resistance form. J Prosthet Dent 1974;32:651–656.
53. Hegdahl T, Silness J. Preparation areas resisting displacement of artificial crowns. J Oral Rehabil 1977;4:201–207.
54. Barkhordar RA, Radke R, Abbasi J. Effect of metal collars on resistance of endodontically treated teeth to root fracture. J Prosthet Dent 1989;61:676–678.
55. Hemmings KW, King PA, Setchell DJ. Resistance to torsional forces of various post and core designs. J Prosthet Dent 1991;66:325–329.
56. Sorensen JA, Engelman MJ. Ferrule design and fracture resistance of endodontically treated teeth. J Prosthet Dent 1990;63:529–536.
57. Morgano SM. Restoration of pulpless teeth: application of traditional principles in present and future contexts. J Prosthet Dent 1996;75:375–380.
58. Assif D, Gorfil C. Biomechanical considerations in restoring endodontically treated teeth. J Prosthet Dent 1994;71:565–567.
59. Nissan J, Parson A, Barnea E, Shifman A, Assif D. Resistance to fracture of crowned endodontically treated premolars restored with ceramic and metal post systems. Quintessence Int 2007;38:e120–123.
60. Coslet JG, Vanarsdall R, Weisgold A. Diagnosis and classification of delayed passive eruption of the dentogigival junction in the adult. Alpha Omegan 1977;70:24–28.
61. Weinberg MA, Eskow RN. An overview of delayed passive eruption. Compend Contin Educ Dent 2000 Jun;21:511–514, 516, 518.

12 State of the Art: Esthetic Perspectives

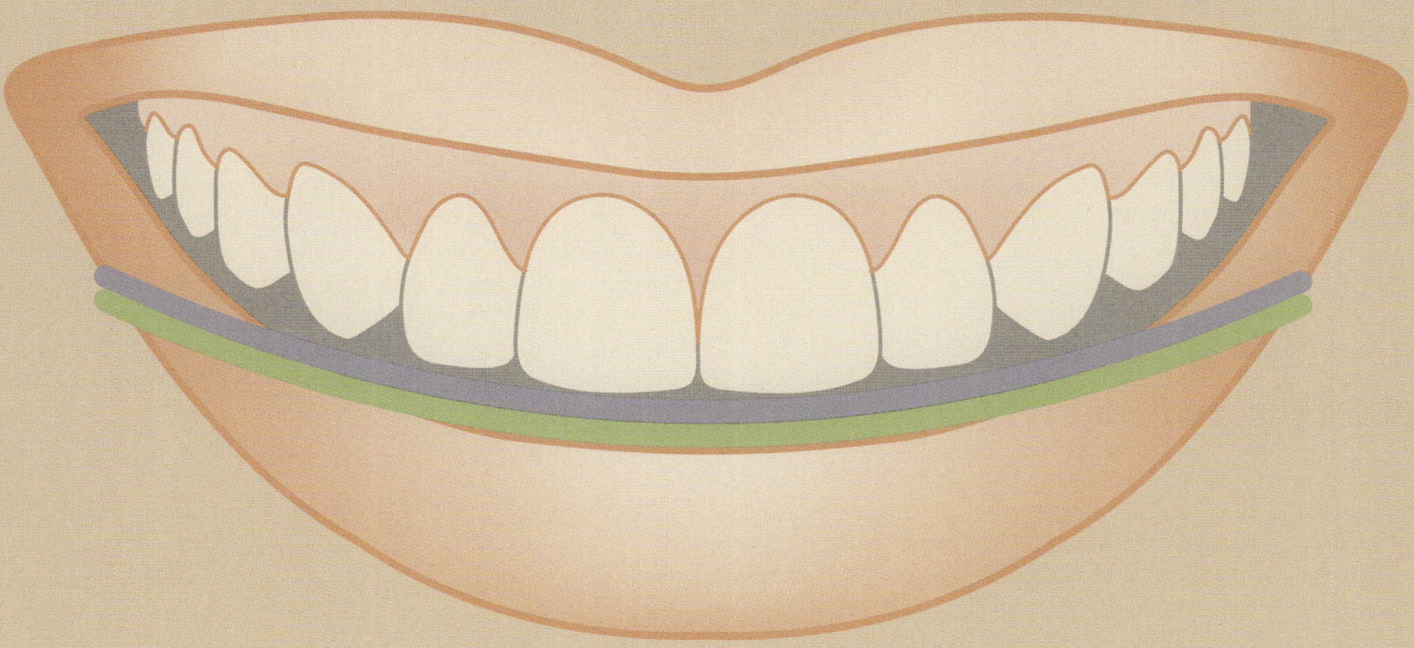

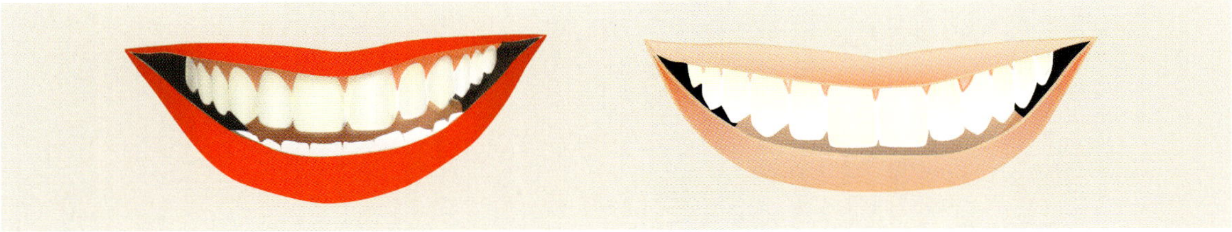

Fig 12-1 Alpha smiles. These have light colored teeth, radiating symmetry with smile lines showing maxillary gingival papillae, gingival line, and esthetic occlusal planes in harmony with upper and lower lip lines.

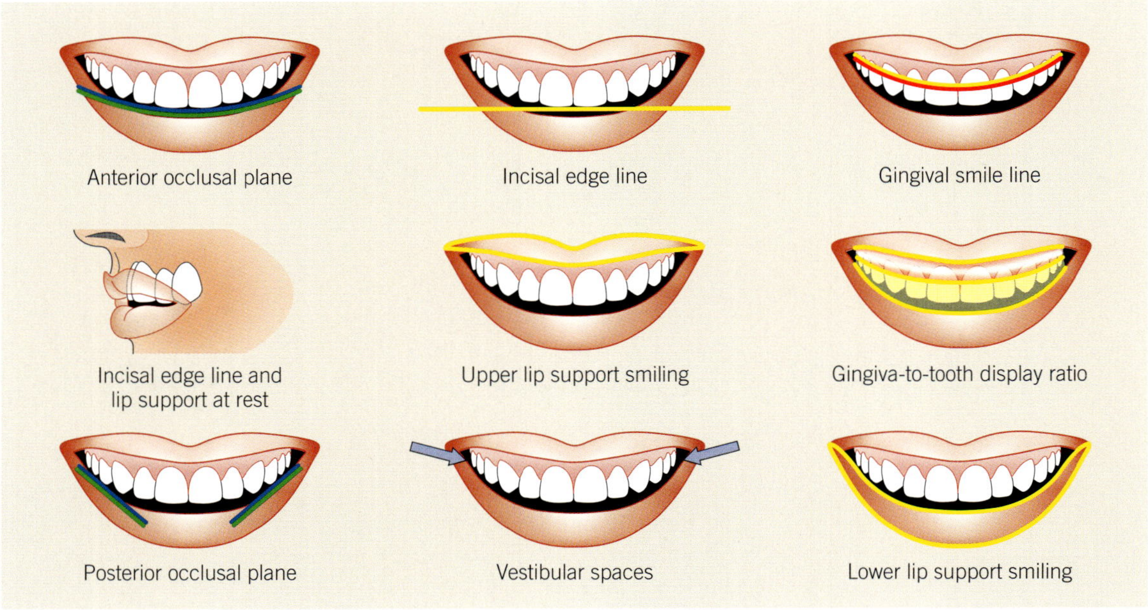

Fig 12-2 Nine esthetic determinants.

Contents

Esthetics and occlusion

Facial factors in individual clinical

Facial factors are significant components of the individual clinical determinants that determine the planning and outcome of oral rehabilitation. They may constitute the interactions of face height, vertical dimension, and orofacial esthetics. Orofacial appearance can include facial morphology, symmetry/asymmetry, proportions, lip support, tooth display, and gingival display. Dental characteristics of tooth display and gingival display in the orofacial window are most apparent on smiling. The dental and gingival characteristics of the smile are important esthetic determinants and are illustrated in Figs 12-1 and 12-2.

Esthetics play an integral role in the interrelation of the individual clinical determinants as they relate to oral rehabilitation. Considerations of esthetics for oral rehabilitation, while being highly subjective and dependent on geographic, cultural, personal, psychosocial, and self-image factors, may still be based on certain principles or norms. The perception of esthetics is based on the recognition of the average as normal and the absence of asymmetry and significant disproportion.[1-4] The perception of a class I appearance is analogous to the class I skeletal and dental model, representing an idealized statistical norm or "alpha" median. Deviations from this artificial norm serve as description of variation as "esthetic variants" (Box 12-1). Classic esthetic texts and presentations are modeled on an idealized smile that is slightly different between male and female.[5-14] These smiles have basic characteristics or determinants, which are illustrated in Figs 12-1 to 12-3. They generally occur in conjunction with idealized normal class I skeletal and dental relations, together with symmetrical facial structures. They can be considered as analogous to the idealized class I skeletal and dental models and are called alpha smiles.

Characteristics of alpha smiles are shown in Figs 12-1 to 12-3. This norm also serves as a therapeutic goal or frame of reference when planning the interrelation of the multiple individual clinical determinants in each case. Esthetic deviations form the alpha median, and their correction or the need to create an esthetically stereotyped alpha norm appearance depends on the patient's desires, clinicians' concepts, abilities, dental technologists, individual clinical determinants, and psychosocial and socioeconomic milieu.

Box 12-1 Esthetic variants according to deviation from the nine esthetic determinants

- Asymmetry of the orofacial window.
- Lack of lip support.
- Diminished/excessive tooth display at rest and smiling.
- Excessive gingival display.
- Asymmetry of form, color, distribution, and alignment of the teeth.
- Disharmony of horizontal and vertical tooth axes planes and gingival lines.
- Excessive/inadequate buccal tooth display and buccal corridor.
- Lip incompetence and disharmonies.

Occlusal gingival and facial planes

Variables of maxillary working guidance inclines and resulting maxillary guiding buccal cusp dimensions can have a significant effect on the esthetic appearance of the smile (Fig 12-4).

14 Treating Severe Tooth Wear and Bruxism

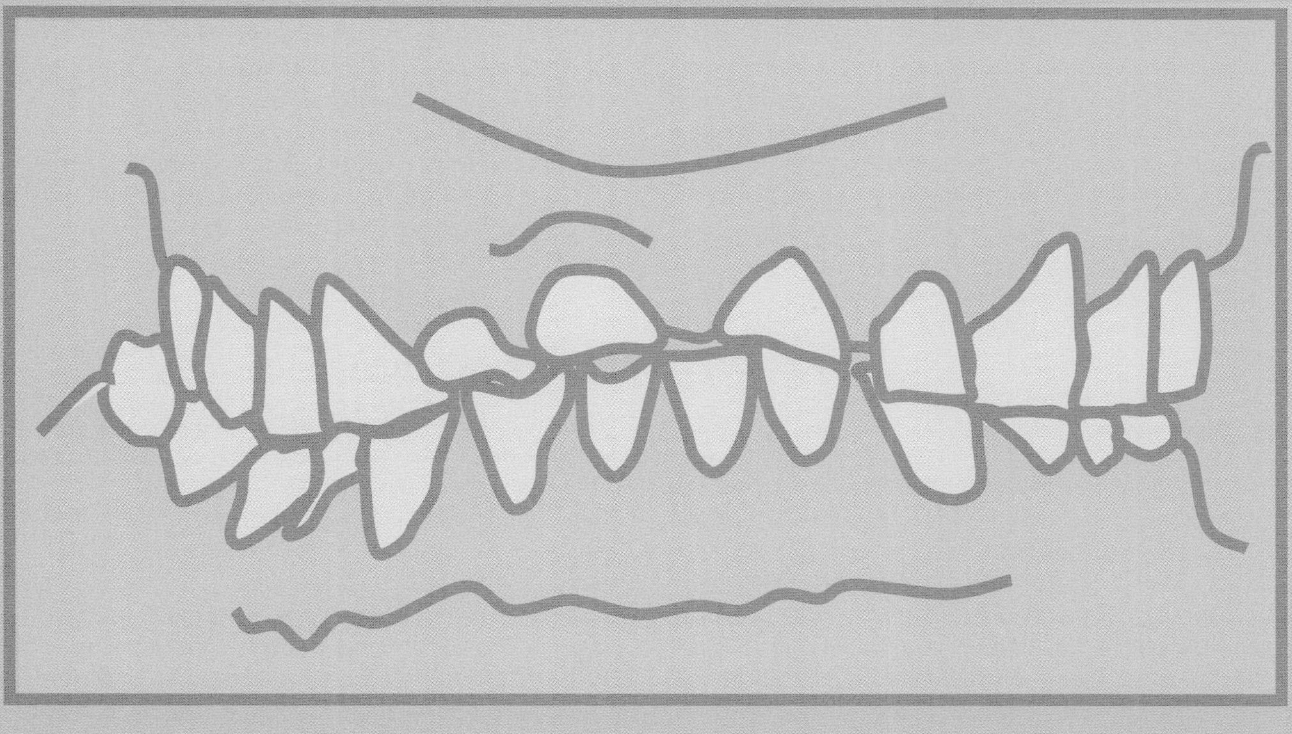

Contents

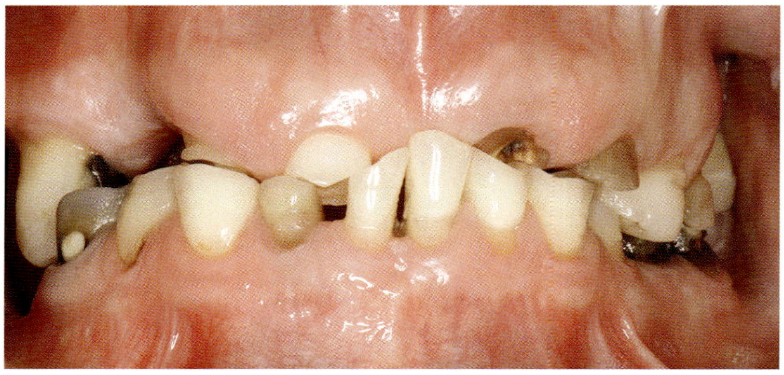

Fig 14-1 Severe loss of tooth substance from occlusal parafunction, bruxism and erosion.

Occlusal parafunction and bruxism

Occlusal parafunction is the conscious or unconscious clenching or grinding of the teeth. It occurs in varying degrees in most individuals. It may occur in the day or at night.[1] Occlusal parafunction and bruxism have been synonymously liked in the literature. In the eighth edition of *The Glossary of Prosthodontic Terms*, bruxism is defined as: "the parafunctional grinding of teeth," and "an oral habit consisting of involuntary rhythmic or spasmodic nonfunctional gnashing, grinding, or clenching of teeth, in other than chewing movements of the mandible, which may lead to occlusal trauma and includes the buccal and lingual surfaces of the teeth."[2] Distinctions were made between nocturnal (nighttime) parafunction and diurnal (daytime) occlusal parafunction.[2,3] These were described as different entities. Recently, the terms sleep bruxism and day time bruxism are more commonly used.[1,4,5]

Loss of occlusal tooth substance results from occlusal parafunction, bruxism, and erosion (Figs 14-1 to 14-3).

Sleep bruxism

Sleep bruxism is currently described as a sleep disorder, as an excessive response to microarousals. Microarousals occur in short 3 to 15 second periods of cortical activation during sleep, in association with increased sympathetic activity. Close to 80% of sleep bruxism episodes occur in clusters of microarousals. A sequence of events preceding grinding has been described.[4,5] Sympathetic activity occurs 4 minutes before grinding, cortical activation takes place 1 minute before, and increased cardiac rhythm and muscle tone takes place at 1 second before.[1,4,5] Sleep bruxism is the most destructive occlusal parafunction.

Occlusal trauma

Occlusal trauma is defined as: "trauma to the periodontium from functional or parafunctional forces causing damage to the attachment apparatus of the periodontium by exceeding its adaptive and reparative capacities. It may be self-limiting or progressive."[2] In the glossary definition "occlusal trauma" refers only to the traumatic effects on the periodontium. The origin of this definition dates back to the period when distinctions were first made between bone loss due to microbial plaque and occlusal parafunction. The resulting semantic confusion arose since the term occlusal trauma could not at that time include the other destructive or traumatic effects of occlusal parafunction, such as tooth wear and restorative breakdown (Figs 14-1 and 14-2).

Etiology

The principal etiological component is central in origin.[1,4,5] Forces generated by occlusal parafunction may be considerable and have been measured in a range of 30 to 80 kg. Most people may grind or clench their teeth during the day and night. The amount and time varies considerable between individuals and in the same individual over different periods of time. When this occurs, these potentially destructive forces are transferred to the teeth, dental restorations, and supporting structures (Fig 14-3).

Stressful events and stress reaction are considered to be risk factors. No single etiological component has been identified in severe bruxers, either in psychological profile or environmental scenarios. Active periods of occlusal parafunction may be diagnosed by the presence of shiny wear facets in enamel porcelain or metal and opposing wear facets aligned in particular mandibular excursions. So-called occlusal disorders have been considered in the past to constitute a significant etiological component[6-9]; however, this is no longer considered to be the case.[3,10-13]

Occlusal interferences

Newly introduced single excursive contacts "interferences" may have an initial irritant effect and cause either avoidance or local grinding, and some temporamandibular (TMD) symptoms.[14-17] This is usually transient. While occlusal elements such as occlusal interferences or steep vertical overlap may not be the direct cause of occlusal parafunction, they constitute the sites of high stress concentration on which this activity occurs. High mechanical stress concentrations on these and other sites of excursive grinding can cause significant wear and damage to the teeth, their restorations, and supporting structures. Observation of temporarily increased tooth grinding in some studies of experimental occlusal interferences was reported[14,15] and no reactions in others.[16] In a controlled study, experimental occlusal interferences did not provoke nocturnal bruxism.[17]

Attrition, erosion, and abrasion

Many authors use the terms tooth wear and erosion interchangeably. Strictly, the definitions relate to different causes. "Tooth wear" is recognized as the general term including erosion, attrition, and abrasion. "Loss of tooth substance" is also used. There is general agreement that "erosion" is caused by the effect of non-bacterial acids on teeth, "attrition" is the result of friction from tooth-to-tooth contact, and "abrasion" is the result of mechanical action from surfaces other than teeth.[18-30]

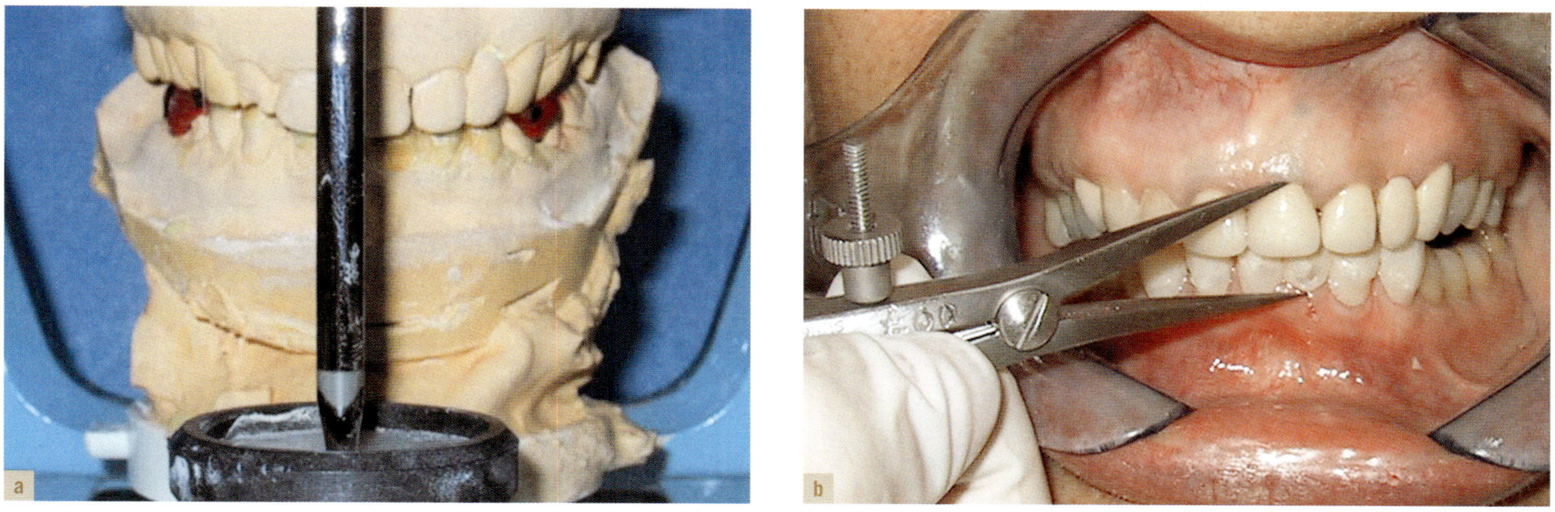

Fig 14-28a and b Evaluation of new vertical dimension of occlusion by assessment of anterior and posterior crown height dimension from diagnostic modeling and measurement of interarch and interocclusal distance.

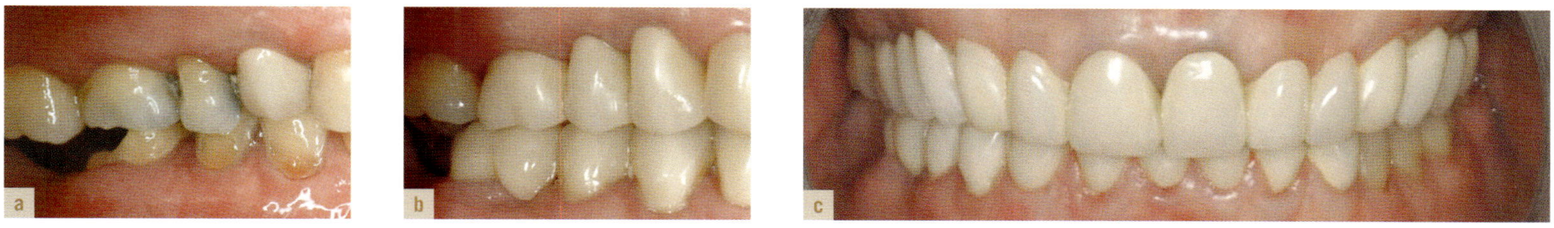

Fig 14-29a Initial OVD. OVD may be increased to achieve sufficient interocclusal clearance for the planned occlusal material. The effect and adaptation to changes in OVD may be evaluated in the provisional restoration. b and c Esthetics, function, cementation, degree of wear, fracture rate, and muscle or joint symptoms are evaluated in the provisional phase. If the OVD is to be increased further, crown height may be increased in both arches, provided that the esthetic occlusal planes are not adversely altered.

Fig 14-30a and b Upper cast mounted with facebow. Lower cast mounted with centric relation record at the correct OVD.

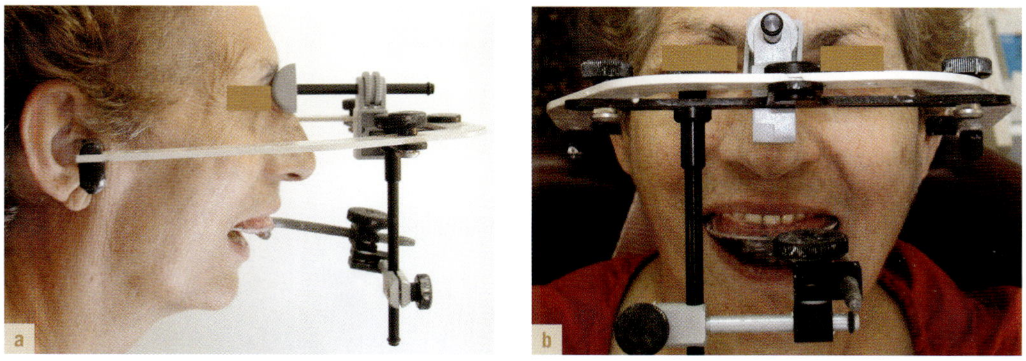

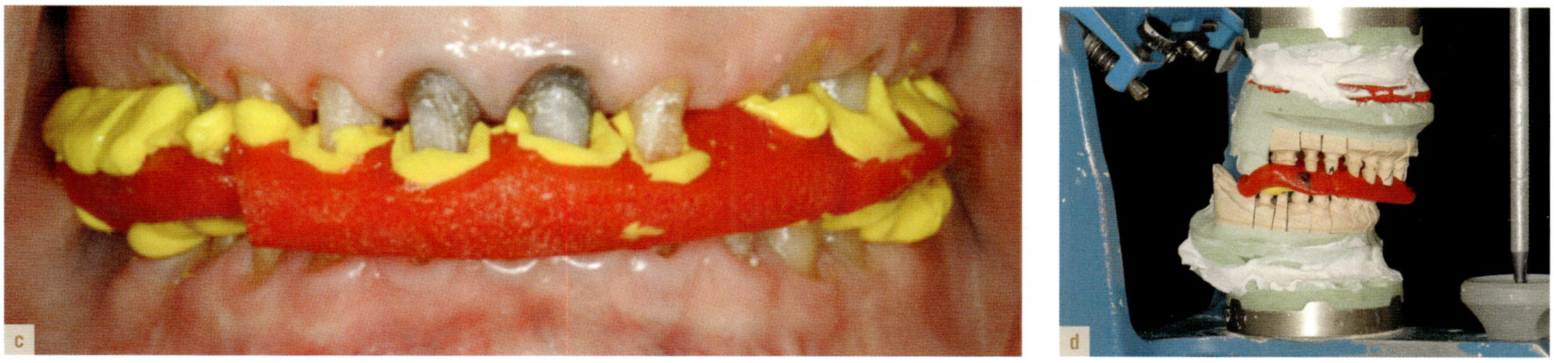

Cross-mounting working casts and casts of provisional restorations

In order to copy the form of the provisional restorations in the final restoration, cross-mounting may be used. Cross-mounting allows the alternate mounting of working casts and casts of provisional restorations. The cast of the mandibular provisional is mounted against the maxillary final working cast. The maxillary provisional cast is mounted against the lower final working cast. The maxillary provisional cast is mounted against the mandibular provisional cast (Fig 14-31). Working and provisional casts are interchangeable and allow the fabrication of buccal and occlusal silicone indices for a wax-up of the final restoration (Fig 14-32).

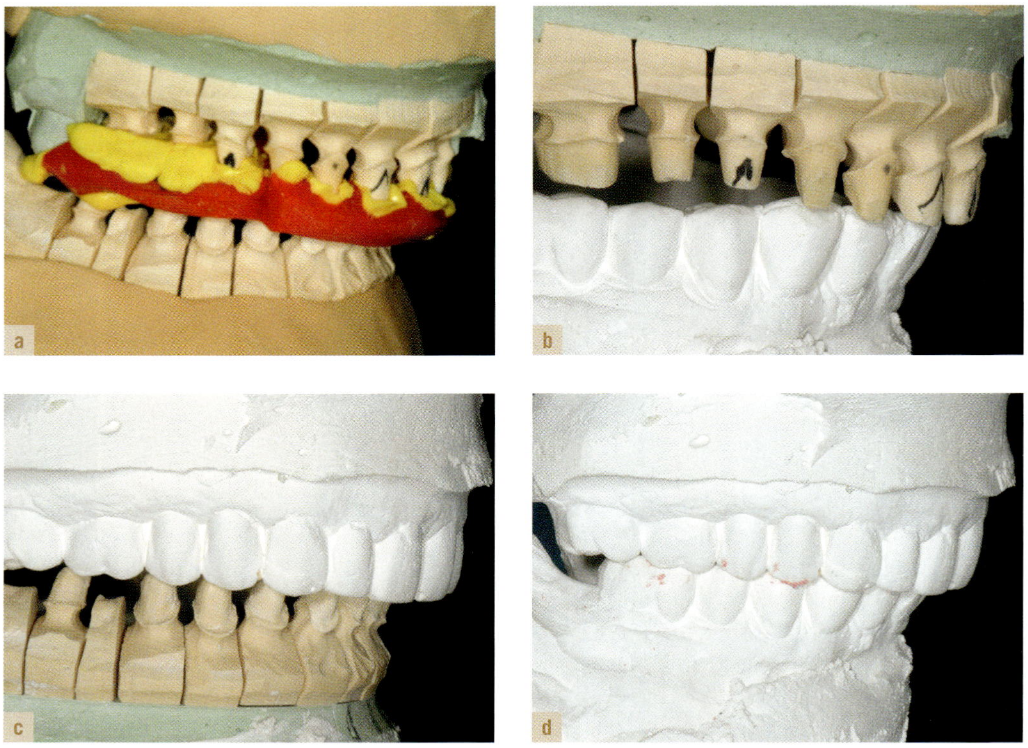

Fig 14-31 Cross-mounting. a Opposing working casts. b Maxillary working cast against mandibular provisional cast. c Mandibular working cast against maxillary provisional cast. d Opposing provisional casts. All mountings are interchangeable.

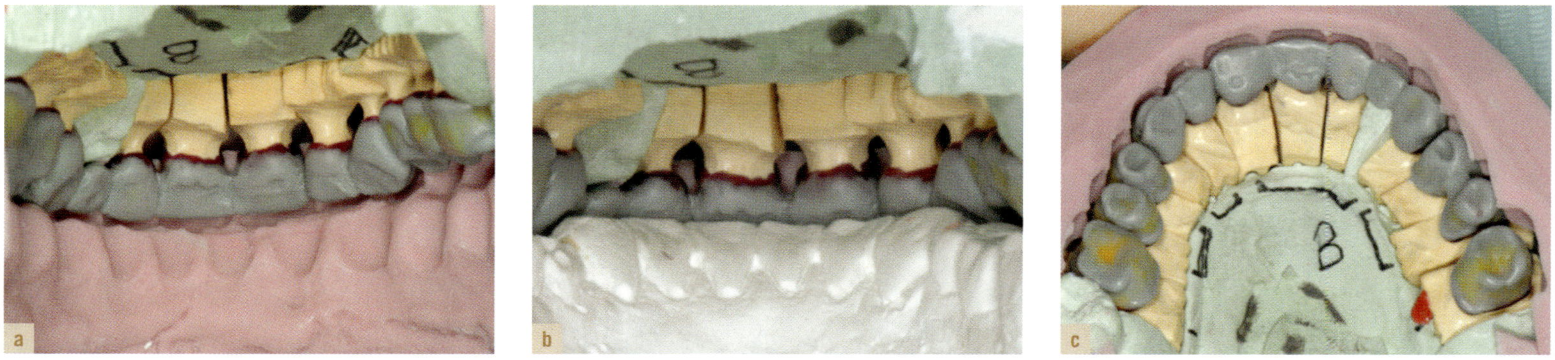

Fig 14-32a to c Wax-up of final restorations. Buccal and occlusal silicone indexes are made from the cross-mounted casts of the provisional restorations against corresponding working casts. Cutback or build-up waxing techniques allow appropriate relation of the wax to the planned occlusal design and for sufficient thickness of porcelain with the necessary metal support.

Wax-up of final restorations

Buccal and occlusal silicone indexes are made from the cross-mounted casts of the provisional restorations against corresponding working casts. Cutback or build-up waxing techniques allow appropriate relation of the wax to the planned occlusal design and for sufficient thickness of porcelain with the necessary metal support (Fig 14-32).

Excursive resistance and abutment connection

Excursive resistance is the resistance to protrusive or lateral excursive forces provided by the abutments and their supporting structures. This applies to both the working and non-working side in the case of a cross-arch splint. Multiple factors influence the decision regarding the joining of adjacent abutments. Interrelating factors of esthetics, interarch distance, resistance retention, OVD, interocclusal clearance, abutment and tooth durability, excursive guidance, and excursive resistance all need to be considered. Lingual abutment preparation walls on the working side and buccal axial walls on the non-working side provide the combined abutment resistance to lateral parafunctional force on the working inclines. Similar considerations apply to the distal abutment preparation inclines that resist torquing forces applied in protrusive contacts and parafunction.

Figure 14-33 illustrates considerations for planning excursive resistance and abutment connection possibilities. To replace a missing left canine in the upper arch, a simple three-unit bridge joining the first premolar and lateral incisor is first considered. The left lateral incisor may not be considered strong enough and can be joined to the adjacent left central incisor. This central incisor has a weakened root from a wide cast dowel post. Further connection to the adjacent non-vital dowel restored right central incisor would reduce the risk of fracture of both weakened central incisor roots and provide increased combined resistance and retention for the restoration of the missing left canine. One option would therefore be to splint two separate anterior segments: right central incisor to the left first premolar, and the right canine to the adjacent lateral incisor.

Alternatively all seven abutments can be joined together in a single unit from the right canine to the left first premolar. The first option was decided upon to minimize cross-arch torquing from both right and left working guidance. The two splinted units of right canine and lateral incisor provide additional support for the lateral incisor, since splints of two units are less liable to decementation. Distal maxillary pairs of right premolars and left second premolar and resected first molar were joined in consideration of the weakened endodontically treated premolars and resected molar roots, to reduce the risk of potential root fracture.

In the mandibular arch, the lower anterior incisors and canines were left lone standing and the right side was connected with two premolars to the hemisected molar root for increased support.

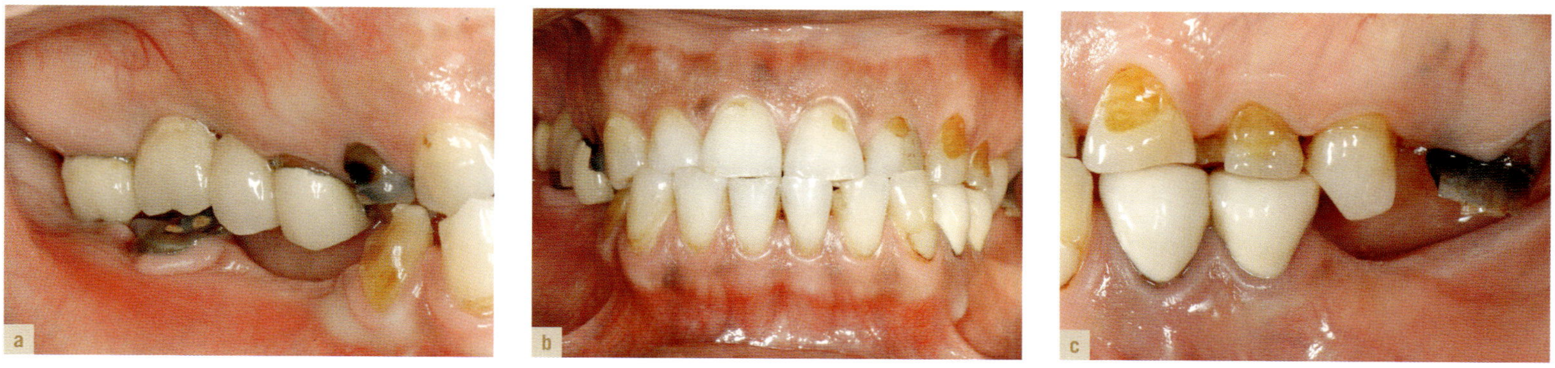

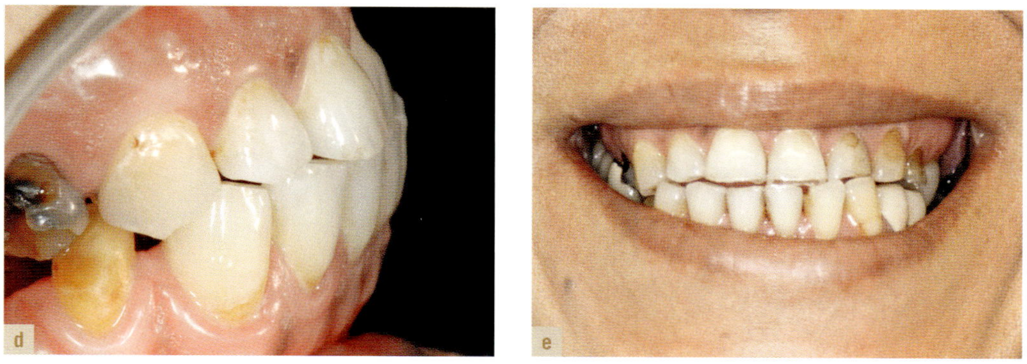

Fig 15-24a to e Loss of posterior support, posterior supereruption, reduced interarch space. Anterior edge-to-edge relation, moderate occlusal wear, loss of OVD, unesthetic appearance.

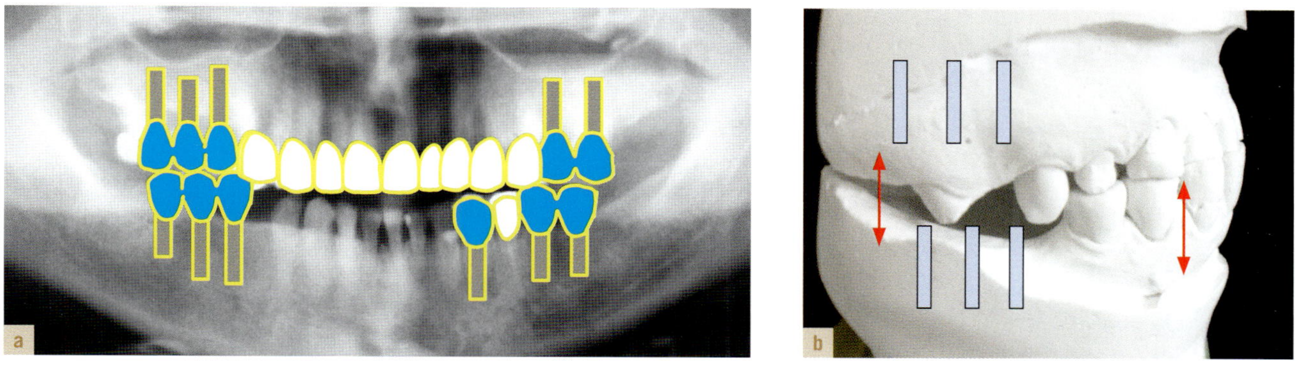

Fig 15-25a and b Treatment plan to restore posterior support with posterior implant-supported restorations. An increase in OVD is necessary to produce adequate posterior crown length.

Case presentation: class III edge-to-edge incisor relation – loss of posterior support

A 43-year-old healthy woman was unhappy with her esthetics and function and wanted fixed restorations. Her diagnosis included a skeletal class III relation, edge-to-edge articulation, moderate tooth wear, an unesthetic appearance, reduced posterior occlusal support, loss of OVD, posterior segmental overeruptions, reduced interarch distance, missing teeth, and faulty and failing restorations. She was a heavy smoker, with night bruxism, dental caries, and chronic periodontitis (Fig 15-24).

Treatment stages

The treatment plan required restoration of lost posterior support with posterior implant-supported restorations. An increase in the OVD was necessary to produce adequate posterior crown length (Fig 15-25). Imaging indicated the need for increased anterior crown length and harmonizing anterior and posterior esthetic planes with anterior and posterior gingival planes (Figs 15-24 and 15-26). Anterior crown length was coordinated with increased OVD for posterior crown length with a diagnostic wax-up and provisional restorations (Fig 15-26). Posterior gingival levels were harmonized with crown lengthening surgery and coordinated posterior implant placement relative to the bone crest and gingival levels. Esthetics, function, and the occlusal plane were tested in provisional restorations with MI in centric relation and anteriors in an edge-to-edge relation with a minimal anterior overlap. The protrusive guidance was generated on incisors, canines, and first premolars. Flat working guidance on canines and premolars on both right and left sides separated non-working contact. Maxillary anterior restorations were restored with ceramic restorations. Posterior restorations were restored with PFM restorations (Figs 15-27 and 15-28).

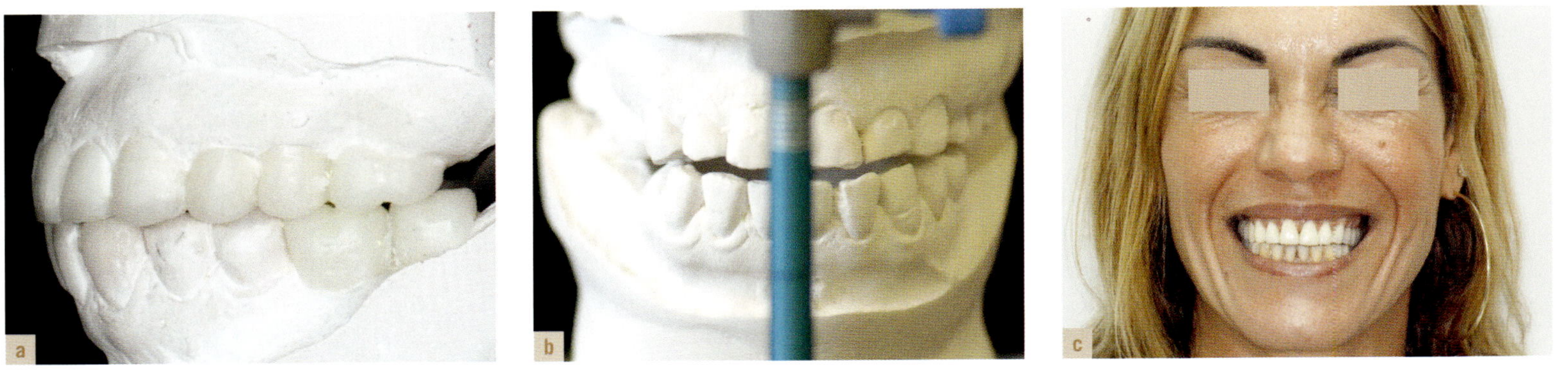

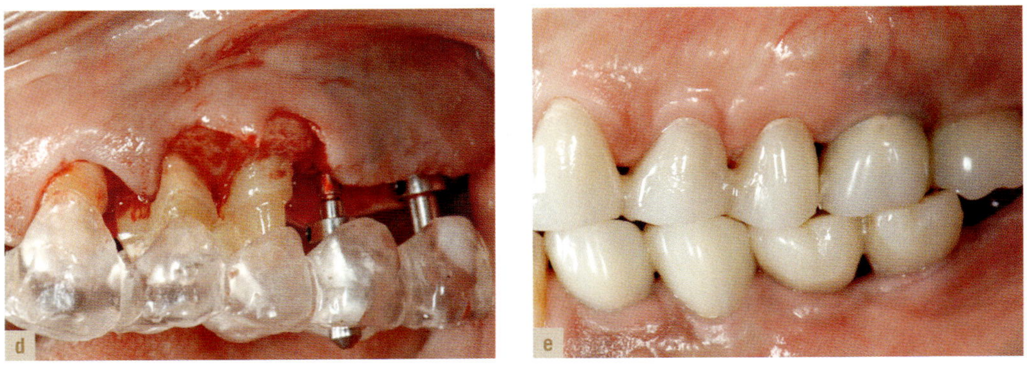

Fig 15-26a Wax-up at increased OVD. b Required anterior crown length at new OVD. c Imaging for anterior tooth display. d Crown lengthening surgery and implant placement to level gingival lines. e Provisional restorations with corrected gingival lines, esthetic occlusal planes, and new functional OVD.

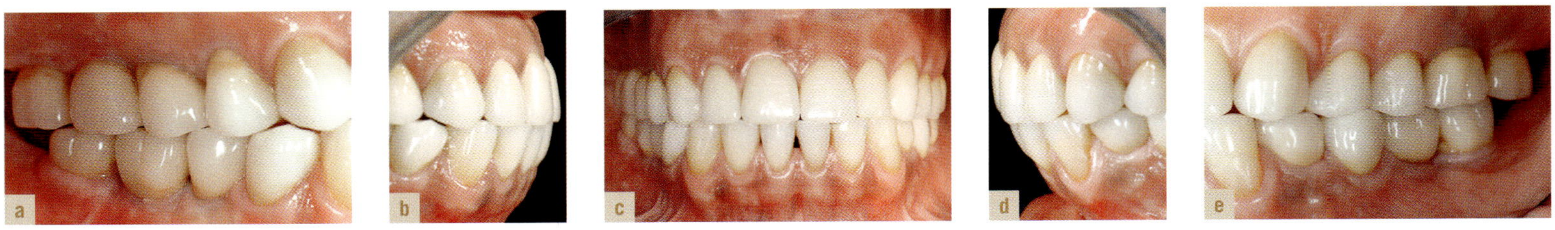

Fig 15-27a to e Final restoration. Posterior support restored. Anterior porcelain restorations in an edge-to-edge relation with very slight anterior overlap. Protrusive guidance on incisors, canines, and first premolars. Right and left working guidance group function.

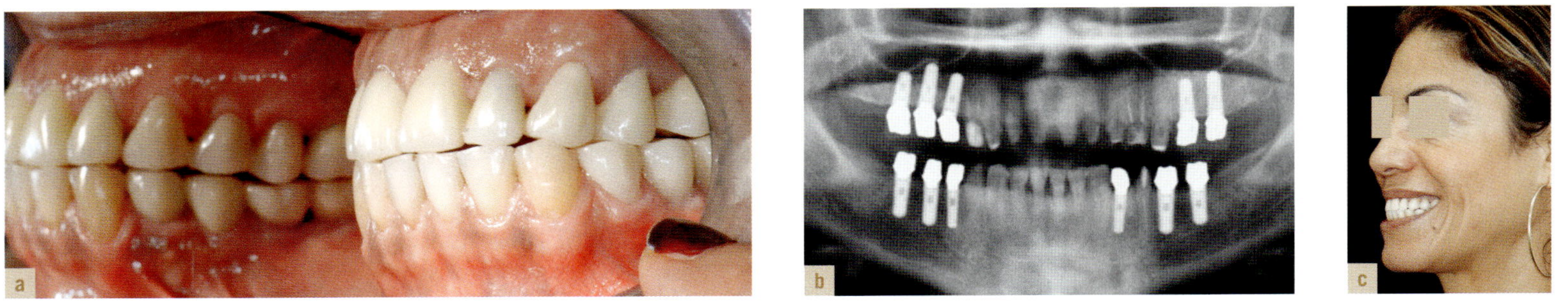

Fig 15-28a Left working guidance separating contralateral non-working side contact. b Final radiograph. c Final appearance. (Images courtesy of Dr E Zensiper.).

Fully edentulous implant-supported restorations

Planning and restoring the fully edentulous arch presents significant challenges to the restorative dentist, surgeon, and technician. The planned restoration needs to be simulated in advance by "predictive modeling" to serve as a template for implant planning, location orientation, and bone augmentation if necessary. The simulated restoration needs to take into account all of the general prosthetic determinants, as well as any other individual determinants that are specific to each case. The individual determinants include skeletal relations, residual ridge relations, vertical dimension, supporting anatomy, interarch distance, esthetic determinants, occlusal plane orientation, tooth display, lip support, and potential implant numbers, dimensions, and orientations (Fig 15-29). All of these must be integrated into this predictive model. Failure to take into consideration any of these factors can lead to severe prosthetic, biomechanical, or esthetic problems that may only become apparent once the implants are in place and the final or temporary restorations are fabricated.

Predictive modeling

This template has to be created in advance and is needed to determine whether implants can and should be placed, how they can be distributed, and how they will bear the forces of function and parafunction. This template or diagnostic model is used to create the form of the radiographic template and then the surgical guide. These diagnostic models may be made in wax or with mounted denture teeth on diagnostic bases seated on the edentulous ridges. In appropriate cases temporary bridges and modified duplicates of successful dentures may be used as the basis and modified where necessary. Using an old denture as the template for a future fixed implant-supported restoration may

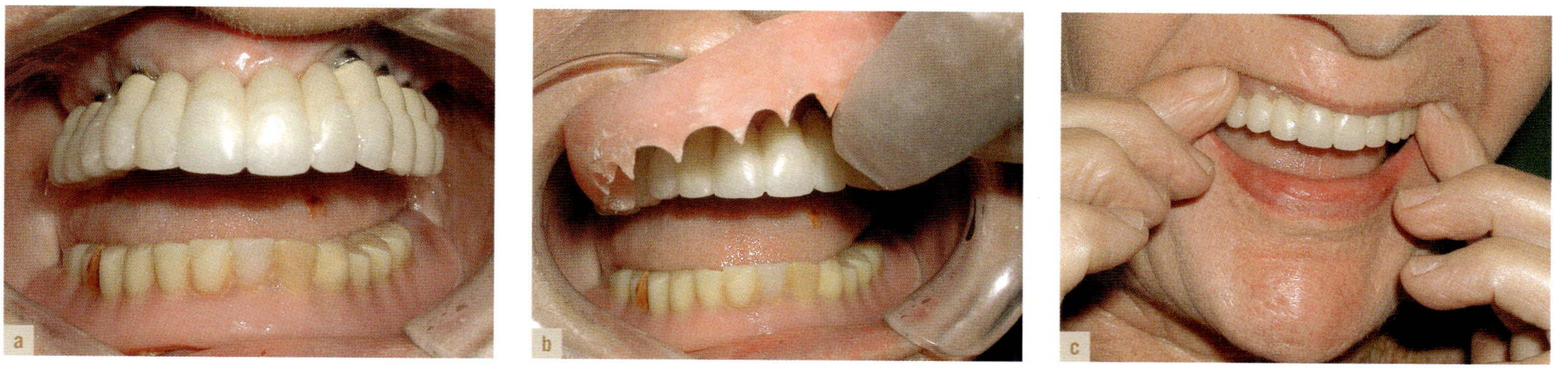

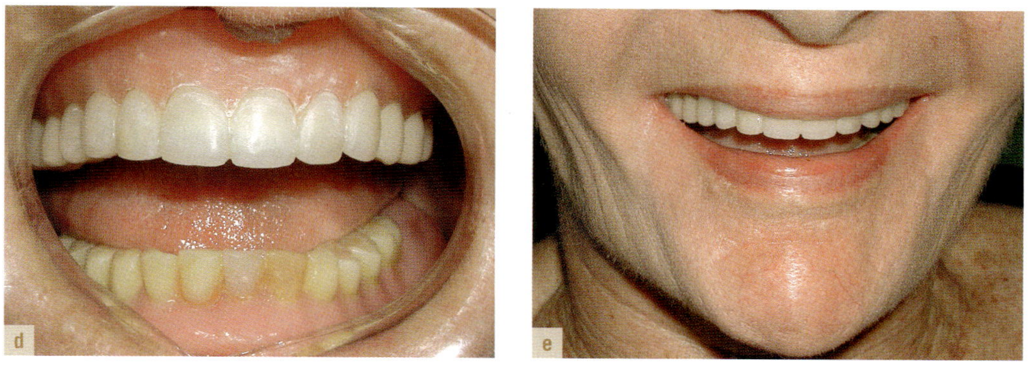

Fig 15-42a to e Fixed upper implant-supported prosthesis. Lack of buccal lip support compensated by the use of a silicone removable buccal flange that can be placed by the patient and removed regularly for oral hygiene. (Images courtesy of Mr O Koenig.)

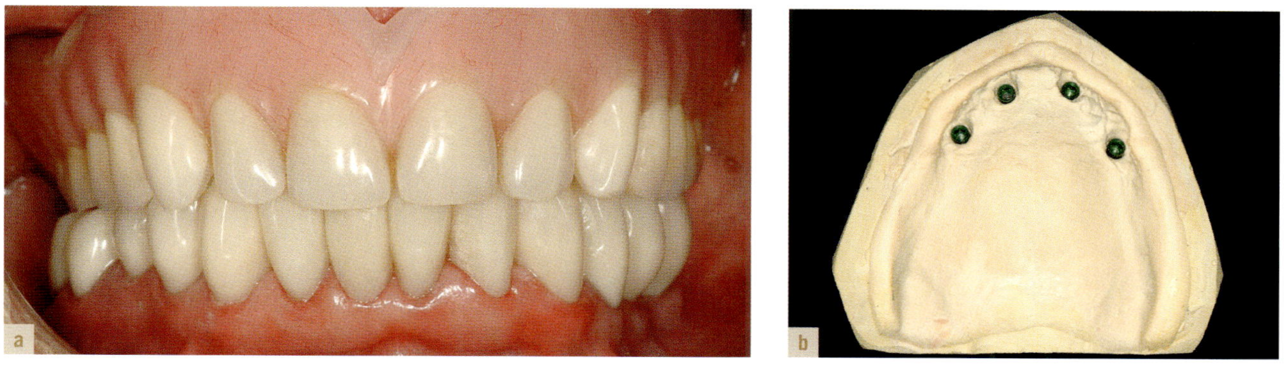

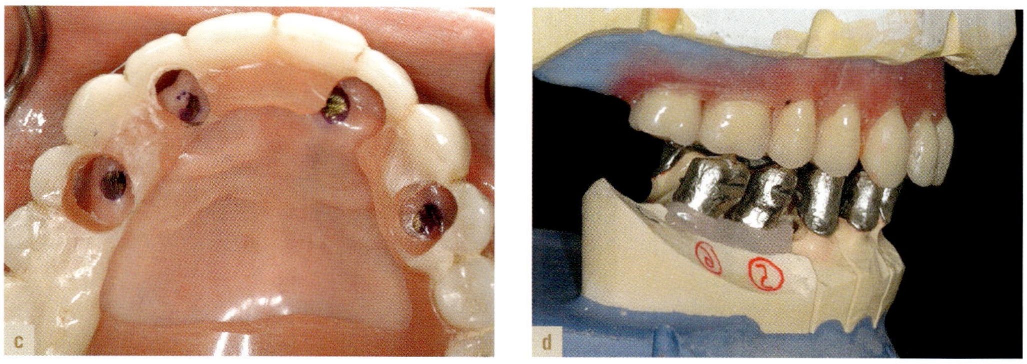

Fig 15-43a to d Maxillary overdenture on four stud attachments. Achieving a balanced occlusion against natural teeth is challenging. Protrusive records were used for condylar guidance setting. Working group function and isolated non-working contacts were obtained. The ability to achieve protrusive balance depends on the vertical and horizontal overlap. (Images courtesy of Dr B Oz Ari.)

modality. Maxillary bars and studs both seem to provide an adequate service with no difference in bone loss.[29] Bars need more vertical space and are more troublesome to maintain. Stud attachments may be made to be solely retentive and non-load bearing with appropriate relief. The posterior load is generally supported by the edentulous ridges. If anterior bar systems are used, the anterior segment becomes implant supported and the posterior segment becomes ridge supported (Figs 15-38 to 15-40). No outcome differences were found between bar and stud attachments after 7 years of loading.[30] Anterior lip support above the teeth can generally only be provided by flanges of removable overdentures (Fig 15-41). Removable silicone buccal flanges may be placed by the patient over fixed restorations and removed for oral hygiene (Fig 15-42).

Occlusion of overdentures

Balanced occlusion has been advocated as an appropriate occlusal scheme for overdentures.[5,31] The original objective of balanced occlusion for fully tissue-supported dentures was to avoid tipping of the posterior aspect in protrusive movements and tipping of the non-working section in lateral tooth-guided movements. Fully balanced occlusion is not always easy to achieve, especially in the presence of an anterior vertical overlap.

Lateral balance is also limited by esthetic factors and either group function or group function with single balancing contacts is more obtainable. The adage of "enter bolus, exit balance" holds true and dentures will tend to tip when closing on a bolus until opposing tooth contact occurs. However, if the initial excursive contact is a balancing contact, this will have a stabilizing effect on the tipped denture bases. The added retentive effect of the stud or bar attachments will tend to stabi-

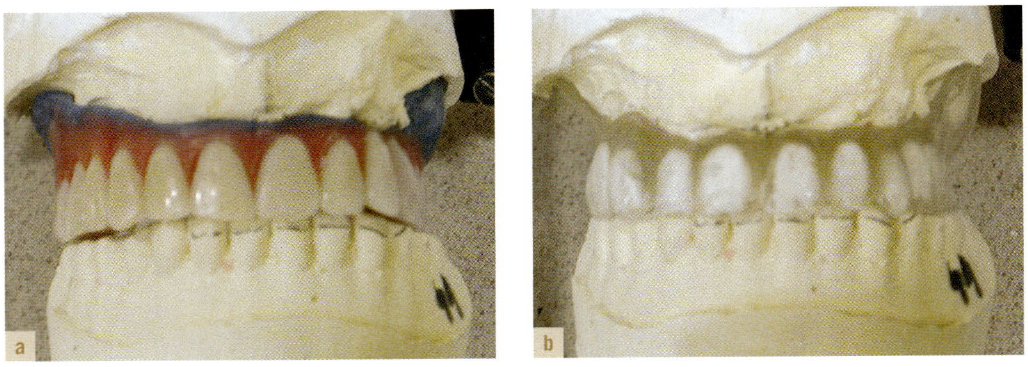

Fig 15-44a to d Diagnostic setup without buccal flanges duplicated to radiographic guide and CT images showing the sagittal and axial relation of the bone to the radiopaque teeth images.

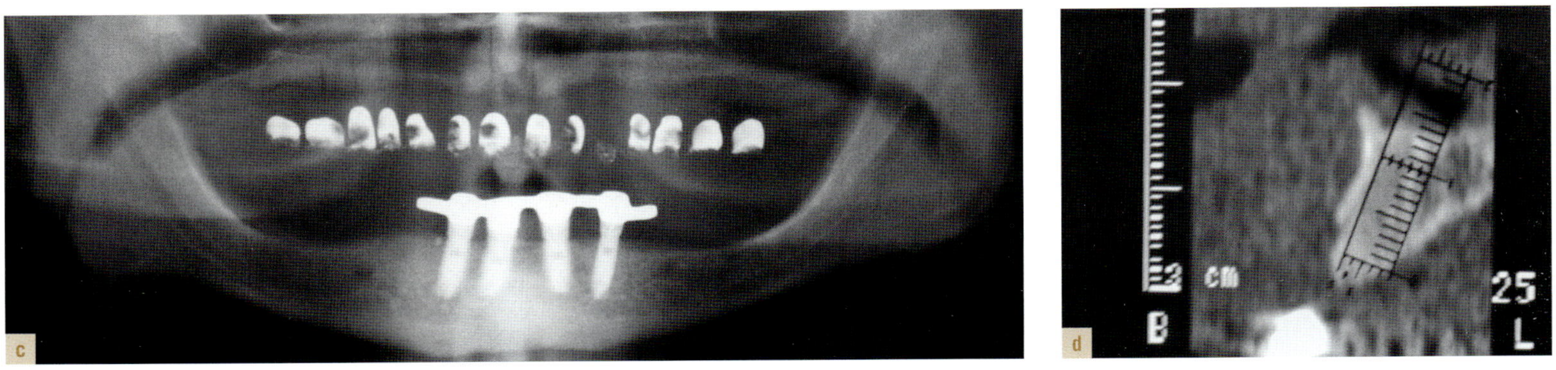

lize the non-working tipping effect. The anterior retention is less affected and anterior closure will often result in posterior tipping (Figs 15-38 and 15-39). This may be offset by obtaining some indirect retention from the anterior attachment housings or bars with the negative effect of creating greater torquing load on the anterior implants. Some clinicians advocate single posterior implants for retention to prevent this tipping effect. Creating a balanced occlusion in a single denture opposing a natural dentition or fixed restoration is often difficult – if not impossible – to achieve due to anterior vertical overlap, posterior cusp height, cuspal inclinations, and occlusal plane orientations. In such cases, group function working guidance and a shallow protrusive anterior guidance minimizing vertical overlap is indicated (Figs 15-43).[32]

Number of implants and anchorage type

Implant-supported overdentures have been used as a viable therapeutic option for many years.[29,31]

Maxillary options are generally used with four anterior implants with either bars or stud attachments and lower mandibular overdentures used with two stud attachments or a connecting bar. Over 10-year survival rates are 80 to 95%.[29,31] Complication rates are greater in the maxilla. Bar attachments have the advantage of joining implants, with the connected section being implant supported. Creating rotational fulcrums is difficult due to posterior tipping on anterior closure. Stud attachments have fewer complications and can be designed to provide solely retention with the edentulous ridges providing the support.[29-37]

Physical and virtual modeling

In order to achieve the predicted implant placement the information incorporated into diagnostic modeled setups must be transferred to radiographic and surgical guides. This may be achieved by physical modeling techniques and by virtual digital technology combined with physical modeling. Physical models are made from duplicates of the diagnostic setups, wax-ups, or provisional restorations or previous dentures (Figs 15-44 to 15-49). Radiopaque material, such as barium sulfate with acrylic, metal strips or gutta percha are incorporated in the radiographic guides. Computed tomograms will then provide 3D images of the supporting osseous structures in relation to the diagnostic modeled teeth. Radiographic guides may be converted into surgical guides or new surgical guides fabricated according to the same principles (Figs 15-45, 15-46, and 15-55). Acrylic modeled surgical guides may be made with holes or grooves from the buccal side to allow for some surgical latitude. These guides must be cut down sufficiently to allow for vertical access and spacing after flap reflection and irrigation (Figs 15-45 and 15-46).

Prosthetic-driven, computer-assisted implant planning, guidance, and restoration

Virtual digital technologies offer several options to achieve virtual diagnostic planning and guided surgical placement (Figs 15-47 to 15-88).[38-41] Many of these still rely on the clinical fabrication of diagnostic modeled setups according to the above principles which are converted into radiopaque guides to allow for virtual implant planning and computer generated surgical guides (Figs 15-53 to 15-70).

Extremely accurate technologies of stereolithographic modeling and computer-aided design and computer-aided manufacturing (CAD/CAM) now allow the creation of accurate bone and soft tissue models, together with accurate surgical guidance models, prosthetic components, and superstructures (Figs 15-47, 15-66, 15-70, 15-82, and 15-84).

Digital, virtual, and analog systems

Advances in digital systems in dentistry allow the creation of virtual images and models based on optical and radiograph 3D scanning. A distinction is made between virtual models and analog or real models. Three-dimensional virtual models may be converted to analog models in various plastics – the most sophisticated being by laser-cured stereolithography. This is termed 3D printing. Laser-cured modeling is carried out in international manufacturing centers. Digital files are sent to these centers, where they are processed and converted into analog models of the jaws and teeth, surgical guides, and also provisional restorations.[38-43]

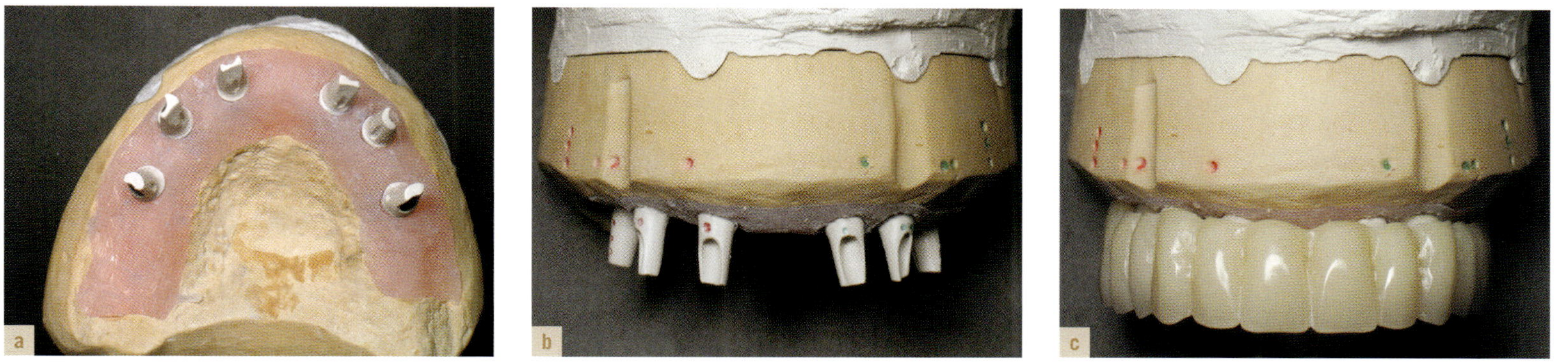

Fig 15-57a and b Temporary abutments placed on mounted casts. c Provisional restoration based on the initial setup.

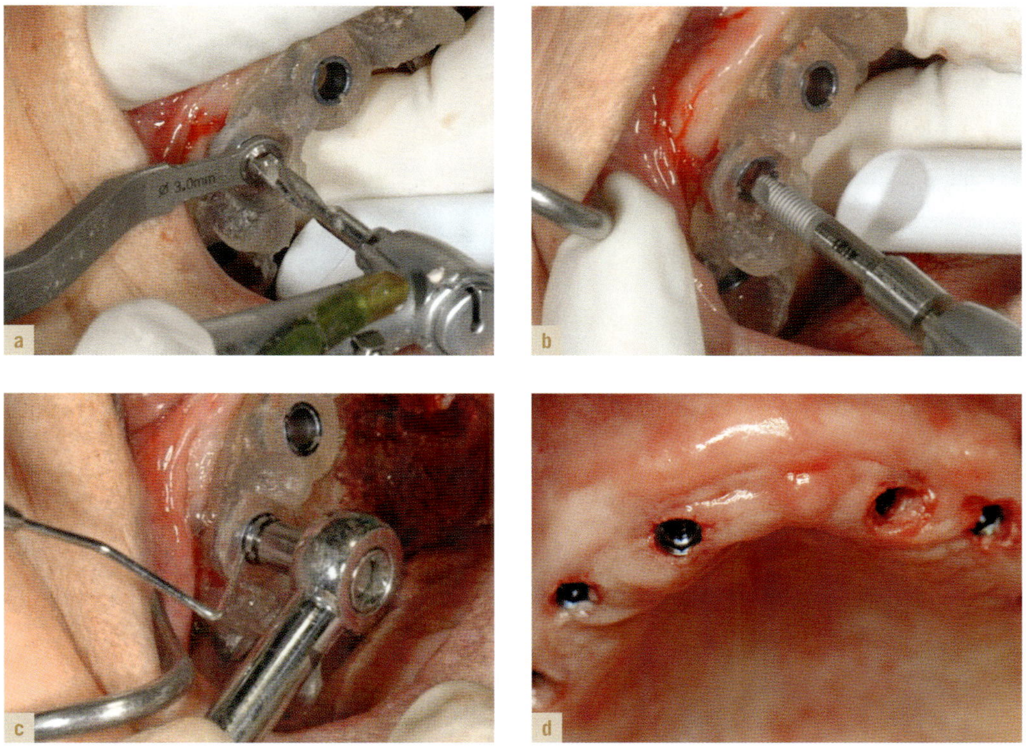

Fig 15-58 Surgical stages. a Site preparation through the tissue-borne surgical guide. b implant placement through surgical guide. c Alignment of grooves in the guide rings and implant mount allows for accurate hex orientation and placement of abutments in predetermined relations for immediate provisional restoration. d Implants in position immediately after removal of the surgical guide.

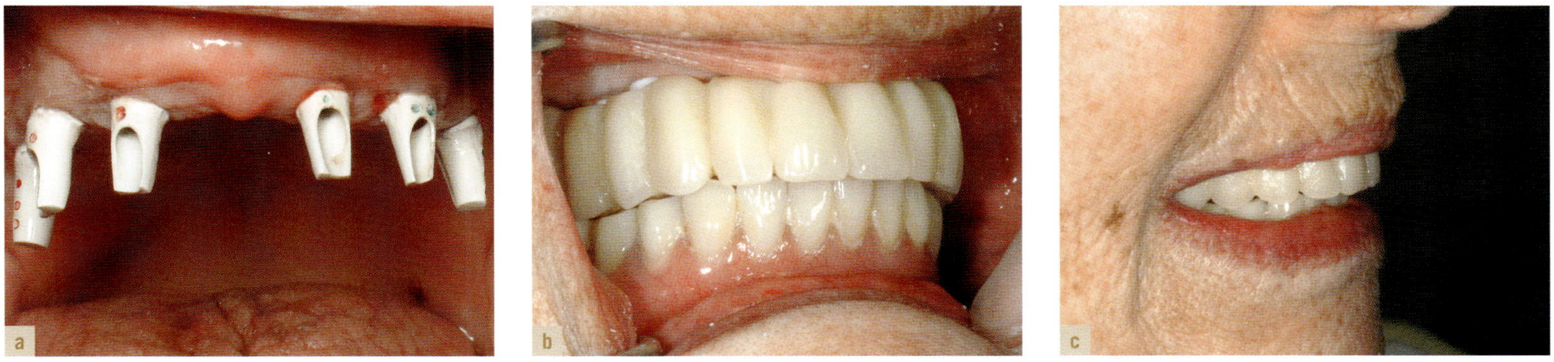

Fig 15-59a Temporary abutments. b and c Immediate provisional bridge with verified occlusal relations, vertical dimension, and esthetic appearance.

surgical guide is manufactured with the fit surface obtained from the stereolithographic model of the jaw (Figs 15-66a). The surgical guide is shown seated on the stereolithographic model of the jaw and in the mouth during surgery (Figs 15-66b and 15-66c). An immediate provisional restoration was fitted following implant placement.

Pre-existing dentures

Pre-existing, well-fitting dentures may be used to create appropriate virtual models of the denture teeth and soft tissue fit surface representing the soft tissue contour of the supporting jaw. These may be duplicated to a radiopaque replica that is scanned by CBCT in the mouth as a single scan.

Alternatively the denture with reference markers may be scanned separately. Reference markers are incorporated into the denture to enable accurate superimposition of the 3D denture image and the 3D radiographic image of the jaw (Fig 15-49). For tissue-supported flapless surgical guides in both single scan and dual scans, the fit surface of the duplicated or original denture is accurately copied in the surgical guide (Figs 15-55 and 15-70). If a bone-supported surgical guide is planned, this is printed from the 3D anatomical surface of the jaw (Fig 15-66).

A radiopaque duplicate of a well-fitting, pre-existing denture can transfer the individual prosthetic determinants in the denture through the radiopaque duplicate to enable software masking, and accurate implant planning in relation to the desired clinical position of the teeth. A clinical case showing all stages from duplication, software design,

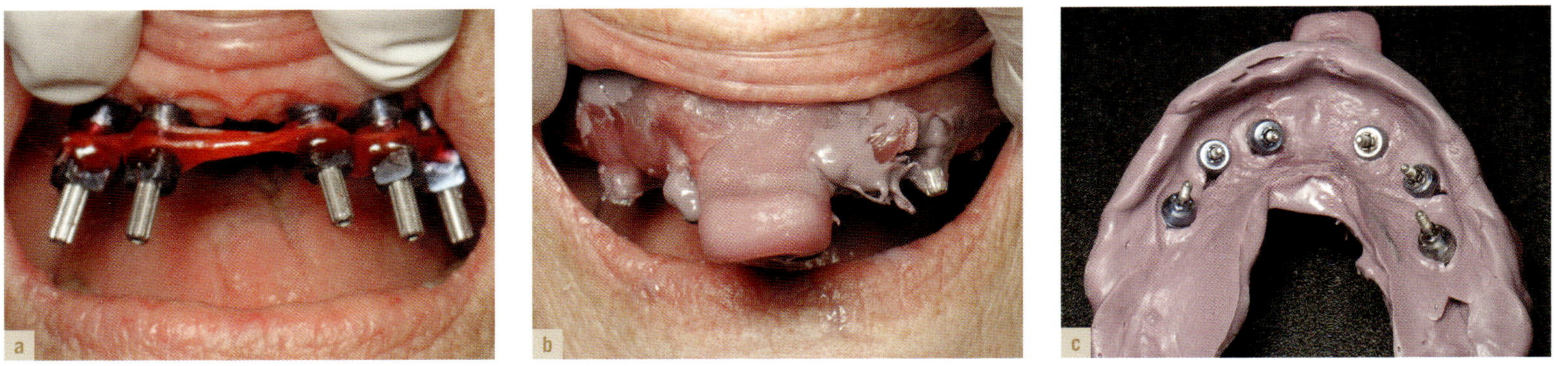

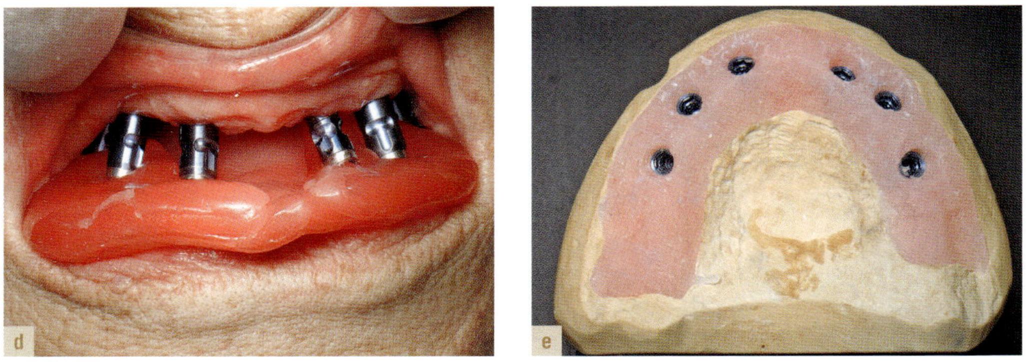

Fig 15-60a to e Impressions and records in MI with fabrication of master cast with implant analogs (after 6 months).

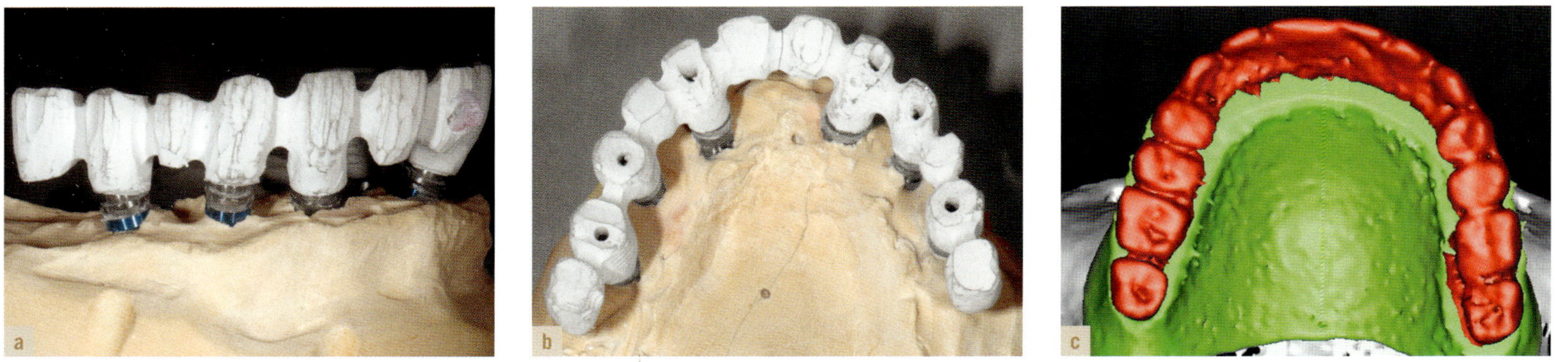

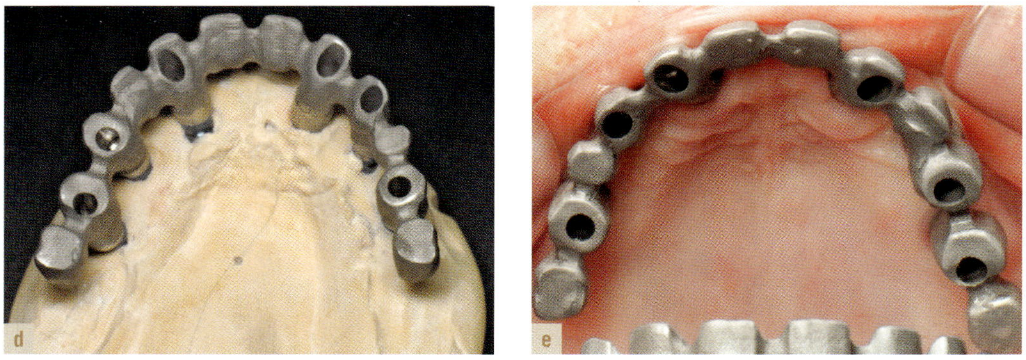

Fig 15-61a and b Plastic acrylic cut back from indexed provisional restoration. c Virtual occlusal image. d and e CAD/CAM metal superstructure .

surgery and prosthetics, to the final restoration is shown in Figs 15-67 to 15-71.

Standing bridges with superimposed virtual teeth

Virtual images of standing teeth may be used in planning cases, for instance, where extraction and immediate implant placement is considered (Figs 15-72 to 15-74). Digital separation of the standing teeth into masks may be accurately achieved by a skilled technician using appropriate software. Natural teeth with no metal scatter will produce clear 3D masks of crowns and roots (Fig 15-76). Pre-existing crowns or bridges containing metal will create radiographic scatter and not enable clear software masks of the crowns. In these cases, superimposition of virtual crowns creates a virtual setup used to plan accurate implant and abutment orientation. The virtual teeth may also be reproduced by CAD/CAM technology into provisional acrylic restorations (Figs 15-72 and 15- 74).

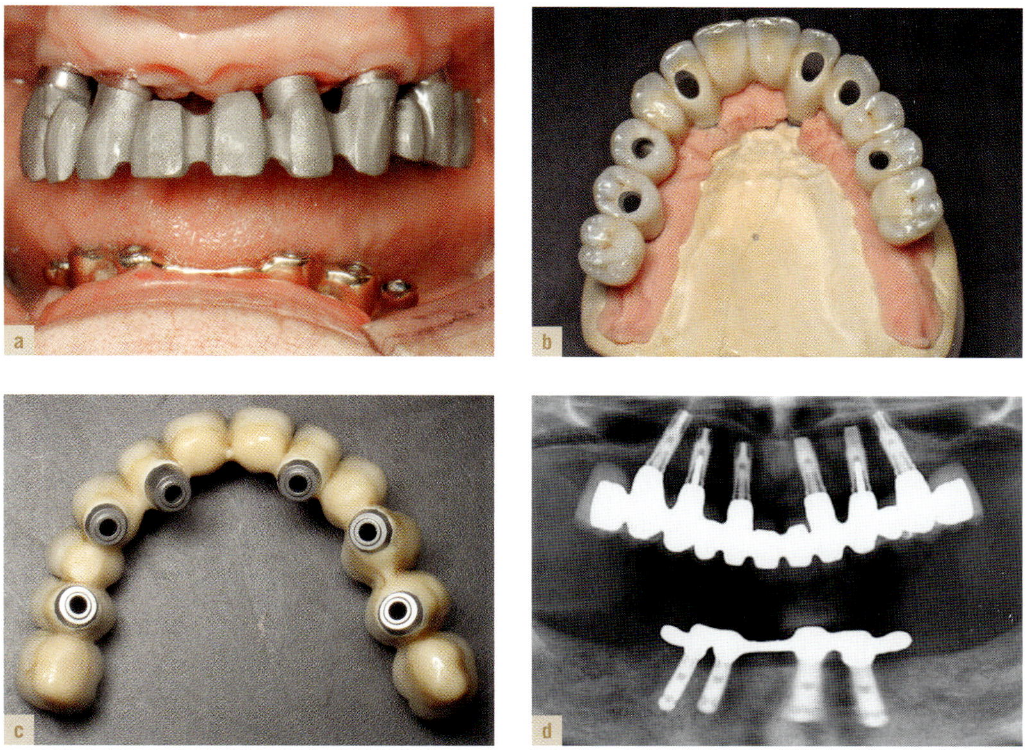

Fig 15-62 CAD/CAM metal superstructure and porcelain, with orthopantomograhic radiograph of completed restorations.

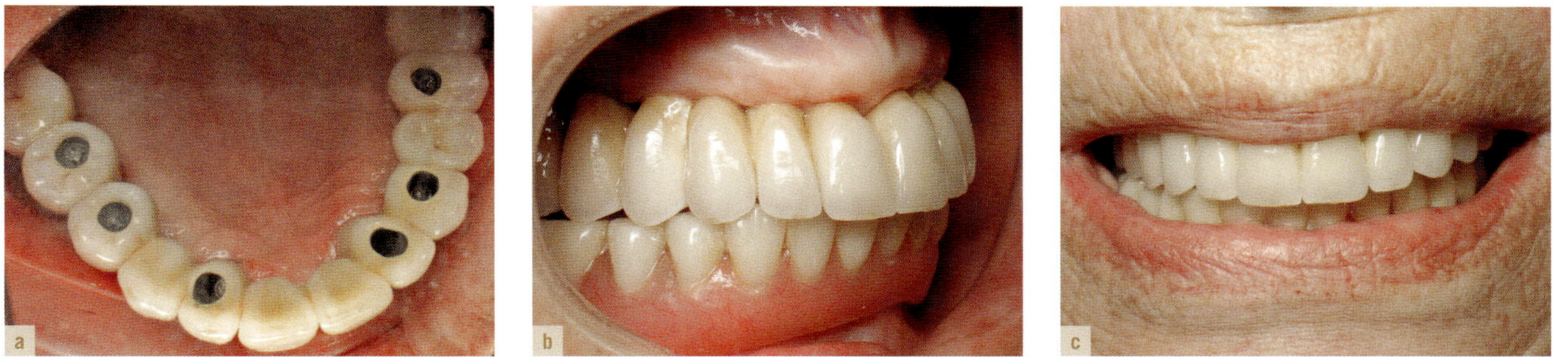

Fig 15-63 Final restoration.

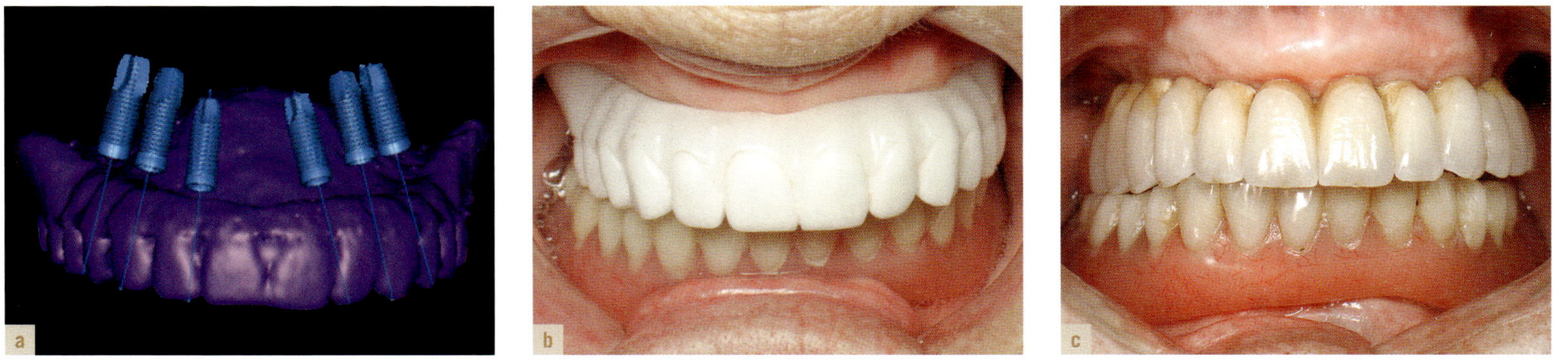

Fig 15-64 Stages of transferring individual esthetic and functional prosthetic determinants, through setup, radiographic guide, and virtual planning, to final restoration. (Images courtesy of Mr R Krauze.)

Optically scanned intraoral virtual model superimposed onto virtual CT model of the jaw

Three-dimensional virtual models of the teeth and soft tissues may be obtained from optically scanned plaster casts. These may be superimposed exactly onto corresponding 3D virtual radiographic models (Fig 15-75). Virtual implants may then be positioned in the virtual models relative to the anatomic structures in the jaw, the adjacent and opposing teeth, and the soft tissue of the edentulous areas (Figs 15-76 and 15-77). The appropriate surgical guide, radiographs of surgery, laboratory, and final clinical stages are shown in Figs 15-77 to 15-79.

Virtual setup

Virtual teeth may be positioned and manipulated in the software to facilitate implant position, dimensions, and inclinations, together with abutment dimensions and inclinations. CBCT scanning with the teeth in occlusion allows the positioning of the virtual teeth in appropriate relation to the opposing dentition. The 3D virtual teeth may be milled in

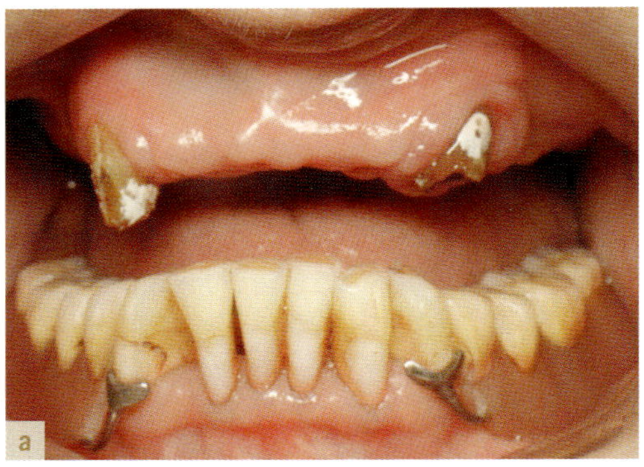
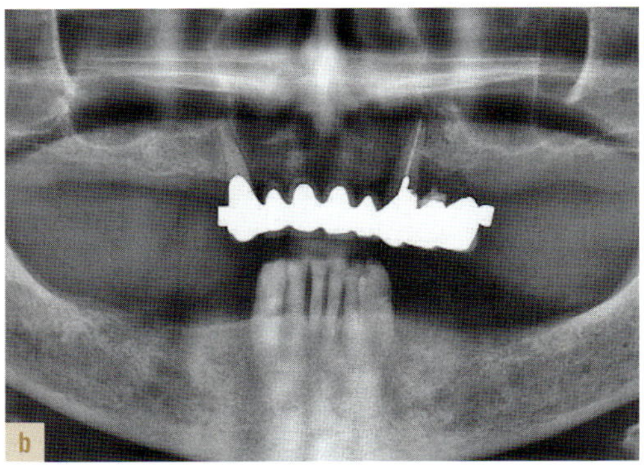
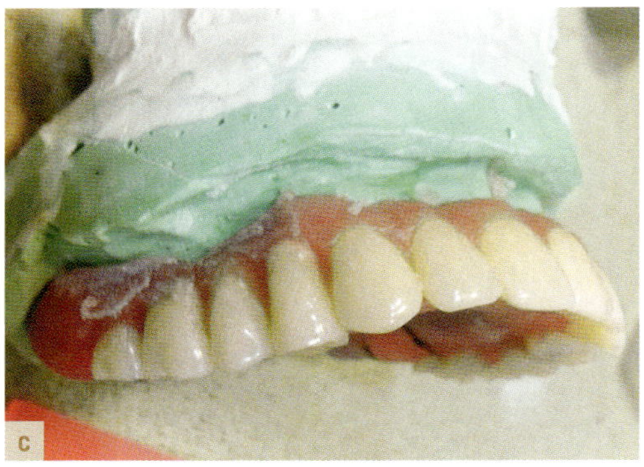
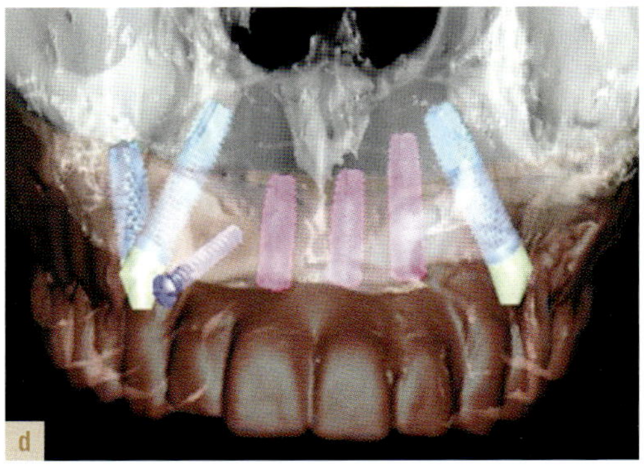

Fig 15-65a Edentulous maxilla – planned fixed implant-supported prosthesis. b Original orthopantomograph. c Setup of denture teeth on a trial base. d Virtual 3D jaw model with planned implants and superimposed optically scanned model of the trial base setup.

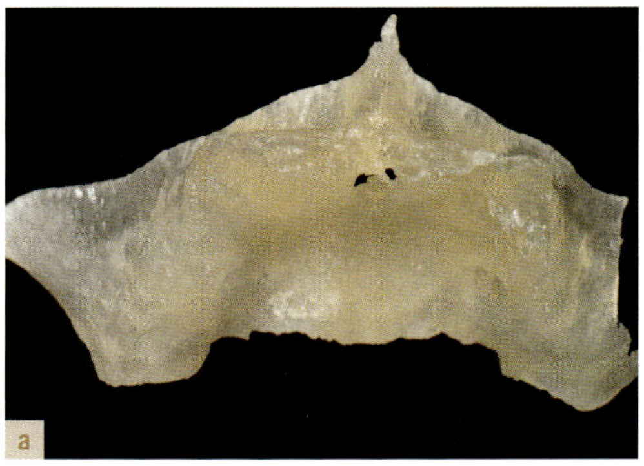
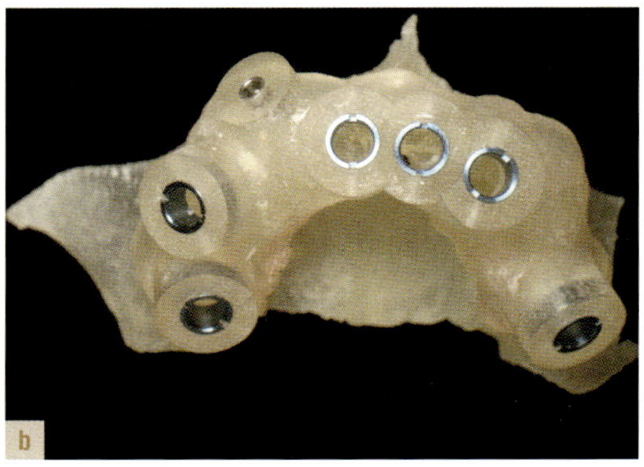
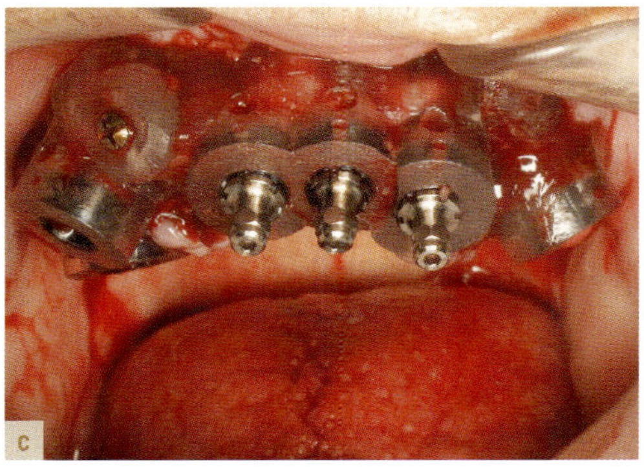
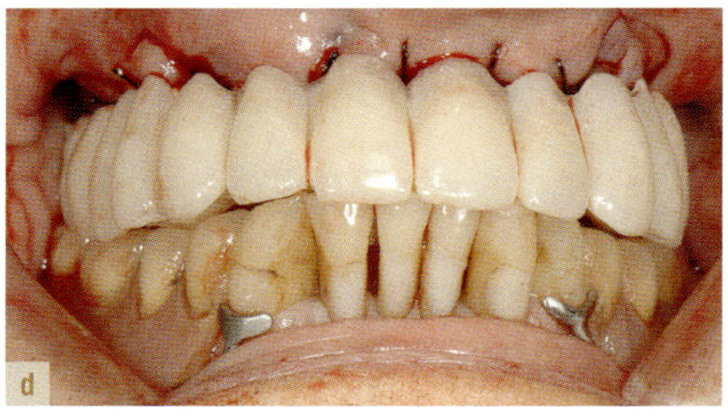
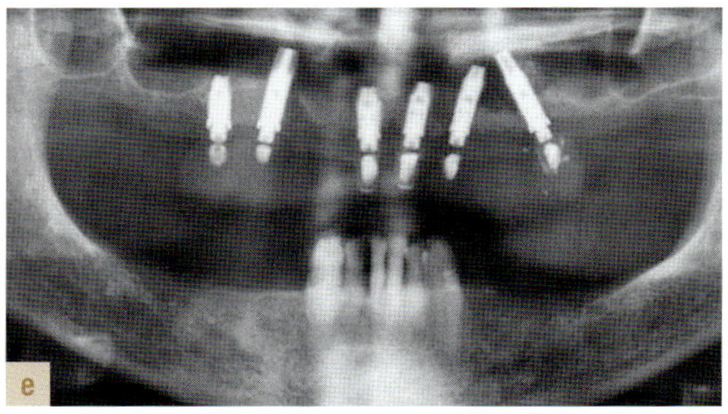

Fig 15-66a Stereolithographic model of the maxillary bone. b Surgical guide seated on the bone model. c Surgical guide seated on the bone with fixation screw and implant mounts of inserted implants. d Maxillary provisional restoration. e Orthopantomograph of implants.

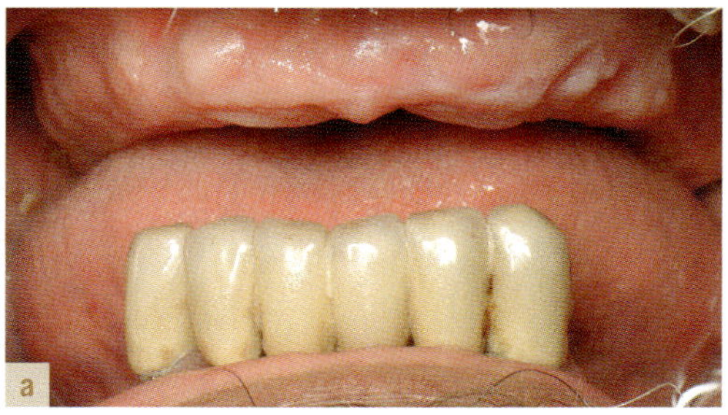
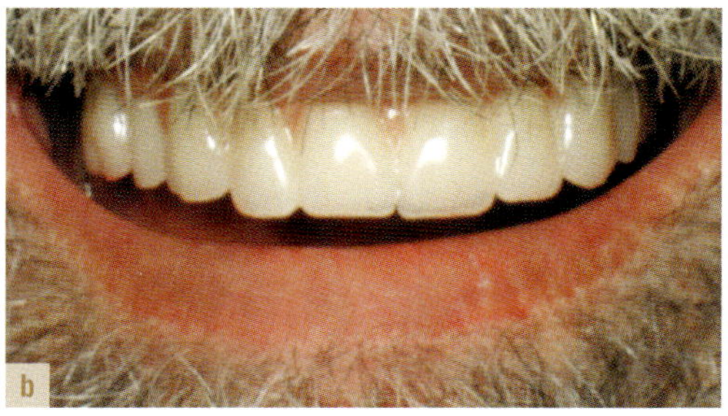

Fig 15-67a Fully edentulous maxilla – planned fixed supported restoration on five implants. b Pre-existing complete denture. c Orthopantomograph. d Radiographic guide. Duplicate of original denture in radiopaque acrylic.

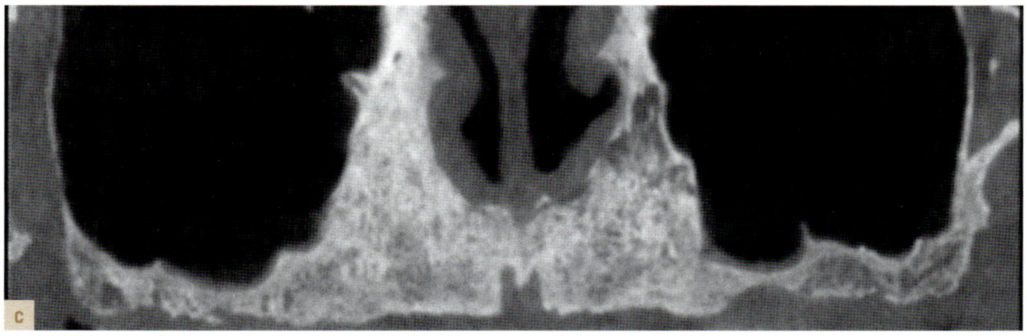
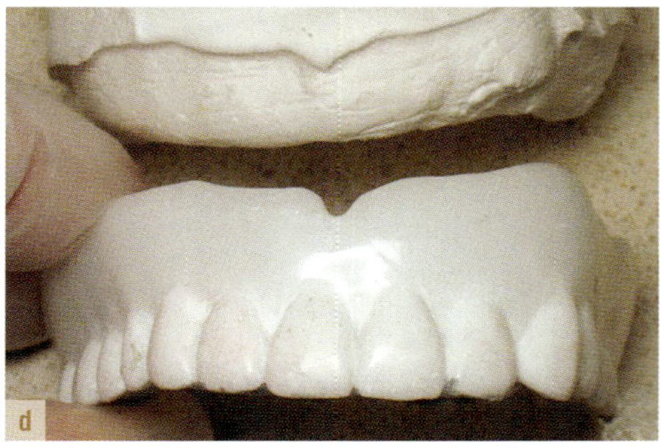